T0195540

Current Issues in Clinical Microbiology

Editors

NICOLE D. PECORA
MATTHEW A. PETTENGILL

CLINICS IN LABORATORY MEDICINE

www.labmed.theclinics.com

Editor-in-Chief
MILENKO JOVAN TANASIJEVIC

December 2020 • Volume 40 • Number 4

ELSEVIER

1600 John F. Kennedy Boulevard • Suite 1800 • Philadelphia, Pennsylvania, 19103-2899

http://www.theclinics.com

CLINICS IN LABORATORY MEDICINE Volume 40, Number 4
December 2020 ISSN 0272-2712, ISBN-13: 978-0-323-73395-3

Editor: Katerina Heidhausen
Developmental Editor: Laura Fisher

Reprints. For copies of 100 or more, of articles in this publication, please contact the Commercial Reprints Department, Elsevier Inc., 360 Park Avenue South, New York, New York 10010-1710. Tel. 212-633-3874, Fax: 212-633-3820, E-mail: reprints@elsevier.com.

Clinics in Laboratory Medicine (ISSN 0272-2712) is published quarterly by Elsevier Inc., 360 Park Avenue South, New York, NY 10010-1710. Months of issue are March, June, September, and December. Business and Editorial offices: 1600 John F. Kennedy Blvd., Suite 1800, Philadelphia, PA 19103-2899. Periodicals postage paid at NewYork, NY and additional mailing offices. Subscription prices are $277.00 per year (US individuals), $571.00 per year (US institutions), $100.00 per year (US students), $349.00 per year (Canadian individuals), $693.00 per year (Canadian institutions), $100.00 per year (Canadian students), $404.00 per year (international individuals), $693.00 per year (international institutions), $185.00 (international students). Foreign air speed delivery is included in all Clinics subscription prices. All prices are subject to change without notice. POSTMASTER: Send address changes to *Clinics in Laboratory Medicine*, Elsevier Health Sciences Division, Subscription Customer Service, 3251 Riverport Lane, Maryland Heights, MO 63043. **Customer Service: 1-800-654-2452 (US). From outside of the US and Canada, call 1-314-447-8871. Fax: 1-314-447-8029. E-mail: journalscustomerservice-usa@elsevier.com (for print support) or journalsonlinesupport-usa@elsevier.com (for online support).**

Clinics in Laboratory Medicine is covered in *EMBASE/Exerpta Medica, MEDLINE/PubMed (Index Medicus), Cinahl, Current Contents/Clinical Medicine, BIOSIS and ISI/BIOMED.*

Printed in the United States of America.

Contributors

EDITOR-IN-CHIEF

MILENKO JOVAN TANASIJEVIC, MD, MBA
Vice Chair for Clinical Pathology and Quality, Department of Pathology, Director of Clinical Laboratories, Brigham and Women's Hospital, Dana-Farber Cancer Institute, Associate Professor of Pathology, Harvard Medical School, Boston, Massachusetts, USA

EDITORS

NICOLE D. PECORA, MD, PhD
Associate Director of Clinical Microbiology, Assistant Professor of Pathology and Laboratory Medicine, University of Rochester Medical Center, Rochester, New York, USA

MATTHEW A. PETTENGILL, PhD, D(ABMM)
Assistant Professor, Scientific Director of Clinical Microbiology, Department of Pathology, Anatomy, and Cell Biology, Thomas Jefferson University, Philadelphia, Pennsylvania, USA

AUTHORS

DIANA ALAME, MD
Medical Director, Clinical Microbiology, Thomas Jefferson University Hospital, Assistant Professor of Pathology, Anatomy and Cell Biology, Sidney Kimmel Medical College at Thomas Jefferson University, Philadelphia, Pennsylvania, USA

MARC W. ALLARD, PhD
US Food and Drug Administration, Center for Food Safety and Applied Nutrition, College Park, Maryland, USA

NIAZ BANAEI, MD
Stanford University School of Medicine, Palo Alto, California, USA

NEIL BLUMBERG, MD
Director of Transfusion Medicine/Blood Bank, Department of Transfusion Medicine/Blood Bank, University of Rochester Medical Center, Rochester, New York, USA

JESSICA L. BOHRHUNTER, PhD
Department of Pathology and Laboratory Medicine, University of Rochester Medical Center, Rochester, New York, USA

CARRIE A. BOWLER, MS
Assistant Professor, Program Manager, Department of Laboratory Medicine and Pathology, Graduate Medical Education, Mayo Clinic, Rochester, Minnesota, USA

ERIC W. BROWN, PhD
US Food and Drug Administration, Center for Food Safety and Applied Nutrition, College Park, Maryland, USA

CHRISTINE CAHILL, RN, MS
Nurse Coordinator, Department of Transfusion Medicine/Blood Bank, Patient Blood Management, University of Rochester Medical Center, Rochester, New York, USA

ANDREW CAMERON, PhD
Department of Pathology and Laboratory Medicine, University of Rochester Medical Center, Rochester, New York, USA

GUOJIE CAO, PhD
US Food and Drug Administration, Center for Food Safety and Applied Nutrition, College Park, Maryland, USA

KAREN C. CARROLL, MD
Division of Medical Microbiology, Department of Pathology, Johns Hopkins School of Medicine, Baltimore, Maryland, USA

TIMOTHY CHAO, MD, PhD
Resident Physician, Department of Pathology, Anatomy, and Cell Biology, Thomas Jefferson University Hospital, Philadelphia, Pennsylvania, USA

JENNIFER DIEN BARD, PhD, D(ABMM)
Director, Microbiology and Virology Laboratories, Department of Pathology and Laboratory Medicine, Children's Hospital Los Angeles, Associate Professor of Pathology (Clinical Scholar), University of Southern California, Keck School of Medicine of USC, Los Angeles, California, USA

JAMES J. DUNN, PhD, D(ABMM)
Director, Medical Microbiology and Virology, Department of Pathology, Texas Children's Hospital, Associate Professor of Pathology and Immunology, Baylor College of Medicine, Houston, Texas, USA

CLAUDINE EL-BEYROUTY, PharmD, BCPS
Advanced Practice Pharmacist, Infectious Diseases, Thomas Jefferson University Hospital, Philadelphia, Pennsylvania, USA

MARK D. GONZALEZ, PhD
Associate Director, Microbiology, Section Director of Infectious Disease Serology, Children's Healthcare of Atlanta, Atlanta, Georgia, USA

DWIGHT J. HARDY, PhD
Director, Clinical Microbiology Laboratories, UR Medicine Labs, Professor of Microbiology and Immunology, Pathology and Laboratory Medicine, University of Rochester Medical Center, Rochester, New York, USA

BRYAN HESS, MD
Medical Director, Antimicrobial Stewardship Program, Assistant Professor of Medicine, Division of Infectious Diseases, Sidney Kimmel Medical College at Thomas Jefferson University, Philadelphia, Pennsylvania, USA

ROMNEY M. HUMPHRIES, PhD, D(ABMM)
Professor, Pathology, Microbiology and Immunology, Vanderbilt University Medical Center, Nashville, Tennessee, USA

ALVARO C. LAGA, MD, MMSc
Assistant Professor, Department of Pathology, Associate Pathologist, Brigham and Women's Hospital, Harvard Medical School, Boston, Massachusetts, USA

ADEL MALEK, PhD
Faculty of Laboratory Medicine, Memorial University, St John's, Newfoundland and Labrador, Canada

DEBRA MASEL, MT, (ASCP) SBB
Chief Supervisor, Department of Transfusion Medicine/Blood Bank, University of Rochester Medical Center, Rochester, New York, USA

ERIN McELVANIA, PhD, D(ABMM)
Director of Clinical Microbiology, Department of Pathology and Laboratory Medicine, Evanston Hospital, NorthShore University HealthSystem, Evanston, Illinois, USA; Clinical Assistant Professor of Pathology, University of Chicago Pritzker School of Medicine, Chicago, Illinois, USA

HEBA H. MOSTAFA, MD, PhD, D(ABMM)
Division of Medical Microbiology, Department of Pathology, Johns Hopkins School of Medicine, Baltimore, Maryland, USA

KIMBERLEE A. MUSSER, PhD
Wadsworth Center, New York State Department of Health, Albany, New York, USA

ANDY NGO, MD
Transfusion Medicine Fellow, Department of Transfusion Medicine/Blood Bank, University of Rochester Medical Center, Rochester, New York, USA

NICOLE D. PECORA, MD, PhD
Associate Director of Clinical Microbiology, Assistant Professor of Pathology and Laboratory Medicine, University of Rochester Medical Center, Rochester, New York, USA

MICHAEL A. PENTELLA, PhD, D(ABMM)
Clinical Professor, College of Public Health, University of Iowa, Iowa City, Iowa, USA; Laboratory Director, State Hygienic Laboratory, University of Iowa, Coralville, Iowa, USA

MATTHEW A. PETTENGILL, PhD, D(ABMM)
Assistant Professor, Scientific Director of Clinical Microbiology, Department of Pathology, Anatomy, and Cell Biology, Thomas Jefferson University, Philadelphia, Pennsylvania, USA

BOBBI S. PRITT, MD, MSc
Professor, ACGME Medical Microbiology Program Director, Department of Laboratory Medicine and Pathology, Division of Clinical Microbiology, Graduate Medical Education, Mayo Clinic, Rochester, Minnesota, USA

MAJED A. REFAAI, MD
Associate Director of Transfusion Medicine/Blood Bank, Department of Transfusion Medicine/Blood Bank, University of Rochester Medical Center, Rochester, New York, USA

PAULA A. REVELL, PhD, D(ABMM)
Associate Director, Medical Microbiology and Virology, Department of Pathology, Texas Children's Hospital, Associate Professor of Pediatrics and Pathology and Immunology, Baylor College of Medicine, Houston, Texas, USA

MAX SALFINGER, MD
University of South Florida College of Public Health, Morsani College of Medicine, Tampa, Florida, USA

LINOJ SAMUEL, PhD, D(ABMM)
Division Head, Clinical Microbiology, Department of Pathology and Laboratory Medicine, Henry Ford Health System, Detroit, Michigan, USA

AKOS SOMOSKOVI, MD, PhD, DSc
Roche Molecular Systems Inc., Pleasanton, California, USA

ERIC STEVENS, PhD
US Food and Drug Administration, Center for Food Safety and Applied Nutrition, College Park, Maryland, USA

SAMANTHA TAFFNER, MS
Department of Pathology and Laboratory Medicine, University of Rochester Medical Center, Rochester, New York, USA

ELITZA S. THEEL, PhD
Associate Professor, CPEP Clinical Microbiology Fellowship Program Director, Department of Laboratory Medicine and Pathology, Division of Clinical Microbiology, Mayo Clinic, Rochester, Minnesota, USA

RUTH TIMME, PhD
US Food and Drug Administration, Center for Food Safety and Applied Nutrition, College Park, Maryland, USA

KATHARINE UHTEG, MS
Division of Medical Microbiology, Department of Pathology, Johns Hopkins School of Medicine, Baltimore, Maryland, USA

MARTIN S. ZAND, MD, PhD
Professor, Department of Medicine, Nephrology (SMD), Co-Director, Clinical and Translational Science Institute, Senior Associate Dean, Clinical Research University of Rochester Medical Center, School of Medicine and Dentistry, University of Rochester Medical Center, Rochester, New York, USA

ADRIAN M. ZELAZNY, PhD
National Institutes of Health, Bethesda, Maryland, USA

JIE ZHENG, PhD
US Food and Drug Administration, Center for Food Safety and Applied Nutrition, College Park, Maryland, USA

Contents

The optimal care of septic patients depends on the successful recovery of clinically relevant microorganisms from blood cultures and the timely reporting of organism identification and antimicrobial susceptibility testing (AST) results. Many preanalytic factors play a critical role in culturing microorganisms, and advancements in blood culture instrument technology have reduced the time to positive results. Additionally, rapid organism identification and AST results directly from positive blood culture broth via new methods help to further shorten the time from empiric to targeted treatment. This article summarizes the current state of blood culture methods, including preanalytic, analytical, and postanalytic factors that are available to clinical microbiology laboratories.

Syndromic panels have allowed clinical microbiology laboratories to rapidly identify bacteria, viruses, fungi, and parasites and are now fully integrated into the standard testing practices of many clinical laboratories. To maximize the benefit of syndromic testing, laboratories must implement strict measures to ensure that syndromic panels are being used responsibly. This article discusses commercially available syndromic panels, the benefits and limitations of testing, and how diagnostic and laboratory stewardship can be used to optimize testing and improve patient care while keeping costs at a minimum.

Planning for a new laboratory is exciting and daunting. The project's success starts with an agreed on vision and scope as defined by key stakeholders. In addition to the work of architects and building professionals, such projects require major investment in upfront thought, time, and commitment from laboratory directors, supervisors, and technologists who will use the space. Incorporating design features critical to efficient and flexible workflow as required to meet growing and changing needs will extend the lifetime of the space. Open floor plans may challenge some sensibilities and biosafety concerns but are the vogue for BSL-2 laboratories.

> Antimicrobial susceptibility testing (AST) is now, more than ever, a critical role of the microbiology laboratory. Several factors limit its application for patient care and antimicrobial resistance epidemiology, including time to results, requirements for pure cultures, and high starting concentration of bacteria. This review discusses the global status of AST and new phenotypic and genotypic methods in late-stage development or that are new to market.

> Recent improvements in next-generation sequencing technologies have enabled clinical laboratories to increasingly pursue pathogen genomics for infectious disease diagnosis. Clinical laboratories can also benefit from whole-genome sequence characterization of cultured isolates, helping to resolve infection prevention questions pertaining to pathogen outbreaks and surveillance. Metagenomic sequencing from primary specimens can also provide laboratories with an unbiased universal test for situations where traditional methods fail to identify infectious etiologies despite, high clinical suspicion. Here, the most useful applications of whole-genome sequence and metagenomic sequencing are summarized, as are the main advantages, limitations, and considerations for building an in-house clinical genomics program.

> Endemic species of coronavirus (HCoV-OC43, HCoV-229E, HCoV-NL63, and HCoV-HKU1) are frequent causes of upper respiratory tract infections. Three highly pathogenic coronaviruses have been associated with outbreaks and epidemics and have challenged clinical microbiology laboratories to quickly develop assays for diagnosis. Their initial characterization was achieved by molecular methods. With the great advance in metagenomic whole-genome sequencing directly from clinical specimens, diagnosis of novel coronaviruses could be quickly implemented into the workflow of managing cases of pneumonia of unknown cause, which will markedly affect the time of the initial characterization and accelerate the initiation of outbreak control measures.

> Biosafety risks are prevalent in all areas of the clinical laboratories. Clinical laboratorians have become accustomed to accepting these risks. When an emerging pathogen appears, the concerns become elevated. Since the appearance of Ebola virus in the United States in 2014, biosafety practices have made progress. A recent Association of Public Health

Laboratories survey shows that clinical laboratories are unprepared for current and emerging biosafety challenges. This article focuses on the biosafety program that clinical laboratory leaders should build to meet the needs of clinical laboratories; biosafety challenges of automated laboratory systems, facilities, personnel, and practices; and the relationship with occupational health.

Point-of-care (POC) or near patient testing for infectious diseases is a rapidly expanding space that is part of an ongoing effort to bring care closer to the patient. Traditional POC tests were known for their limited utility, but advances in technology have seen significant improvements in performance of these assays. The increasing promise of these tests is also coupled with their increasing complexity, which requires the oversight of qualified laboratory-trained personnel.

Infants and young children are uniquely susceptible to primary viral and bacterial infections, predisposing them to responses of greater frequency and severity than in adults. Etiologies and manifestations of infections in pediatric patients are often different than those in adults. It can be challenging for clinical laboratories to implement appropriate microbiologic methods for rapid and accurate diagnoses in this population. Laboratorians should be cognizant of the distinctive features of children to provide comprehensive pediatric clinical microbiology services. This article discusses laboratory aspects of several clinically significant pediatric pathogens that cause severe harm to patients and impact public health responses.

Misuse of antibiotics, including unnecessary use or inappropriate selection, may result in side effects and poor outcome in individual patients, as well as contribute to the spread of antimicrobial resistance. Antimicrobial stewardship programs exist to reduce such misuse of antibiotics and ill effect in order to promote patient outcome. The importance of diagnostics, antibiogram data, possible interventions, and impact are reviewed. It is essential for clinical microbiologists and other health care members to understand the field and scope of antimicrobial stewardship, actively participate in, and understand the value they bring to supporting their institution's efforts.

Formal medical and public health microbiology (MPHM) fellowship programs play a key role in preparing future clinical microbiology laboratory directors for their leadership and management responsibilities. Given the continually evolving MPHM field, fellowships must remain adaptable to changes in the field, providing trainees with the opportunity to engage with newly emerging diagnostic modalities, while continuing to emphasize the "bread and butter" techniques of clinical microbiology. This article discusses the key components of a fellowship program and provides recommendations for incorporating educational best practices.

Although tuberculosis is slowly decreasing, nontuberculous mycobacterial lung disease is significantly increasing. We describe new methods and applications for faster turnaround times in the diagnosis of tuberculosis and nontuberculous mycobacterial lung disease and have included the latest mycobacterial taxonomy. Although the focus is mainly on molecular assays, we also discuss improvements of acid-fast bacilli smear microscopy and stress the need for performing minimal inhibitory concentration determinations especially for tuberculosis. Additionally, important considerations for negative nucleic acid amplification assay results used for releasing tuberculosis suspects from airborne infection isolation rooms saving precious resources for the health care system, are also included.

This article describes the potential for one health surveillance of foodborne pathogens and disease using the revolutionary methodologies of whole genome sequencing. Whole genome sequencing of viral and bacterial pathogens is a natural fit to a one health perspective because these pathogens reside and are shared by humans, animals, and the environment and their genomes are compared easily regardless of where or from what host the pathogen was isolated. A genome provides a huge amount of data that can be analyzed for numerous applications. Sharing data coordinates surveillance efforts across the various disciplines.

Anatomic pathology is an important resource for detection and exclusion of infectious diseases in tissue specimens. Detection of a microorganism (i.e. bacteria, fungi, parasite) in tissue sections is frequently the beginning of a work-up and occasionally sufficient for definitive microbiologic identification. Close correlation with cultures and ancillary testing in the microbiology laboratory is of paramount importance in arriving at a diagnosis and identify with certitude causative pathogen(s). This review will discuss the adequacy and limitations of histopathology in the diagnosis of infectious diseases, describe potential pitfalls, and discuss the appropriate use of molecular diagnostics in formalin-fixed, paraffin embedded tissues.

SARS-CoV-2 (also known as COVID-19) has been an unprecedented challenge in many parts of the medical field with blood banking being no exception. COVID-19 has had a distinctly negative effect on our blood collection nationwide forcing blood banks, blood centers, and the US government to adopt new policies to adapt to a decreased blood supply as well as to protect our donors from COVID-19. These policies can be seen distinctly in patient blood management and blood bank operations. We are also faced with developing policies and procedures for a nontraditional therapy, convalescent plasma; its efficacy and safety is still not completely elucidated as of yet.

The entire spectrum of diagnostic testing, from reagent supply to test performance, has been a major focus during the coronavirus disease 2019 (COVID-19) pandemic. The hope for serologic testing is that it will provide both epidemiologic information about seroprevalence as well as individual information about previous infection. This information is particularly helpful for high-risk individuals who may be outside of the viral shedding window, such as children with suspected multisystem inflammatory syndrome. It is not yet understood whether serologic testing can be interpreted in terms of protective immunity. These concerns must be addressed using highly sensitive and specific tests.

CLINICS IN LABORATORY MEDICINE

SERIES OF RELATED INTEREST

Surgical Pathology Clinics
Available at: https://www.surgpath.theclinics.com/

THE CLINICS ARE NOW AVAILABLE ONLINE!
Access your subscription at:
www.theclinics.com

Preface

2020: A Year for Clinical Microbiology

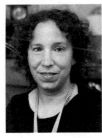
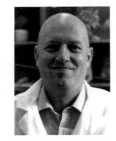

Nicole D. Pecora, MD, PhD   Matthew A. Pettengill, PhD
Editors

We had originally intended this issue to provide an update in many dynamic areas of clinical microbiology practice, including the introduction of groundbreaking technologies and major logistical challenges, such as laboratory consolidation and design. As the issue started to come together, authored primarily by active clinical microbiology lab directors, we were collectively confronted with the COVID-19 pandemic. The warnings that we have heard over the past decade about the potential for a pandemic in the highly interconnected global economy were suddenly proven to be prescient, and yet, despite all of those warnings, we were nationally unprepared for the magnitude of the event. Every aspect of our operations was impacted, and as a group, we became deeply involved in global supply chain logistics, the intricacies of the FDA regulatory process and Emergency Use Authorizations, biosafety and risk assessments, and the test validation and performance measures for the diagnosis of a completely novel pathogen on a massive scale, virtually overnight.

We would like to extend our appreciation to all of the authors in this issue for their dedication and for producing high-quality and pertinent content despite being pulled in a hundred other directions at this time. We feel a great sense of pride to be a part of the clinical microbiology professional community. Clinical laboratory science was at the forefront of the COVID-19 pandemic as part of a global discussion of diagnostic test logistics, performance measures, and result interpretation. We endeavored to incorporate many of these lab practice concerns into the topics discussed in this issue.

Several topics of enduring importance to the practice of clinical microbiology are included: updates for modern blood culture methodologies, mycobacterial diagnostics, antimicrobial susceptibility testing, and special pediatric diagnostic considerations. In recent years, technological advances have brought considerable changes to the lab in the form of syndromic panel development, diagnostic genomics, and point-of-care molecular testing, which are carefully considered in separate sections.

Clin Lab Med 40 (2020) xiii–xiv
https://doi.org/10.1016/j.cll.2020.09.001
0272-2712/20/© 2020 Published by Elsevier Inc.   labmed.theclinics.com

Clinical microbiologists are often consulted on infectious diseases topics outside of the laboratory walls within our departments of pathology, with our infectious diseases colleagues, and in our larger scientific community, which is why we have included updates on infectious diseases diagnostics in surgical pathology, antimicrobial stewardship, and genomics in One Health, respectively.

We also include an article on the design of a central laboratory, which is an increasingly common theme in modern health care systems. COVID-19 required laboratories to be nimble when it came to validating and running many platforms at once. Several testing options required the use of molecular techniques and equipment (extractors, thermocyclers, and so forth) that are normally exclusively used for laboratory-developed tests. The utility of a laboratory design that is not restricted to a single platform and an operation with the skill set, space, and equipment to develop molecular and serological tests have never been more clear than during this pandemic. Similarly, the training of future lab directors is a topic as changing as the profession itself, and this article highlights the variety of experiences that must go into their preparation. The experience of COVID-19 has put a spotlight on how a diverse training that is strong in both basic science and management is necessary to meet the challenges facing a laboratory leader. The topics of biosafety and clinical virology were dramatically impacted by the COVID-19 pandemic, and these articles reflect this new emphasis. Lastly, 2 articles were added to specifically address the unique considerations of COVID-19 in blood bank laboratory practice, and the development of serologic assays for SARS-CoV-2/COVID-19.

We hope that this issue provides useful and thought-provoking content. We are honored to bring together the work of such an accomplished group of individuals and can only expect that the field will change at such a pace that we will be looking for the next clinical microbiology updates issue in short order.

Nicole D. Pecora, MD, PhD
UR Medicine Central Laboratories
211 Bailey Road
West Henrietta, NY 14586, USA

Matthew A. Pettengill, PhD
Department of Pathology, Anatomy, and Cell
Biology
Thomas Jefferson University
117 South 11th Street
Pavilion Building, Suite 207
Philadelphia, PA 19107-4998, USA

E-mail addresses:
Nicole_pecora@urmc.rochester.edu (N.D. Pecora)
matthew.pettengill@jefferson.edu (M.A. Pettengill)

Modern Blood Culture
Management Decisions and Method Options

Mark D. Gonzalez, PhD[a], Timothy Chao, MD, PhD[b],
Matthew A. Pettengill, PhD[c],*

KEYWORDS

- Blood culture • Bloodstream infections • Contamination • Sepsis

KEY POINTS

- Considerable improvements can be made in preanalytical aspects of blood culture collection that impact patient care.
- There are newer methods developed in recent years to improve time to reporting blood culture isolate identification and antibiotic susceptibility patterns.
- The successful utilization of rapid identification and antimicrobial susceptibility results requires coordination with antimicrobial stewardship programs.

INTRODUCTION

One of the most important functions of the clinical microbiology laboratory is the detection and characterization of organisms causing bloodstream infections. Several preanalytical considerations have a considerable impact on downstream results for blood cultures. The laboratory, with input from key stakeholders, selects blood culture media types and provides guidance on collection methods and collection site sterilization, the volume of blood to be collected, and downstream testing options for positive blood cultures. This article provides an update on recent data and developments in each of these areas.

SELECTION OF MEDIA AND ADDITIVE TYPES FOR BLOOD CULTURE

Most modern media formulations are similar, a base of soybean casein digest (trypticase soy broth) with sodium polyanethol sulfonate (SPS) as an anticoagulant. The

[a] Microbiology, Section Director of Infectious Disease Serology, Children's Healthcare of Atlanta, 1405 Clifton Road, Northeast, Atlanta, GA 30322, USA; [b] Department of Pathology, Anatomy, and Cell Biology, Thomas Jefferson University Hospital, 132 South 10th Street, Room 285, Philadelphia, PA 19107, USA; [c] Department of Pathology, Anatomy, and Cell Biology, Thomas Jefferson University, 117 South 11th Street, Pavilion Building Suite 207, Philadelphia, PA 19107-4998, USA
* Corresponding author.
E-mail address: matthew.pettengill@jefferson.edu
Twitter: @tim_hf_chao (T.C.)

Clin Lab Med 40 (2020) 379–392
https://doi.org/10.1016/j.cll.2020.07.001
0272-2712/20/© 2020 Elsevier Inc. All rights reserved.

headspace of the bottles consists of CO_2 and N_2 for anaerobic bottles and ambient air supplemented with CO_2 for aerobic bottles. Anaerobic bottles also include reducing agents. Two major decisions are whether to utilize bottles with polymeric resin beads to neutralize antibiotics, and if one's laboratory serves a pediatric population whether to use pediatric-specific bottles (aerobic only, modified media formulation, lower media volume, and lower SPS concentration). Resins can neutralize select antibacterial agents (including common empirically utilized antibiotics such as piperacillin-tazobactam, vancomycin, and some cephalosporins), but have lower to no ability to neutralize other agents (eg, carbapenems and fluoroquinolones).[1–3] Resins improve the yield of blood cultures for patients who are on antibiotics at the time of blood collection; this has clear advantages for initial blood cultures but also results in more positive cultures for patients subsequently on therapy, and thus more laboratory expense. The clinical significance of subsequent positive cultures in bottles with resins is unclear. Pediatric bottles have been compared with standard aerobic bottles in vitro,[4] and also compared with aerobic and anaerobic bottles in clinical evaluations.[5–7] Bloodstream infections in children are rarely caused by strict anaerobes. In the largest study to date that included aerobic and anaerobic culture in a pediatric population, only 15 of 723 clinically significant isolates (2.1%) were strict anaerobes isolated from anaerobic bottles.[8] Bacteremia with strict aerobes may be more common in this population.[9] This does not mean, however, that utilizing anaerobic bottles could not contribute to increased sensitivity for pediatric cultures. A more recent study demonstrated improved yield with 1 mL of blood divided evenly between aerobic (BACTEC Peds Plus/F) and anaerobic bottles (68/72, 94.4%) compared with 1 mL added to 1 pediatric bottle (56/72, 77.7%).[5] The additionally detected organisms using the combination of aerobic and anaerobic bottles were mostly facultative anaerobes rather than strict anaerobes. Studies to date have either not specifically evaluated fastidious organisms (such as *Neisseria*) or are too small to expect a meaningful number of such isolates to occur in clinical evaluations; thus it is not clear if the modified media formulation or reduced SPS would offer advantages for these types of organisms in a larger study or clinical use. It seems that loading the entire volume into a pediatric bottle or dividing it evenly between a pediatric aerobic bottle and a standard anaerobic bottle are both reasonable and justifiable approaches to pediatric blood culture.

PREVENTING CONTAMINATION OF BLOOD CULTURES

Contamination of blood cultures has a big impact on patient care and hospital resources. Several key factors that can reduce contamination rates have been clearly demonstrated. Skin sites for collection should be disinfected with an alcohol-containing disinfectant, and blood should not be collected from an intravascular device unless specifically requested out of concern it is the source of bacteremia. Additionally, ongoing education should be provided to phlebotomy staff and other blood collectors, and methods or devices that divert an initial volume of blood can significantly reduce blood culture contamination rates.[10–12] In fact, it is possible to make so much progress relative to historic baselines that a group of experts on the topic recently proposed changing the longstanding performance standard for US health care institutions, currently set at less than 3% of blood cultures contaminated, with the proposal to consider lowering this expectation to less than 1% contamination.[10] As noted, the use of commercial diversion devices reduced contamination rates,[11] which in models is projected to lead to considerable cost savings and reductions in patient length of stay.[13,14] In 2 recent studies, blood culture contamination was reduced without using expensive commercial diversion devices, by diverting a small amount of blood using vacutainer tubes by changing the test draw order, which could also be accomplished for blood cultures alone by simply discarding the diverted portion.[15,16]

VOLUME OF BLOOD COLLECTED FOR CULTURE

The volume of blood collected for blood culture is the single most important variable in the ability of the microbiology laboratory to detect microorganisms causing bloodstream infections.[17,18] The American Society for Microbiology (ASM) and the Infectious Diseases Society of America (IDSA) jointly recommend 2 to 4 collections per septic episode, with each collection consisting of 20 to 30 mL divided among 2 or 3 bottles.[19] Thus, at a minimum, 40 mL total volume should be cultured per septic episode, with 2 important exceptions. The IDSA recommends that for neutropenic patients, blood collected for culture should be limited to 1% of total blood volume (usually approximately 70 mL/kg) in patients weighing less than 40 kg.[20] The other exception is pediatric patients, for whom there are various recommendations for blood culture volumes based on age or weight, with those from IDSA cited here.[19] The volume of blood collected and number of bottles collected can be increased without increasing the number of collections by increasing the volume at each collection to 30 mL in 3 bottles (2 aerobic bottles and 1 anaerobic bottle in this study) instead of 20 mL, which could improve causative microorganism recovery without significantly increasing costs.[21]

Although blood collection happens outside of the laboratory, ensuring that adequate volume is collected is the direct responsibility of laboratory administration. The College of American Pathologists (CAP) requires that accredited laboratories have a system in place to evaluate adult blood culture volume and communicate these data at regular intervals to clinical staff responsible for blood collection. Laboratory-initiated education and quality improvement projects can lead to marked improvements in blood volume submitted. One group found that targeted education in intensive care units (ICUs) led to 30% to 60% sustained improvement in blood volume submitted on average.[22] Another recent study found that a rigorous quality improvement program that included group education, targeted communications, and bottle marking led to not only considerably increased blood volume (increased from 2.3 mL average per bottle before implementation to 8.6 mL after implementation) but most importantly a 20% improved yield of true pathogens in blood culture.[23]

BLOOD CULTURE SYSTEMS AND ALTERNATIVE BLOOD CULTURING METHODS

Numerous improvements in blood culture incubation and monitoring have occurred over time, culminating in the current continuous-monitoring blood culture system (CMBCS). Three US Food and Drug Administration (FDA)-cleared CMBCS are available, including BACTEC (Becton-Dickinson, Sparks, MD, USA), BacT/Alert (bioMérieux, Inc., Durham, North Carolina) and VersaTREK (Thermo Scientific, Waltham, Massachusetts). Key features are summarized in **Table 1**. All 3 systems detect microbial growth via some form of gas detection but utilize distinct methods. Delays in getting bottles onto the CMBCS can result in delayed positive results or false-negative results. In a 30-month retrospective study of 50,955 blood cultures, where cultures were only loaded onto the CMBCS during the morning to late afternoon or otherwise held on the hospital floor at room temperature, 13.0% were positive while the laboratory was open, but only 10.8% were positive when the laboratory was closed.[24]

Table 1
Summary of current continuous-monitoring blood culture system features

Blood Culture System	Method for Monitoring Growth	Bottle Types	Additional Information	FDA-Cleared Indications	Max Fill Volume
BacT/ALERT	Colorimetric change caused by drop in pH from increased CO_2 levels	BacT/ALERT FA PLUS	Aerobic media with adsorbent polymeric resin beads	Blood or SBF	10 mL
		BacT/ALERT FN PLUS	Anaerobic media with adsorbent polymeric resin beads	Blood or SBF	10 mL
		BacT/ALERT PF PLUS	Pediatric, standard aerobic	Blood	4 mL
		BacT/ALERT SA	Standard aerobic	Blood or SBF	10 mL
		BacT/ALERT SN	Standard anaerobic	Blood or SBF	10 mL
		BacT/ALERT BPA	Aerobic media	Platelets	10 mL
		BacT/ALERT BPN	Anaerobic media	Platelets	10 mL
BACTEC	Change in fluorescence caused by a drop in pH from increased CO_2 levels	BACTEC Plus Aerobic	Aerobic media with adsorbent polymeric resin beads	Blood	10 mL
		BACTEC Plus Anaerobic	Anaerobic media with adsorbent polymeric resin beads	Blood	10 mL
		BACTEC Peds Plus	Pediatric, aerobic media w/ adsorbent polymeric resin beads	Blood	5 mL
		BACTEC Lytic Anaerobic	Anaerobic media with detergent to lyse RBCs and WBCs	Blood	10 mL
		BACTEC Standard Aerobic	Standard aerobic	Blood	10 mL
		BACTEC Standard Anaerobic	Standard anaerobic	Blood	7 mL
		BACTEC Myco/F Lytic	Mycobacterial/fungal media	Blood	5 mL
VersaTREK	Measures pressure changes caused by gas consumption or production	REDOX 1	Aerobic	Blood or SBF	10 mL
		REDOX 2	Anaerobic	Blood or SBF	10 mL
		REDOX 1 EZ Draw	Aerobic, direct blood inoculation	Blood or SBF	5 mL
		REDOX 2 EZ Draw	Anaerobic, direct blood inoculation	Blood or SBF	5 mL
		VersaTREK Myco	Mycobacterial media	Blood, SBF or processed specimen	1 mL

Abbreviation: SBF, sterile body fluids.

The current BACTEC CMBCS model is the BACTEC FX, which is available in different sizes depending on the capacity required. Bottles for the BACTEC system contain fluorometric sensors that fluoresce in the presence of CO_2 via acidification. Specialized media (BACTEC Myco/F Lytic) for improved recovery of *Mycobacteria* and fungi are available.

The current BacT/Alert system models include the BacT/Alert 3D and the recently introduced BacT/Alert VIRTUO. Both systems detect CO_2 production via a colorimetric system present in the bottom of the bottles that changes color with pH. The BacT/ALERT VIRTUO system automates bottle loading and unloading, helping to maintain temperature stability. During the loading process, the instrument scans the bar-coded labels, determining the fill-level in the bottles, while on the instrument an improved algorithm shortens the time to positive detection. In 1 study comparing the BacT/ALERT VIRTUO with the BacT/ALERT 3D, 115 clinical isolates were inoculated into blood cultures, and although both systems demonstrated similar detection rates, the BacT/ALERT VIRTUO reduced time to detection by approximately 20%.[25] Similarly, a reduced time to detection was observed with BacT/ALERT VIRTUO in a multicenter study with clinical specimens, which was statistically significant for gram-negative bacilli and enterococci.[26] The type of BacT/ALERT bottle used determines the maximal volume inoculated. Additionally there are BacT/ALERT bottles FDA-cleared for sterile body fluids and platelet sterility testing (see **Table 1**).

Unlike the other CMBCS, microbial growth detection by the VersaTREK system requires an adapter to be affixed onto the bottles before instrument loading. This adapter allows the instrument to monitor pressure changes in CO_2, O_2, H_2, and N_2 caused by gas production or consumption by growing microorganisms. Additionally, the VersaTREK system is FDA-cleared for culturing mycobacteria from blood, processed specimens, and sterile body fluids, and for *Mycobacterium tuberculosis* susceptibility testing.

There are numerous studies comparing the CMBCS and media types. Recent examples will be highlighted. Overall, the CMBCS perform similarly in many aspects with some differences. One study compared the BacT/ALERT VIRTUO and BACTEC FX system using contrived bottles with differing (125 CFU/mL, 30 CFU/mL, and 5 CFU/mL) microorganism concentrations, for a total of 405 comparisons.[27] Although both systems flagged positive for all cultures at 125 CFU/mL and 30 CFU/mL, the BacT/ALERT VIRTUO demonstrated a lower false-negative rate (5.2%) at 5 CFU/mL compared with the BACTEC FX (8.1%), but no statistically significant difference was noted in the time to detection.[27] In contrast, another simulated study inoculated 2610 bottles with 30 CFU/mL of 330 clinical relevant species and compared the BacT/ALERT Virtuo, BacT/ALERT 3D and the BACTEC FX system. Although all 3 systems flagged positive for 99.6% of all cultures, the median time to positivity for the BacT/ALERT VIRTUO was significant shorter.[28] A previous study comparing the BacT/ALERT 3D and VersaTREK using patient specimens found no overall difference in time to positivity or isolation of microorganisms, but there was a higher false-positive rate with the VersaTREK system (ie, 1.6% vs 0.7% for aerobic bottles).[29] However, the VersaTREK demonstrated a statistically significant higher recovery of streptococci and enterococci.[29]

As noted, monitoring and feedback to collectors of inadequate blood culture volumes is a CAP requirement, and the BacT/Alert and BACTEC can assist in volume determination. The BacT/Alert Virtuo scans the sample level to determine the inoculated volume. An evaluation of the BacT/Alert Virtuo volume monitoring of 1141 bottles was compared with weight-based volume determination.[30] Although the results between the BacT/Alert Virtuo and weight-based volume strongly correlated (r = 0.87), the BacT/Alert Virtuo tended to overestimate volumes (median difference of 1.4 mL for the aerobic bottle and 0.2 mL for the anaerobic bottle). Software for the BACTEC FX, BD EpiCenter, determines the mean blood volume from at least 25 culture-negative aerobic bottles by measuring red blood cell metabolic activity. This measurement method means that low hematocrit levels and delays in getting bottles on the instrument can give inaccurate results. One study compared the BACTEC FX to weight-based volume determination, initially found that the BACTEC FX had a mean underestimation of 1.4 mL but this was reduced to a mean underestimation of 0.3 mL with a software upgrade.[31] However, this improved software demonstrated a mean overestimation of 2.8 mL with plastic BACTEC bottles,[31] but further updates were planned to adjust for plastic bottles.

In addition to the CMBCS, some laboratories use lysis centrifugation methods to culture blood for molds and mycobacteria. Note that CMBCS are the preferred method for recovery of *Candida* species and *Cryptococcus* species. In a 10-year retrospective study, the Isolator system recovered the lipid requiring *Malassezia* species. and isolated dimorphic and filamentous fungi not recovered in CMBCS.[32] However, this same study found that the Isolator rarely provided results not available by other methods, and there were many instances of fungal isolates deemed to be clinically insignificant.[32]

INCUBATION TIME

Blood cultures are routinely incubated for 4 to 7 days with CMBCS. Studies indicate that 98% to 99% of true pathogens are detected within 5 days of incubation relative to longer incubation times.[17] Five days of incubation appear to be optimal for balancing increased recovery versus occupying incubator space unnecessarily and delaying final reporting for negative cultures. It may be reasonable, however, to shorten incubation times to 4 days or even 3 days if equipment failure or a surge of demand for blood cultures (eg, during the COVID-19 pandemic) leads to a sudden demand for more CMBCS space than laboratory infrastructure can accommodate. Several studies demonstrated only modest reductions in true pathogen recovery with 3 to 4 days of incubation relative to longer times.[33–35] Although routine incubation beyond 5 days is not necessary with CMBCS, even for HACEK organisms,[36] it may be justified to hold cultures for a longer period of time on request in select cases.

PROCESSING POSITIVE BLOOD CULTURES: STAINING METHODS AND IMPACT OF GRAM STAIN CALL TIME

The first analytical step in processing a positive blood culture is probably the most impactful step for patient care: the Gram stain. Studies have demonstrated that for therapeutic interventions, the reporting of Gram stain results to the patient care team was more impactful than reporting final antimicrobial susceptibility testing (AST) results.[37] The timing of Gram stain reporting matters too. In many clinical microbiology laboratories it can be difficult to provide highly skilled Gram stain readers on off shifts for rapid turnaround of positive blood culture Gram stains. Gram stain turn-around time for blood cultures was shown in a relatively small study to correlate with mortality, with increased mortality among patients with delayed Gram stain reporting.[38] Infrastructure can also be developed to allow for remote consultative review of blood culture Gram stains so that more experienced readers can assist technologists at remote laboratory sites if needed to improve accuracy.[39] Some microorganisms stain poorly or not all with Gram reagents, and for positive blood cultures with negative Gram stains there are alternative stains, such as acridine orange, which can be employed in addition to repeating Gram stains.

RAPID IDENTIFICATION FROM POSITIVE BLOOD CULTURES: MOLECULAR TESTING

There are several commercial, FDA-cleared, molecular tests available for the rapid identification (<2 hours) of organisms in positive blood culture bottles. These tests may target a single organism (eg, *Staphylococcus aureus*), or large panels of organisms tested simultaneously (gram-negative and gram-positive bacteria on the same test) or organized by Gram stain results "Panels and Syndromic Testing in Clinical Microbiology". Molecular testing direct from blood culture bottles is sometimes negatively impacted by residual microbial nucleic acid in commercial blood culture media (sterile, but not always genetically inert), leading to false-positive results; this has led to product recalls for issues related to false-positive *Enterococcus* and *Proteus* identification in recent years. Blood culture molecular identification panels generally also include genetic markers of resistance for such targets as *mecA* when *Staphylococcus* is detected, *vanA/vanB* when *Enterococcus* is detected, and ESBL or carbapenemase genes such as KPC when gram-negative rods are detected "Panels and Syndromic Testing in Clinical Microbiology".

RAPID IDENTIFICATION FROM POSITIVE BLOOD CULTURES: MASS SPECTROMETRY

Bacteria and yeast in positive blood culture bottles may also be directly identified using matrix-assisted laser desorption ionization time-of-flight mass spectrometry (MALDI-TOF MS),[40,41] a technology commonly employed for identification of bacteria and yeast colonies. Whereas colony growth can be tested directly, organisms in blood culture broth must be processed to separate the organism from blood cells for testing, and various methods have been evaluated.[42] Identification accuracy for direct MALDI-TOF from blood culture bottles is typically better for gram-negative bacteria than for gram-positive bacteria, and can be improved by a short incubation on agar (smudge plate, 4–8 hours, 84%–97% with correct identification) prior to MALDI-TOF analysis.[43,44]

RAPID, DIRECT, PHENOTYPIC ANTIMICROBIAL SUSCEPTIBILITY TESTING OPTIONS

The Accelerate PhenoTestBC kit used in conjunction with the Accelerate Pheno system (APS) is the first FDA-cleared in vitro diagnostic test for pathogen identification and quantitative AST directly from positive blood cultures.[45] The APS uses multiplexed fluorescence in situ hybridization (FISH) to identify on-panel microbes based on the colocalization of target-specific probes with a universal bacterial probe in the same cell. The minimum inhibitory concentration (MIC) is calculated from analyzing the cellular morphokinetic growth pattern in the presence of antimicrobial agents. The APS assay can provide pathogen identity and quantitative AST phenotype within 2 and 7 hours, respectively. However, whether this rapid turnaround time (TAT) translates into more favorable clinical outcomes remains to be determined.[46,47]

Studies using the APS assay have reported pathogen identification sensitivities ranging from 91.2% to 100% and specificities ranging from 97.3% to 100% for organisms on the panel.[45,48–54] However, 1 study reported an overall false-positive rate as high as 9.5%, of which 42.1% is mitigated by having prior negative Gram stain.[45] Therefore, confirmatory Gram stain should be performed before performing the APS assay. AST results have demonstrated essential agreements (EAs) ranging from 94.5% to 97.6% and categorical agreements (CAs) ranging from 86% to 97.9% compared with routine methods. Importantly, lower CA values have been observed for *Pseudomonas* species and *Acinetobacter* species.[48,52,55] Because assay performance varies depending on the pathogen, laboratories should decide on which organisms to perform the APS assay to best complement existing techniques and improve resulting times. Although this assay has high sensitivity for target organisms, in 1 study only 58.1% to 88.7% of clinical samples analyzed by this assay received any pathogen identification.[56] This low overall sensitivity highlights the need to perform routine methods in parallel with the APS assay.

There is much interest in the application of FDA-approved automated AST platforms intended for use on isolated colonies, such as the BD Phoenix and Biomérieux VITEK2 systems, directly on positive blood culture samples. The Phoenix and VITEK 2 systems are capable of performing colorimetric-based biochemical identification and turbidimetric-based quantitative AST with TATs of 3 to 16 hours. Studies report variable performance of the Phoenix system depending on the species involved and the method of microbial extraction. For instance, the identity concordance of direct inoculation compared with standard procedure ranges from 82% with saponin-based to 92.9% to 95.2% with serum separation tube (SST)-based extraction methods.[57–59] AST results using the Phoenix system similarly vary, with an overall CA of 77% and 95.4% to 99% when using saponin- and SST-based methods, respectively.[57,58] Studies of direct phenotypic AST using the VITEK 2 system compared with standard techniques have similarly reported high identity concordance rates of 82.2% to 95.8% and AST CAs of 94.6% to 99.2% for gram-negative bacilli (GNB).[60–63] Performance for gram-positive cocci (GPC) may not be as reliable.[60] However, parallel MALDI-TOF MS identification and VITEK 2 for AST can provide reasonably accurate results for GNB and GPC.[64,65] Investigations comparing direct AST results using the VITEK 2 and Phoenix systems have also reported high CAs, ranging from 92.4% to 99.5%.[66,67]

The European Committee on Antimicrobial Susceptibility Testing (EUCAST) recently published a rapid AST (RAST) method based on direct disk diffusion (dDD) testing of positive blood cultures on Mueller-Hinton (MH) or Mueller-Hinton Fastidious agar plates.[68] Zone diameter breakpoints after 4, 6, and 8 hours of incubation for 8 common bacterial species and relevant antibiotics are provided. Typical workflow begins with a Gram stain of positive blood culture, followed by inoculating the appropriate subculture plates and a RAST plate with the antibiotic disks of choice. Inhibition zone diameters after 4, 6, and 8 hours on the RAST plate can then be interpreted. In general, the EUCAST RAST method has CAs of greater than 90% when compared with standard method.[68,69] Similarly, a Clinical and Laboratory Standards Institute (CLSI) committee has recently released some promising preliminary results.[70] Given their low costs and ease of use, standardized dDD methods may eventually allow more laboratories to perform direct phenotypic ASTs.

OTHER DIRECT ENZYME-BASED TARGETED ANTIMICROBIAL SUSCEPTIBILITY TESTING METHODS

Detection of bacterial antimicrobial resistance enzymatic activity is widely used for the qualitative phenotypic AST on isolated bacteria. Because these assays are relatively cheap and simple, many have explored their use directly on positive blood cultures to test for the presence of β-lactamase and/or carbapenemase-producing gram-negative bacteria, which are of great clinical concern internationally.[71–74] Colorimetric methods usually start with microbial extraction from positive blood cultures using lysis centrifugation or a short subculture on solid media. The ideal choice of hemolytic agent varies depending on the assay. For example, 10% SDS is more compatible with the β-CARBA test, while 5% saponin is with the Carba NP and NeoRapid CARB tests.[73]

Variations of CLSI's modified carbapenem inactivation method (mCIM) have also been used for bacteria with ESBL and carbapenemase activity directly from positive blood cultures.[71,73,74] Briefly, bacteria are extracted from blood cultures and incubated with either a meropenem or a cephalosporin disk at 35°C to 37°C for approximately 2 hours. Zinc supplementation can be used for metallo-β-lactamase activity detection.[73] The impregnated disk is then applied on an MH plate that is inoculated either freshly or 2 hours previous with a 0.5 McFarland suspension of a standard antibiotic-susceptible strain. The inhibition zone is read and interpreted after 6 to 22 hours of incubation.

Overall, both colorimetric and mCIM-based methods demonstrate high specificities (≥90%) and sensitivities (80%–100%) for the detection of β-lactamase and/or carbapenemase-producing *Enterobacterales* extracted directly from aerobic blood culture bottles.[71–74] Resulting times between 20 minutes to 6.5 hours have been reported for colorimetric methods, and between 8 to 24 hours for mCIM-based methods. Although these early results are generally promising, more studies must be done to standardize methodology and result interpretation before clinical use.

STEWARDSHIP/UTILIZATION

By March of 2020, the US Centers for Medicare and Medicaid Services required all acute care hospitals to implement antimicrobial stewardship programs (ASPs).[75] ASPs ensure that patients receive appropriate antimicrobial regimens, which improves patient outcomes, reducing adverse events (eg, toxicity, antibiotic resistance, or *Clostridioides difficile* infection), and allows for optimal resource utilization. To meet these goals, the US Centers for Disease Control and Prevention recommend that ASPs work with the microbiology laboratory on diagnostic stewardship and implementation of rapid diagnostic testing (RDT).[76] In regards to blood cultures, the IDSA recommends that ASPs advocate for RDT from positive blood cultures to optimize therapy and improve outcomes.[77]

Once blood cultures flag positive, it is through the use of RDTs, such as those described previously, that timely microorganism identification and potentially antimicrobial susceptibility/resistance information, via genotypic or phenotypic methods, can be quickly provided to clinicians. However, the impact of RDTs on patient outcomes requires ASP intervention. In a meta-analysis that included 31 observational studies (5920 patients) and various RDTs, it was found that RDTs had a mortality benefit but only in the presence of ASPs.[78] This mortality benefit was found with both gram-positive and gram-negative infections.[78] In addition to the mortality benefit of RDTs in combination with ASPs, this combination is also cost-effective. A cost-effectiveness evaluation of RDTs with or without ASPs was compared to conventional laboratory methods with ASP involvement.[79] It was found that the use of molecular RDTs with ASP had an 80% chance of being cost-effective, while it was only a 41.1% change without an ASP.[79] Thus it is imperative for laboratories to work with their ASPs to maximize the benefits of RDTs from positive blood cultures.

DISCLOSURE

The authors do not have any external funding or conflicts of interest.

REFERENCES

1. Chen IH, Nicolau DP, Kuti JL. Effect of clinically meaningful antibiotic concentrations on recovery of *Escherichia coli* and *Klebsiella pneumoniae* isolates from

anaerobic blood culture bottles with and without antibiotic binding resins. J Clin Microbiol 2019;57(12):e01344.

2. Chen IH, Nicolau DP, Kuti JL. Recovery of gram-negative bacteria from aerobic blood culture bottles containing antibiotic binding resins after exposure to beta-lactam and fluoroquinolone concentrations. J Clin Microbiol 2019;57(10). e00849-19.

3. Flayhart D, Borek AP, Wakefield T, et al. Comparison of BACTEC PLUS blood culture media to BacT/Alert FA blood culture media for detection of bacterial pathogens in samples containing therapeutic levels of antibiotics. J Clin Microbiol 2007;45(3):816–21.

4. Lancaster DP, Friedman DF, Chiotos K, et al. Blood volume required for detection of low levels and ultralow levels of organisms responsible for neonatal bacteremia by use of bactec peds plus/F, Plus Aerobic/F Medium, and the BD Bactec FX System: an in Vitro Study. J Clin Microbiol 2015;53(11):3609–13.

5. Yaacobi N, Bar-Meir M, Shchors I, et al. A prospective controlled trial of the optimal volume for neonatal blood cultures. Pediatr Infect Dis J 2015;34(4):351–4.

6. Messbarger N, Neemann K. Role of anaerobic blood cultures in neonatal bacteremia. J Pediatric Infect Dis Soc 2018;7(3):e65–9.

7. Gross I, Gordon O, Abu Ahmad W, et al. Yield of anaerobic blood cultures in pediatric emergency department patients. Pediatr Infect Dis J 2018;37(4):281–6.

8. Zaidi AK, Knaut AL, Mirrett S, et al. Value of routine anaerobic blood cultures for pediatric patients. J Pediatr 1995;127(2):263–8.

9. Dien Bard J, McElvania TeKippe E. Diagnosis of bloodstream infections in children. J Clin Microbiol 2016;54(6):1418–24.

10. Doern GV, Carroll KC, Diekema DJ, et al. A comprehensive update on the problem of blood culture contamination and a discussion of methods for addressing the problem. Clin Microbiol Rev 2019;33(1). e00009-19.

11. Rupp ME, Cavalieri RJ, Marolf C, et al. Reduction in blood culture contamination through use of initial specimen diversion device. Clin Infect Dis 2017;65(2):201–5.

12. Weinstein MP. Blood culture contamination: persisting problems and partial progress. J Clin Microbiol 2003;41(6):2275–8.

13. Skoglund E, Dempsey CJ, Chen H, et al. Estimated clinical and economic impact through use of a novel blood collection device to reduce blood culture contamination in the emergency department: a cost-benefit analysis. J Clin Microbiol 2019;57(1). e01015-18.

14. Geisler BP, Jilg N, Patton RG, et al. Model to evaluate the impact of hospital-based interventions targeting false-positive blood cultures on economic and clinical outcomes. J Hosp Infect 2019;102(4):438–44.

15. Lalezari A, Cohen MJ, Svinik O, et al. A simplified blood culture sampling protocol for reducing contamination and costs: a randomized controlled trial. Clin Microbiol Infect 2020;26(4):470–4.

16. Zimmerman FS, Karameh H, Ben-Chetrit E, et al. Modification of blood test draw order to reduce blood culture contamination: a randomized clinical trial. Clin Infect Dis 2019. https://doi.org/10.1093/cid/ciz971.

17. Cockerill FR 3rd, Wilson JW, Vetter EA, et al. Optimal testing parameters for blood cultures. Clin Infect Dis 2004;38(12):1724–30.

18. Mermel LA, Maki DG. Detection of bacteremia in adults: consequences of culturing an inadequate volume of blood. Ann Intern Med 1993;119(4):270–2.

19. Miller JM, Binnicker MJ, Campbell S, et al. A guide to utilization of the microbiology laboratory for diagnosis of infectious diseases: 2018 update by the

Infectious Diseases Society of America and the American Society for Microbiology. Clin Infect Dis 2018;67(6):813–6.

20. Freifeld AG, Bow EJ, Sepkowitz KA, et al. Clinical practice guideline for the use of antimicrobial agents in neutropenic patients with cancer: 2010 update by the infectious diseases society of America. Clin Infect Dis 2011;52(4):e56–93.

21. Patel R, Vetter EA, Harmsen WS, et al. Optimized pathogen detection with 30-compared to 20-milliliter blood culture draws. J Clin Microbiol 2011;49(12): 4047–51.

22. Zaleski M, Erdman P, Adams J, et al. Establishing a long-term model for analysis and improvement of underfilled blood culture volumes. Am J Clin Pathol 2019; 151(2):164–70.

23. Khare R, Kothari T, Castagnaro J, et al. Active monitoring and feedback to improve blood culture fill volumes and positivity across a large integrated health system. Clin Infect Dis 2020;70(2):262–8.

24. Venturelli C, Righi E, Borsari L, et al. Impact of pre-analytical time on the recovery of pathogens from blood cultures: results from a large retrospective survey. PLoS One 2017;12(1):e0169466.

25. Altun O, Almuhayawi M, Luthje P, et al. Controlled evaluation of the new BacT/ alert virtuo blood culture system for detection and time to detection of bacteria and yeasts. J Clin Microbiol 2016;54(4):1148 51.

26. Jacobs MR, Mazzulli T, Hazen KC, et al. Multicenter clinical evaluation of BacT/ alert virtuo blood culture system. J Clin Microbiol 2017;55(8):2413–21.

27. Park J, Han S, Shin S. Comparison of growth performance of the BacT/ALERT VIRTUO and BACTEC FX blood culture systems under simulated bloodstream infection conditions. Clin Lab 2017;63(1):39–46.

28. Menchinelli G, Liotti FM, Fiori B, et al. In vitro Evaluation of BACT/ALERT(R) VIRTUO(R), BACT/ALERT 3D(R), and BACTEC FX automated blood culture systems for detection of microbial pathogens using simulated human blood samples. Front Microbiol 2019;10:221.

29. Mirrett S, Hanson KE, Reller LB. Controlled clinical comparison of VersaTREK and BacT/ALERT blood culture systems. J Clin Microbiol 2007;45(2):299 302.

30. Lee S, Kim S. Accuracy of BacT/alert virtuo for measuring blood volume for blood culture. Ann Lab Med 2019;39(6):590–2.

31. Coorevits L, Van den Abeele AM. Evaluation of the BD BACTEC FX blood volume monitoring system as a continuous quality improvement measure. Eur J Clin Microbiol Infect Dis 2015;34(7):1459–66.

32. Campigotto A, Richardson SE, Sebert M, et al. Low utility of pediatric isolator blood culture system for detection of fungemia in children: a 10-year review. J Clin Microbiol 2016;54(9):2284–7.

33. Bourbeau PP, Foltzer M. Routine incubation of BacT/ALERT FA and FN blood culture bottles for more than 3 days may not be necessary. J Clin Microbiol 2005; 43(5):2506–9.

34. Bourbeau PP, Pohlman JK. Three days of incubation may be sufficient for routine blood cultures with BacT/Alert FAN blood culture bottles. J Clin Microbiol 2001; 39(6):2079–82.

35. Wilson ML, Mirrett S, Reller LB, et al. Recovery of clinically important microorganisms from the BacT/Alert blood culture system does not require testing for seven days. Diagn Microbiol Infect Dis 1993;16(1):31–4.

36. Petti CA, Bhally HS, Weinstein MP, et al. Utility of extended blood culture incubation for isolation of *Haemophilus, Actinobacillus, Cardiobacterium, Eikenella,* and

Kingella organisms: a retrospective multicenter evaluation. J Clin Microbiol 2006; 44(1):257–9.

37. Munson EL, Diekema DJ, Beekmann SE, et al. Detection and treatment of bloodstream infection: laboratory reporting and antimicrobial management. J Clin Microbiol 2003;41(1):495–7.

38. Barenfanger J, Graham DR, Kolluri L, et al. Decreased mortality associated with prompt Gram staining of blood cultures. Am J Clin Pathol 2008;130(6):870–6.

39. Martinez RM. Remote technical review of blood culture gram stains at a large integrated healthcare network. J Appl Lab Med 2019;3(4):733–4.

40. Spanu T, Posteraro B, Fiori B, et al. Direct maldi-tof mass spectrometry assay of blood culture broths for rapid identification of *Candida* species causing bloodstream infections: an observational study in two large microbiology laboratories. J Clin Microbiol 2012;50(1):176–9.

41. Lagace-Wiens PR, Adam HJ, Karlowsky JA, et al. Identification of blood culture isolates directly from positive blood cultures by use of matrix-assisted laser desorption ionization-time of flight mass spectrometry and a commercial extraction system: analysis of performance, cost, and turnaround time. J Clin Microbiol 2012;50(10):3324–8.

42. Saffert RT, Cunningham SA, Mandrekar J, et al. Comparison of three preparatory methods for detection of bacteremia by MALDI-TOF mass spectrometry. Diagn Microbiol Infect Dis 2012;73(1):21–6.

43. Chen Y, Porter V, Mubareka S, et al. Rapid identification of bacteria directly from positive blood cultures by use of a serum separator tube, smudge plate preparation, and matrix-assisted laser desorption ionization-time of flight mass spectrometry. J Clin Microbiol 2015;53(10):3349–52.

44. Mitchell SL, Alby K. Performance of microbial identification by MALDI-TOF MS and susceptibility testing by VITEK 2 from positive blood cultures after minimal incubation on solid media. Eur J Clin Microbiol Infect Dis 2017;36(11):2201–6.

45. Pancholi P, Carroll KC, Buchan BW, et al. Multicenter evaluation of the Accelerate PhenoTest BC Kit for rapid identification and phenotypic antimicrobial susceptibility testing using morphokinetic cellular analysis. J Clin Microbiol 2018;56(4). e01329-17.

46. Ehren K, Meissner A, Jazmati N, et al. Clinical impact of rapid species identification from positive blood cultures with same-day phenotypic antimicrobial susceptibility testing on the management and outcome of bloodstream infections. Clin Infect Dis 2020;70(7):1285–93.

47. Juttukonda LJ, Katz S, Gillon J, et al. Impact of a rapid blood culture diagnostic test in a children's hospital depends on gram-positive versus gram-negative organism and day versus night shift. J Clin Microbiol 2020;58(4). e01400-19.

48. Bowler SL, Towne JW, Humphries RM, et al. Evaluation of the accelerate pheno system for identification of *Acinetobacter* clinical isolates and minocycline susceptibility testing. J Clin Microbiol 2019;57(3). e01711-18.

49. Burnham JP, Wallace MA, Fuller BM, et al. Clinical effect of expedited pathogen identification and susceptibility testing for gram-negative bacteremia and candidemia by use of the accelerate pheno(TM) System. J Appl Lab Med 2019;3(4): 569–79.

50. Charnot-Katsikas A, Tesic V, Love N, et al. Use of the accelerate pheno system for identification and antimicrobial susceptibility testing of pathogens in positive blood cultures and impact on time to results and workflow. J Clin Microbiol 2018;56(1). e01166-17.

51. De Angelis G, Grossi A, Menchinelli G, et al. Rapid molecular tests for detection of antimicrobial resistance determinants in gram-negative organisms from positive blood cultures: a systematic review and meta-analysis. Clin Microbiol Infect 2020;26(3):271–80.
52. Descours G, Desmurs L, Hoang TLT, et al. Evaluation of the Accelerate Pheno system for rapid identification and antimicrobial susceptibility testing of Gram-negative bacteria in bloodstream infections. Eur J Clin Microbiol Infect Dis 2018;37(8):1573–83.
53. Lutgring JD, Bittencourt C, McElvania TeKippe E, et al. Evaluation of the accelerate pheno system: results from two academic medical centers. J Clin Microbiol 2018;56(4). e01672-17.
54. Schneider JG, Wood JB, Smith NW, et al. Direct antimicrobial susceptibility testing of positive blood cultures: a comparison of the Accelerate Pheno and VI-TEK(R) 2 systems. Diagn Microbiol Infect Dis 2019;95(3):114841.
55. Calderaro A, Buttrini M, Martinelli M, et al. Rapid microbial identification and phenotypic antimicrobial susceptibility testing directly from positive blood cultures: a new platform compared to routine laboratory methods. Diagn Microbiol Infect Dis 2020;96(3):114955.
56. Trotter AJ, Aydin A, Strinden MJ, et al. Recent and emerging technologies for the rapid diagnosis of infection and antimicrobial resistance. Curr Opin Microbiol 2019;51:39–45.
57. Lupetti A, Barnini S, Castagna B, et al. Rapid identification and antimicrobial susceptibility profiling of gram-positive cocci in blood cultures with the Vitek 2 system. Eur J Clin Microbiol Infect Dis 2010;29(1):89–95.
58. Beuving J, Verbon A, Gronthoud FA, et al. Antibiotic susceptibility testing of grown blood cultures by combining culture and real-time polymerase chain reaction is rapid and effective. PLoS One 2011;6(12):e27689.
59. Funke G, Funke-Kissling P. Use of the BD PHOENIX Automated Microbiology System for direct identification and susceptibility testing of gram-negative rods from positive blood cultures in a three-phase trial. J Clin Microbiol 2004;42(4):1466–70.
60. Chen JR, Lee SY, Yang BH, et al. Rapid identification and susceptibility testing using the VITEK 2 system using culture fluids from positive BacT/ALERT blood cultures. J Microbiol Immunol Infect 2008;41(3):259–64.
61. Munoz-Davila MJ, Yague G, Albert M, et al. Comparative evaluation of Vitek 2 identification and susceptibility testing of gram-negative rods directly and isolated from BacT/ALERT-positive blood culture bottles. Eur J Clin Microbiol Infect Dis 2012;31(5):663–9.
62. Bruins MJ, Bloembergen P, Ruijs GJ, et al. Identification and susceptibility testing of Enterobacteriaceae and Pseudomonas aeruginosa by direct inoculation from positive BACTEC blood culture bottles into Vitek 2. J Clin Microbiol 2004;42(1):7–11.
63. Ling TK, Liu ZK, Cheng AF. Evaluation of the VITEK 2 system for rapid direct identification and susceptibility testing of gram-negative bacilli from positive blood cultures. J Clin Microbiol 2003;41(10):4705–7.
64. Romero-Gomez MP, Gomez-Gil R, Pano-Pardo JR, et al. Identification and susceptibility testing of microorganism by direct inoculation from positive blood culture bottles by combining MALDI-TOF and Vitek-2 Compact is rapid and effective. J Infect 2012;65(6):513–20.
65. De Angelis G, Posteraro B, Menchinelli G, et al. Antimicrobial susceptibility testing of pathogens isolated from blood culture: a performance comparison of

Accelerate Pheno and VITEK(R) 2 systems with the broth microdilution method. J Antimicrob Chemother 2019;74(Suppl 1):i24–31.

66. Gherardi G, Angeletti S, Panitti M, et al. Comparative evaluation of the Vitek-2 Compact and Phoenix systems for rapid identification and antibiotic susceptibility testing directly from blood cultures of gram-negative and gram-positive isolates. Diagn Microbiol Infect Dis 2012;72(1):20–31.

67. Horing S, Massarani AS, Loffler B, et al. Rapid antibiotic susceptibility testing in blood culture diagnostics performed by direct inoculation using the VITEK(R)-2 and BD Phoenix platforms. Eur J Clin Microbiol Infect Dis 2019;38(3):471–8.

68. Jonasson E, Matuschek E, Kahlmeter G. The EUCAST rapid disc diffusion method for antimicrobial susceptibility testing directly from positive blood culture bottles. J Antimicrob Chemother 2020;75(4):968–78.

69. Jasuja JK, Zimmermann S, Burckhardt I. Evaluation of EUCAST rapid antimicrobial susceptibility testing (RAST) for positive blood cultures in clinical practice using a total lab automation. Eur J Clin Microbiol Infect Dis 2020;39(7):1305–13.

70. Chandrasekaran S, Abbott A, Campeau S, et al. Direct-from-blood-culture disk diffusion to determine antimicrobial susceptibility of gram-negative bacteria: preliminary report from the clinical and laboratory standards institute methods development and standardization working group. J Clin Microbiol 2018;56(3). e01678-17.

71. Bianco G, Boattini M, Iannaccone M, et al. Direct beta-lactam inactivation method: a new low-cost assay for rapid detection of carbapenemase- or extended-spectrum-beta-lactamase-producing Enterobacterales directly from positive blood culture bottles. J Clin Microbiol 2019;58(1). e01178-19.

72. Lima-Morales D, Avila H, Soldi T, et al. Rapid detection of carbapenemase production directly from blood culture by colorimetric methods: evaluation in a routine microbiology laboratory. J Clin Microbiol 2018;56(9). e00325-18.

73. Meier M, Hamprecht A. Rapid detection of carbapenemases directly from positive blood cultures by the beta-CARBA test. Eur J Clin Microbiol Infect Dis 2019;38(2):259–64.

74. Sfeir MM, Satlin MJ, Fauntleroy KA, et al. Blood-modified carbapenem inactivation method: a phenotypic method for detecting carbapenemase-producing Enterobacteriaceae directly from positive blood culture broths. J Clin Microbiol 2020;58(2). e01377-19.

75. Federal_Register. Medicare and Medicaid programs; regulatory provisions to promote program efficiency, transparency, and burden reduction; fire safety requirements for certain dialysis facilities; hospital and critical access hospital (CAH) changes to promote innovation, flexibility, and improvement in patient care. Fed Regist 2019;84:51732–834.

76. CDC. The Core Elements of Hospital Antibiotic Stewardship Programs: 2019. 2019. Available at: https://www.cdc.gov/antibiotic-use/core-elements/hospital. html.

77. Barlam TF, Cosgrove SE, Abbo LM, et al. Implementing an antibiotic stewardship program: guidelines by the Infectious Diseases Society of America and the society for Healthcare Epidemiology of America. Clin Infect Dis 2016;62(10):e51–77.

78. Timbrook TT, Morton JB, McConeghy KW, et al. The effect of molecular rapid diagnostic testing on clinical outcomes in bloodstream infections: a systematic review and meta-analysis. Clin Infect Dis 2017;64(1):15–23.

79. Pliakos EE, Andreatos N, Shehadeh F, et al. The cost-effectiveness of rapid diagnostic testing for the diagnosis of bloodstream infections with or without antimicrobial stewardship. Clin Microbiol Rev 2018;31(3). e00095-17.

Panels and Syndromic Testing in Clinical Microbiology

Jennifer Dien Bard, PhD, D(ABMM)[a,b,*],
Erin McElvania, PhD, D(ABMM)[c,d]

KEYWORDS

- Syndromic panel • Respiratory panel • Bloodstream infection panel
- Gastroenteritis panel • Meningitis panel • Encephalitis panel
- Diagnostic stewardship • Laboratory stewardship

KEY POINTS

- Syndromic testing allows clinicians to rapidly test for a broad number of pathogens, generally with greater sensitivity and specificity than traditional methods.
- With the ease of testing has come the overuse of testing.
- Diagnostic stewardship is necessary to ensure proper use of syndromic testing and correct interpretation of the results in the context of the patient.

INTRODUCTION

In 2011, the first respiratory syndromic panel was cleared by the US Food and Drug Administration (FDA). In less than 10 years' time, syndromic panel testing has expanded to multiple commercial assays for detection of respiratory, blood, gastrointestinal (GI), acute meningitis and encephalitis (ME), and lower respiratory tract infections (LRTIs) and in doing so it has revolutionized the clinical microbiology laboratory. Syndromic panels have been embraced by clinical microbiology laboratories who appreciate the low hands-on time and integrated work flow these assays provide. They have also been embraced by clinicians who love the rapid turnaround time and broad number of targets, many of which they had not been able to routinely

[a] Department of Pathology and Laboratory Medicine, Children's Hospital Los Angeles, 4650 Sunset Boulevard MS#32, Los Angeles, CA 90027, USA; [b] University of Southern California, Keck School of Medicine; [c] Department of Pathology and Laboratory Medicine, Evanston Hospital, NorthShore University HealthSystem, 2650 Ridge Avenue, Evanston, IL 60201, USA; [d] University of Chicago Pritzker School of Medicine
* Corresponding author. Department of Pathology and Laboratory Medicine, Children's Hospital Los Angeles, 4650 Sunset Boulevard MS#32, Los Angeles, CA 90027.
E-mail address: jdienbard@chla.usc.edu
Twitter: @dienbard (J.D.B.); @e_mcelvania (E.M.)

Clin Lab Med 40 (2020) 393–420
https://doi.org/10.1016/j.cll.2020.08.001
0272-2712/20/© 2020 Elsevier Inc. All rights reserved.

labmed.theclinics.com

test for before syndromic panels. However, with these advances have come complications—the high cost of testing, overtesting, and confusing results that do not have a clear link to patient care, such as multiple positive results or targets of unknown significance. In this article, we discuss the commercially available syndromic panels, the benefits and limitations of testing, and how diagnostic and laboratory stewardship can be used to optimize testing and improve patient care while keeping costs under control.

DETECTION OF BLOODSTREAM PATHOGENS

Detection of bloodstream infections (BSI) is one of the most important functions of the microbiology laboratory. Because these infections cause great morbidity and mortality, placing patients on optimal treatment as quickly as possible is a high priority.[1] Syndromic testing of positive blood culture broth provides rapid pathogen identification for the majority of bacteria that cause BSIs as well as common contaminants that do not require treatment.[2] In addition, several syndromic blood panels detect antimicrobial resistance genes and 1 assay provides rapid phenotypic susceptibility results. **Table 1** provides a list of FDA-cleared syndromic panels for diagnosis of BSIs. These assays provide bacterial identification 18 to 24 hours earlier than conventional culture and identification methods. The limited susceptibility information is available 48 hours earlier than traditional phenotypic susceptibility results. Syndromic panels for BSIs represent an adjunct test and do not replace culture or complete antimicrobial susceptibility testing. The exception is the Accelerate PhenoTest BC (Accelerate Diagnostics, Tucson, AZ), which provides identification and complete phenotypic susceptibility results in 9 hours.[3]

Limitations of these assays include no detection of off-target pathogens, a lack of full susceptibility information, cost, and false-positive results. Not every bloodstream pathogen is represented as a target organism on syndromic panels and for these off-target organisms no identification is provided. The scope of antimicrobial resistance information provided depends on the targets present on the syndromic panel. Resistance markers provided for gram-positive organisms are largely sufficient for optimal antimicrobial treatment. For gram-negative organisms, most panels provide only partial information. For the PhenoTest BC, the antibiotics tested are set by the manufacturer and may or may not meet the needs of your patient population or hospital drug formulary. In many cases, traditional identification and susceptibility testing, and the associated delay, is still required to provide all of the information needed for patient care. Syndromic panels are expensive, especially compared with other testing performed in the microbiology laboratory and the cost may be a challenge to implement these assays into your institution. This issue is somewhat less important with syndromic tests for BSIs because only positive blood culture broth is tested and the infections being treated are of critical importance. Recently there have been reports of false-positive *Proteus* and *Escherichia coli* results caused by nonviable DNA in the blood culture broth of some blood culture bottles.[2] These false-positive results cause patients to be treated for bacterial infections they do not have and potentially mistreated for bacteria that is present in their blood.

Although all laboratories have reported decreased turnaround time to results using syndromic blood culture panels, the results of outcome studies measuring their effect on patient care and hospital finances has been mixed. The biggest benefits are seen with the detection of highly resistant organisms such as multidrug-resistant gram-negative bacteria or vancomycin-resistant enterococci.[4-7] Empiric therapy is often ineffective against these organisms, so rapid identification and antibiotic escalation

Table 1
Multiplex blood culture panels, FDA-cleared

Assay	Turnaround Time	Throughput	Targets	Antimicrobial Resistance
BioFire FilmArray BCID Panel	1 h	1 test module per instrument (v2.0) 2–12 test modules per instrument (Torch)	Bacterial targets Enterococcus spp. Listeria monocytogenes Staphylococcus spp. Staphylococcus aureus Streptococcus spp. Streptococcus agalactiae Streptococcus pyogenes Streptococcus pneumoniae Acinetobacter baumannii Haemophilus influenzae Neisseria meningitidis Pseudomonas aeruginosa Enterobacteriaceae Enterobacter cloacae complex Escherichia coli Klebsiella oxytoca Klebsiella pneumoniae Proteus spp. Serratia marcescens Fungal Targets Candida albicans Candida glabrata Candida krusei Candida parapsilosis Candida tropicalis	Methicillin resistance detection mecA Vancomycin resistance detection vanA vanB Carbapenemase detection KPC

(continued on next page)

Table 1
(continued)

Assay	Turnaround Time	Throughput	Targets	Antimicrobial Resistance
GenMark ePlex BCID-GP Panel	1.5 h	3–24 test modules per instrument	Bacterial targets *Bacillus cereus group* *Bacillus subtilis group* *Corynebacterium* *Cutibacterium acnes (Propionibacterium acnes)* *Enterococcus spp.* *Enterococcus faecalis* *Enterococcus faecium* *Lactobacillus spp.* *Listeria spp.* *L monocytogenes* *Micrococcus* *Staphylococcus spp.* *Staphylococcus aureus* *Staphylococcus epidermidis* *Staphylococcus lugdunensis* *Streptococcus spp.* *Streptococcus agalactiae* *Streptococcus anginosus group* *Streptococcus pneumoniae* *Streptococcus pyogenes* Other targets Pan gram-negative Pan *Candida*	Methicillin resistance detection mecA Vancomycin resistance detection vanA vanB

| GenMark ePlex BCID-GN Panel | 1.5 h | 3–24 test modules per instrument | Bacterial targets
A baumannii
Bacteroides fragilis
Citrobacter spp.
Cronobacter sakazakii
Enterobacter spp. (non-cloacae complex)
Enterobacter cloacae complex
E coli
Fusobacterium nucleatum
Fusobacterium necrophorum
H influenzae
K oxytoca
K pneumoniae group
Morganella morganii
N meningitidis
Proteus spp.
Proteus mirabilis
P aeruginosa
Salmonella spp.
Serratias spp.
S marcescens
Stenotrophomonas maltophilia
Other targets
Pan gram positive
Pan Candida | ESBL detection
CTX-M
Carbapenemase detection
IMP
KPC
NDM
OXA (OXA-23 and OXA-48)
VIM |

(continued on next page)

Table 1
(continued)

Assay	Turnaround Time	Throughput	Targets	Antimicrobial Resistance
GenMark ePlex BCID-FP Panel	1.5 h	3–24 test modules per instrument	Fungal targets Candida albicans Candida auris Candida dubliniensis Candida famata Candida glabrata Candida guilliermondii Candida kefyr Candida krusei Candida lusitaniae Candida parapsilosis Candida tropicalis Cryptococcus gattii Cryptococcus neoformans Fusarium Rhodotorula	—
Luminex Verigene Gram-Positive Blood Culture Test (BC-GP)	2 h	1 test module per instrument (v1.0) 6 test modules per instrument (v2.0)	Bacterial targets S aureus Staphylococcus epidermidis Staphylococcus lugdunensis S agalactiae S pneumoniae S pyogenes	Methicillin resistance detection mecA Vancomycin resistance detection vanA vanB

Test	Time	Throughput	Targets	Resistance/other detection
			Enterococcus faecalis E faecium	ESBL detection
			Streptococcus anginosus	CTX-M
			Staphylococcus spp.	Carbapenemase detection
			Streptococcus spp.	IMP
			Listeria spp.	KPC
Luminex Verigene Gram-Negative Blood Culture Test (BC-GN)	2 h	1 test module per instrument (v1.0)	Bacterial targets	NDM
		6 test modules per instrument (v2.0)	E coli	OXA
			K pneumoniae	VIM
			K oxytoca	
			P aeruginosa	
			Acinetobacter spp.	
			Citrobacter spp.	
			Enterobacter spp.	
			Proteus spp.	
T2 Biosystems T2Candida Panel	3–5 h	1 test per instrument	Fungal targets	
			C albicans	
			C tropicalis	
			C krusei	
			C glabrata	
			C parapsilosis	
T2Biosystems T2Bacteria Panel	5 h	1 test per instrument	Bacterial targets	
			E faecium	
			S aureus	
			K pneumoniae	
			P aeruginosa	
			E coli	

(continued on next page)

Table 1
(continued)

Assay	Turnaround Time	Throughput	Targets	Antimicrobial Resistance

Accelerate Pheno	2 h for identification
	7 h for phenotypic antimicrobial susceptibility testing
		1 test per instrument	Bacterial targets
			  E faecium
			  E faecalis
			  Coagulase-negative Staphylococcus spp.
			  S aureus
			  S lugdunensis
			  Streptococcus spp.
			  E coli
			  Klebsiella spp.
			  Enterobacter spp.
			  Proteus spp.
			  Citrobacter spp.
			  S marcescens
			  P aeruginosa
			  A baumannii
			Fungal Targets
			  C albicans
			  C glabrata
				Phenotypic susceptibility results

Abbreviation: ESBL, extended spectrum beta-lactamase.

can decrease mortality, hospital length of stay, and hospital costs. For routine bacteria causing BSI, which constitutes the majority of positive blood cultures, patients are receiving effective empiric therapy and syndromic panel results do not affect antimicrobial selection, patient mortality, hospital length of stay, or hospital costs.[4,6,8,9] Passive reporting of syndromic blood culture panel information results in rapid antibiotic escalation, but deescalation and discontinuation of unnecessary antimicrobials is much slower if it happens at all.[10,11] The biggest lesson these outcome studies have taught us is the critical value of antimicrobial stewardship programs in the timely optimization or discontinuation of antibiotics.[12]

Most syndromic blood culture assays use positive blood culture broth as their test medium. That means that a blood culture must incubate for 12 to 48 before becoming positive and testing commences. To identify bloodstream pathogens more rapidly, it would be ideal to eliminate the incubation period and test for pathogens directly from whole blood. T2 Biosystems (Lexington, MA) T2Candida and T2Bacteria panels are 2 FDA-cleared culture-independent assays for detection of BSIs. Although more rapid than culture-based syndromic panels, these assays have limited targets and do not provide susceptibility information, so traditional blood culture is still required. Although not yet FDA cleared, metagenomic next-generation sequencing of microbial cell free DNA is gaining traction as an unbiased method of bacterial, viral, fungal, and parasitic pathogen detection (Karius, Redwood City, CA).[13] Results can be difficult to interpret because this test is often positive for multiple organisms. Although testing is performed directly from plasma, it must be sent to a reference laboratory, which dramatically impacts the turnaround time of results. In the largest outcome study to date, microbial cell-free DNA testing led to minimal impact on patient management.[14] Culture-independent bloodstream pathogen assays are very expensive, even more so than those that use positive blood culture broth as their testing medium. Issues such as who should be tested, for what indications, and how frequently are not settled. Diagnostic stewardship is necessary to optimize the benefits of these tests while keeping the costs under control and clinical microbiology laboratory directors should be involved in testing approval and results interpretation in close collaboration with our infectious disease colleagues.

MENINGITIS/ENCEPHALITIS SYNDROMIC PANEL

Infections of the central nervous system, including ME, cause potentially life-threatening diseases with a myriad of infectious causes in both the pediatric and adult population. There is a dire need for improved diagnostic for ME to address the short-comings of conventional microbiological approaches such as Gram stain and culture.

The FilmArray Meningitis/Encephalitis panel (FA-ME, BioFire Diagnostics, Salt Lake City, UT) (**Table 2**) remains the only syndromic ME panel despite being cleared by the FDA in 2015 for in vitro diagnostic use. There is a paucity of outcome studies evaluating the clinical utility of a multiplexed panel for ME compared with current standard of care testing. One clear-cut benefit of FA-ME is the significant improvement in herpes simplex virus (HSV) turnaround time, which can lead to decreased acyclovir exposure.[15,16] Early diagnosis of aseptic meningitis through detection of enterovirus or parechovirus can allow providers to avoid antibiotics and possibly negate the need for hospital admissions.[17] Limited data have been published on the economic benefits and patient outcomes associated with the FA-ME, but the data we have report hospital cost savings and decreased length of stay.[18,19] Prospective studies investigating the impact of the FA-ME panel on antimicrobial selection, patient outcomes, and

Table 2
Multiplex meningitis encephalitis panel, FDA cleared

Assay	Turnaround Time	Throughput	Bacterial Targets	Viral Targets	Fungal Targets
BioFire FilmArray Meningitis/Encephalitis Panel	1 h	1 test module per instrument (v2.0) 2–12 test modules per instrument (Torch)	*Escherichia coli* K1 *Haemophilus influenzae* *Listeria monocytogenes* *Neisseria meningitidis* *Streptococcus agalactiae* *Streptococcus pneumoniae*	Cytomegalovirus Enterovirus HSV 1 HSV 2 HHV-6 Human parechovirus Varicella zoster virus	*Cryptococcus neoformans/ gattii*

hospital economics is necessary to determine the true benefits of the syndromic panel. In this study, the potential negative impact of a large panel test should also be assessed.

Despite some clear benefits of the FA-ME panel, there are also concerns.[20] Primary among them is the risk of false-positive and false-negative results with the HSV-1 target.[21,22] Yet the performance was noted to be comparable with or superior to alternate HSV polymerase chain reaction (PCR) tests in other studies.[23,24] A recent meta-analysis on the performance of the FA-ME panel reported a negative predictive value of 99.7% after adjudication of the false-negative results.[25] It is important to assess the clinical sensitivity of FA-ME panel to determine the significance of these potentially weak positives detected by alternate PCR and the majority of studies reporting HSV-1 false-negative results have not pursued this point. Nevertheless, in patients with a high suspicion for HSV infection such as neonates, HSV PCR from blood and lesions is indicated before discontinuation of acyclovir. Additional testing recommendations through interpretative comments and/or direct communications with providers in these situations may assist with correct interpretation of test results.

Providers must also be aware that the FA-ME panel is not a standalone test. For instance, the diagnosis of cryptococcal meningitis in patients at high risk for cryptococcosis should consist of culture and cryptococcal antigen testing (both cerebrospinal fluid [CSF] and serum) in conjunction with the FA-ME. A multifactorial approach that include all 3 tests increases the diagnostic yield because false-negative CSF cryptococcal antigen testing results have also been reported.[26] A recent multicenter study of 1384 patients confirmed that the performance of the FA-ME panel for *Cryptococcus* highly correlated with culture at a sensitivity of 96.4%.[27] The sensitivity was lower compared with cryptococcal antigen testing, but the majority of FA-ME false negatives were from patients with chronic cryptococcal meningitis on antifungal therapy, indicating a dependence on organism burden.

The clinical specificity of human herpesvirus (HHV)-6 detection by the FA-ME panel is an ongoing conundrum that requires further investigation to differentiate between self-limiting primary infection, HHV-6 reactivation, chromosomal integrated HHV-6, or true HHV-6 central nervous system infections. The primary concern is the misdiagnosis of HHV-6 infections and unnecessary exposure to ganciclovir or foscarnet as reported in an adult-only study.[28] Contrary to the 40% rate of unnecessary therapy reported, a recent study of 25 HHV-6 positive pediatric patients reported only 8% of patients (2/25) were unnecessarily treated with intravenous ganciclovir for approximately 24 hours.[29] A 20% rate of central nervous system infections was also reported, of which all had abnormal radiographic findings and the majority were immunocompetent.[29] Key tips to the interpretation of positive HHV-6 result include but are not limited to the presence of central nervous system symptoms, abnormal radiographic findings, and additional HHV-6 detection from alternate sources. A quantitative HHV-6 viral load of greater than 300,000 copies/mL in peripheral blood may point to chromosomal integrated HHV-6 rather than true infection, as well as consistently high HHV-6 viral load despite antiviral therapy.[29] Testing for chromosomal integrated HHV-6 by droplet digital PCR is available at the University of Washington.

As with any laboratory tests, there are advantages and disadvantages to the FA-ME panel and optimal use is best achieved through collaboration between the laboratory and providers to maximize the benefits of the test while recognizing the potential challenges that may be specific to each individual patient case. An important question that warrants further investigation is which patient population would FA-ME panel have the highest diagnostic yield? A recent study of 705 inpatients with FA-ME testing reported that 31.9% of patients tested had little or no suspicion for central nervous system infection supporting the need for potential test restrictions in patients with clear index of suspicion for central nervous system infections.[28] CSF testing restriction using parameters such as CSF pleocytosis have been proposed in the past.[30] However, a recent pediatric study on 1025 CSF samples tested by FA-ME determined that restricting based on immune status and abnormal CSF parameters (glucose, protein, and pleocytosis) would have resulted in missed diagnostic opportunities, particularly in the cases of viral central nervous system infections.[31] Nonetheless, further work to identify more appropriate parameters is warranted because the positivity rate was only 11.8% in the patient cohort, indicating a high potential for test restrictions to identify the most pertinent patients to test. Last, the FA-ME panel does not detect the most common pathogens attributed to ventriculoperitoneal shunt infections and thus should not be performed on ventriculoperitoneal shunt samples. The panel is also only FDA-cleared for CSF specimens obtained by lumbar puncture.

DETECTION OF UPPER RESPIRATORY INFECTION

Before the advent of syndromic panels, routine respiratory viral testing was limited to influenza and respiratory syncytial virus (RSV). Syndromic multiplex PCR panels allowed laboratories to rapidly provide highly sensitive and specific test results for a broad range of viruses and bacteria causing upper respiratory illness. **Table 3** provides a list of FDA-cleared syndromic panels for the diagnosis of upper respiratory illnesses. Owing to the ease of testing, these panels have been widely adopted in clinical microbiology laboratories. Testing a broad range of targets has taught us about the prevalence and clinical significance of many viruses. We are now aware that human metapneumovirus often causes severe disease and that rhinoviruses are ubiquitous, but we are still learning about the clinical significance of some of the targets and their infectious potential in otherwise healthy patients.

Coupled with the benefits of multiplex panels are several limitations of cost, overtesting, and difficulty with results interpretation. Syndromic respiratory panels are very expensive compared with traditional methods of respiratory viral testing. The ease of testing has resulted in massive overtesting, passing on the high costs to the patient, insurance company, or hospital with little benefit to patient care. PCR detection of nucleic acids does not rely on viable organism for detection, which increases the sensitivity over traditional methods. Conversely, patients shed virus long after symptoms of upper respiratory illness have resolved and will remain PCR positive if tested. For this reason, repeat testing and test of cure should not be performed. The widespread use of syndromic panel testing has demonstrated that many patients are positive for multiple targets, and because results are qualitative it is not always obvious which pathogen is responsible for a patient's symptoms. Panels that include targets for coronaviruses HKU1, NL63, 229E, and OC43 have recently resulted in confusion with clinicians and patients mistakenly believing they are positive for severe acute respiratory syndrome coronavirus-2.

Outcome studies have been performed in an effort to quantify the benefit (or limitations) of syndromic respiratory panels. For viral targets on respiratory syndromic panels, only influenza, RSV and adenovirus have an associated antiviral therapy. Theoretically, the detection of other viral targets could benefit patients by decreasing the clinician's suspicion of bacterial infection and either preventing initiation or promoting discontinuation of antibiotic therapy. So how are upper respiratory syndromic panels affecting patient care? Results are mixed, with some studies showing a decrease in antibiotic therapy, decreased length of hospital stay, or decreased additional tests and imaging studies,[32] whereas other studies showed no benefit.[33] Many

Table 3
Multiplex upper respiratory panels, FDA cleared

Assay	Turnaround Time	Throughput	Set up	Bacterial Targets	Viral Targets
Applied BioCode Respiratory Pathogen Panel (RPP)	4 h	96-well plate format	Batched	*Bordetella pertussis* *Chlamydia pneumoniae* *Mycoplasma pneumoniae*	Influenza A, A/H1, A/H3, A/H1-2009 Influenza B RSV A/B Parainfluenza virus 1, 2, 3, and 4 Human metapneumovirus Human rhinovirus/enterovirus Parainfluenza virus 1, 2, 3, and 4
BioFire FilmArray Respiratory Panel 2 (RP2)	45 min	1 test module per instrument (v2.0) 2–12 test modules per instrument (Torch)	On demand	*B pertussis* *Bordetella parapertussis* *C pneumoniae* *M pneumoniae*	Influenza A, A/H1, A/H3, A/H1-2009 Influenza B RSV Parainfluenza virus 1, 2, 3, and 4 Human metapneumovirus Human rhinovirus Adenovirus Coronavirus HKU1, NL63, 229E, and OC43 MERS coronavirus[a]

(continued on next page)

Table 3
(continued)

Assay	Turnaround Time	Throughput	Set up	Bacterial Targets	Viral Targets
BioFire FilmArray Respiratory Panel EZ (CLIA-waived)	1 h	1 test module per instrument	On demand	*B pertussis* *C pneumoniae* *M pneumoniae*	Influenza A, A/H1, A/H3, A/H1-2009 Influenza B RSV Parainfluenza virus Human metapneumovirus Human rhinovirus/enterovirus[a] Adenovirus Coronavirus
GenMark ePlex Respiratory Pathogen Panel (RP)	1.5 h	3–24 test modules per instrument	On demand	*C pneumoniae* *M pneumoniae*	Influenza A, A/H1, A/H3, A/H1-2009 Influenza B RSV A and B Parainfluenza virus 1, 2, 3, and 4 Human metapneumovirus Human rhinovirus/enterovirus Adenovirus Coronavirus
Genmark eSensor XT-8 Respiratory Viral Panel	5 h	8–24 test modules per instrument	Batched		Influenza A, A/H1, A/H3, A/H1-2009 Influenza B RSV A and B Parainfluenza virus 1–3 Human metapneumovirus Human rhinovirus/enterovirus Adenovirus B/E and C

Test	Time	Format	Throughput	Bacterial targets	Viral targets
Luminex Verigene Respiratory Pathogens Flex Test (RP Flex)	2 h	1 test module per instrument (v1.0), 6 test modules per instrument (v2.0)	On demand	*B pertussis*, *Bordetella parapertussis/B bronchiseptica*, *Bordetella holmesii*	Influenza A, and subtypes A/H1, A/H3; Influenza B; RSV A and B; Human rhinovirus; Parainfluenza virus 1, 2, and 3; Human metapneumovirus; Adenovirus
Luminex NxTAG Respiratory Pathogen Panel	5 h	96-well plate format	Batched	*C pneumoniae*, *M pneumoniae*	Influenza A, A/H1, A/H3; Influenza B; RSV A and B; Human rhinovirus/enterovirus; Parainfluenza virus 1, 2, 3, and 4; Human metapneumovirus; Adenovirus; Coronavirus HKU1, NL63, 229E, and OC43; Human bocavirus
Luminex NxTAG RVP FAST v2	3.5 h	96-well plate format	Batched		Influenza A, A/H1, A/H3; Influenza B; RSV; Human rhinovirus/enterovirus; Parainfluenza virus 1, 2, 3, and 4; Human metapneumovirus; Adenovirus; Coronavirus HKU1, NL63, 229E, and OC43

Abbreviation: MERS, Middle East respiratory syndrome.
[a] Available on RP2 PLUS (not an FDA-approved target).

of the studies found benefits only for patients with positive influenza results,[34,35] showing that limited testing may be sufficient for most patients. Diagnostic steward- ship is needed to identify patients who would benefit from broad syndromic panels to maximize their impact on patient care.

LOWER RESPIRATORY TRACT INFECTION SYNDROMIC PANEL

LRTIs encompass a broad spectrum of syndromes including community-acquired pneumonia, hospital-acquired pneumonia, and ventilator-acquired pneumonia and are associated with significant morbidity and mortality, especially in hospitalized pa- tients. Infectious agents, including bacteria, fungi, and viruses associated with LRTIs, may vary depending on patient's immune status and exposure history. An etiologic diagnosis through laboratory workup followed by appropriate therapeutic manage- ment in patients with LRTIs have been associated with a significant decrease in mortality.[36]

The status of culture as a gold standard for LRTI diagnosis is in question. Traditional quantitative or semiquantitative culture methods aim at differentiating between true pathogens and normal respiratory flora. At best, a culture is considered adequate and there are a number of factors that are contributory to its demise as the gold stan- dard, including prior antibiotic exposure, poor growth of fastidious bacteria, and sub- jective interpretation of significant versus insignificant growth.[37] Hence, new and improved approaches to LRTI diagnosis in the clinical laboratory are needed and welcomed.

The shift in diagnostic paradigm first occurred with the development of molecular assays to detect viral pathogens and agents of atypical pneumonia years ago and have since been well-accepted as a superior approach compared with culture for these groups of organisms. There are currently 2 FDA-cleared syndromic panel for the diagnosis of LRTIs: the Unyvero LRT test (Curetis, Holzgerlingen, Germany) was the first to receive FDA clearance followed by FilmArray Pneumonia (PN)/Pneumonia plus (PNplus) panel (BioFire Diagnostics) (**Table 4**). A major difference between the 2 FDA-cleared panels is the semiquantitative capability offered only by the FilmArray PN panel for bacteria (excluding atypical pathogens).

To date, there are no prospective studies evaluating the clinical impact of either FDA-cleared syndromic molecular panel testing in patients with LRTIs. A nonrandom- ized interventional study on 49 patients with nosocomial pneumonia was published using the CE-marked version of the Unyvero assay. The difference in time to result was significant at 4 hours versus up to 96 hours for controls, and antimicrobial therapy was modified within 5 to 6 hours in 67% of patients. The cohort was not compared against a standard of care only control group.[38] Further studies are necessary to determine the potential positive and negative effects of such panels on the diagnosis and management of both adult and pediatric patients with LRTIs. The impact on anti- microbial stewardship and infection prevention would be important metrics to capture.

There are certainly challenges associated with the LRTI syndromic panels that require careful consideration before implementation in clinical laboratories. First, these panels function as an adjunct to traditional respiratory culture and susceptibility testing, and laboratories must determine the best reporting approach that would be complementary to culture results. As mentioned elsewhere in this article, the FilmArray PN panel best mimics the current standard of care reporting structure by providing semiquantitative values in 10-log increments. Laboratories must determine what would be classified as quantitatively significant compared with semiquantitative

Table 4
Multiplex lower respiratory panels, FDA cleared

Assay	Turnaround Time	Set UP	Throughput	Bacterial Targets	Viral/Fungal Targets	Antibiotic Resistance Genes
BioFire FilmArray Pneumonia *plus* Panel	1 h	On Demand	1 test module per instrument (v2.0) 2–12 test modules per instrument (Torch)	*Acinetobacter calcoaceticus-baumannii complex*	Influenza A	Methicillin resistance
				Enterobacter cloacae	Influenza B	mecA/mecC and MREJ
				Escherichia coli	Adenovirus	ESBL
				Haemophilus influenzae	Coronavirus	CTX-M
				Klebsiella aerogenes	Parainfluenza virus	Carbapenemases
				Klebsiella oxytoca	RSV	KPC
				Klebsiella pneumoniae group	Human rhinovirus/ enterovirus	NDM
				Moraxella catarrhalis	Human metapneumovirus	Oxa-48-like
				Proteus spp.	Middle East respiratory syndrome coronavirus[a]	VIM
				Pseudomonas aeruginosa		IMP
				Serratia marcescens		
				Staphylococcus aureus		
				Streptococcus agalactiae		
				Streptococcus pneumoniae		
				Streptococcus pyogenes		
				Legionella pneumophila		
				Mycoplasma pneumoniae		
				Chlamydia pneumoniae		

(continued on next page)

Table 4
(continued)

Assay	Turnaround Time	Throughput	Set UP	Bacterial Targets	Viral/Fungal Targets	Antibiotic Resistance Genes
Curetis Unyvero Lower Respiratory Tract Panel	4–5 h	2 test modules per instrument	On Demand	*Acinetobacter* spp. *C pneumoniae* *Citrobacter freundii* *Enterobacter cloacae complex* *E coli* *H influenzae* *K oxytoca* *K pneumoniae* *Klebsiella variicola* *L pneumophila* *M catarrhalis* *Morganella morganii* *M pneumoniae* *P* spp. *P aeruginosa* *S marcescens* *S aureus* *Stenotrophomonas maltophilia* *S pneumoniae*	*Pneumocystis jirovecii*	Penicillin resistance TEM Methicillin resistance mecA, mecC, and MREJ ESBL CTX-M Carbapenemases KPC NDM Oxa-23, 24, 48, 58 VIM

Abbreviation: MREJ, mec right extremity junction.
a Middle East Respiratory Syndrome coronavirus will only be available on the Pneumonia Panel *plus*.

culture, particularly at low abundance. Because the Unyvero LRT panel offers no quantitative values, interpretation of significance would be more difficult.

Although comprehensive, the current panels are by no means representative of all potential pathogens, particularly the bacterial targets, and a negative result may not necessarily prompt deescalation of antibiotic therapy. On the other hand, increased detection of on-target bacteria owing to increased sensitivity of molecular testing may result in excessive misinterpretation of bacterial colonization as true infection, leading to unnecessary antibiotic therapy. Studies conducted on both FDA-cleared panels reported more than 70% increases in bacterial target detected[39,40] and the clinical significance of this warrant careful evaluation that must be interpreted in the context of clinical symptoms and other laboratory findings. Concurrently, the inability to compare and determine the significance of organisms detected against the presence of other off-target oropharyngeal flora makes interpretation of panel result all the more difficult. Laboratories should continue to be diligent stewards by screening respiratory samples microscopically to determine whether the sample has been significantly contaminated with pharyngeal flora and, if so, neither molecular testing nor culture should be pursued. Other challenges include associating the correct pathogen with the correct resistance marker, particularly for the gram-negative bacteria, because the detection of a resistance marker is not linked to a specific pathogen. However, the FilmArray PN panel does prevents the nonspecific detection of mecA in *Staphylococcus* spp. other than *Staphylococcus aureus* through inclusion of the staphylococcal cassette chromosome mec right extremity junction that links the staphylococcal cassette chromosome mec cassette with the *S aureus* genome. Nonetheless, selection of targeted antimicrobial therapy in many of the cases still requires follow-up culture and susceptibility testing.

Based on these challenges, laboratories that wish to implement a syndromic molecular panel to aid in the diagnosis of LRTIs must be thoughtful when considering the reporting and interpretation of the results. Both panel and culture results must be reported in a cohesive manner to avoid confusion and misinterpretation. An integrative reporting approach with inclusion of personalized expert comments by the laboratory director to aid in the interpretation of the result may be helpful, as would consultation with an infectious disease specialist. A pragmatic approach may be to offer testing on bronchoalveolar lavage fluid first, because the sample types are considered a higher quality specimen and less prone to contamination with normal oropharyngeal flora.

DETECTION OF GASTROINTESTINAL INFECTIONS

Syndromic panels for GI infections have the same benefits seen with respiratory syndromic panels. They rapidly provide highly sensitive and specific detection of a broad range of GI[41–44] pathogens. **Table 5** provides a list of FDA-cleared syndromic panels for diagnosis of GI infections. GI syndromic panels are particularly helpful because there is significant clinical overlap between pathogens causing GI disease. The broad range of targets has highlighted the high prevalence of pathogens such as norovirus, which was not routinely tested for before syndromic panels, despite being one of the most common causes of acute gastroenteritis. Owing to the increased sensitivity and rapid turnaround time, outbreaks of *Cyclospora* have been identified more rapidly, allowing for timely investigation and source identification by public health officials.[45]

The limitations of syndromic GI panels are the inclusion of several targets of questionable clinical significance, including enteropathogenic *E coli*, which is among the most frequent positive targets when present.[41,46] Owing to the large number of targets present on some syndromic GI panels, specimens are frequently positive for

Table 5
Multiplex GI panels, FDA-cleared

Assay	Turnaround Time	Throughput	Set up	Bacterial Targets	Viral Targets	Parasitic Targets
Applied BioCode GI Pathogen Panel (GPP)	4 h	96-well plate format	Batched	Campylobacter spp. Clostridium difficile toxin A and B Salmonella spp. Shigella/enteroinvasive E coli Shiga-like toxin producing E coli E coli O157 Enterotoxigenic E coli Enteroaggregative E coli Vibrio vulnificus, V. parahaemolyticus, and V. cholerae Yersinia enterocolitica	Norovirus GI and GII Rotavirus A Adenovirus F40/41	Giardia lamblia Cryptosporidium spp. Entamoeba histolytica
BDMax Enteric Bacterial Panel	3 h	24 tests per instrument	Batched	Salmonella spp. Campylobacter spp. Shigella spp./ enteroinvasive E coli Shiga toxin 1 and 2		
BDMax Extended Enteric Bacterial Panel	3.5 h	24 tests per instrument	Batched	Plesiomonas shigelloides Vibrio vulnificus, V parahaemolyticus, and V cholerae Enterotoxigenic E coli Y enterocolitica		

Assay	Time	Throughput	Testing	Bacteria	Viruses	Parasites
BDMax Enteric Viral Panel	3 h	24 tests per instrument	Batched		Norovirus GI and GII, Rotavirus A, Adenovirus F40/41, Sapovirus, Human astrovirus	
BDMax Enteric Parasite Panel	4.5 h	24 tests per instrument	Batched			*G lamblia*, *Cryptosporidium* spp., *E histolytica*
BioFire bioMérieux FilmArray GI Panel	1 h	1 test module per instrument (v2.0) 2–12 test modules per instrument (Torch)	On demand	*Campylobacter* spp., *C difficile*, *P shigelloides*, *Salmonella* spp., *Vibrio* spp., Enteroaggregative *E coli*, Enteropathogenic *E coli*, Enterotoxigenic *E coli*, Shiga-toxin like producing *E coli*, *E coli* O157, *Shigella* spp./enteroinvasive *E coli*	Adenovirus 40/41, Astrovirus, Norovirus GI and GII, Rotavirus, Sapovirus	*Cryptosporidium*, *Cyclospora cayetanensis*, *E histolytica*, *Giardia*
Hologic Prodesse ProGastro SSCS Assay	4 h	96 tests per plate	Batched	*Campylobacter* spp., *Salmonella* spp., Shiga toxin 1 and 2, *Shigella* spp.		
Luminex Verigene Enteric Pathogens Test	2 h	1 test module per instrument (v1.0) 6 test modules per instrument (v2.0)	On demand	*Campylobacter* spp., *Salmonella* spp., *Shigella* spp., *Vibrio* spp., *Y enterocolitica*, Shiga toxin 1 and 2	Norovirus GI and GII, Rotavirus	

(continued on next page)

Table 5
(continued)

Assay	Turnaround Time	Throughput	Set up	Bacterial Targets	Viral Targets	Parasitic Targets
Luminex xTAG GI Pathogen Panel	5 h	96 tests per plate	Batched	*Campylobacter* spp. *C difficile* *E coli* O157 Enterotoxigenic *E coli* Shiga-toxin like producing *E coli* *Salmonella* spp. *Shigella* spp. *Vibrio cholera*	Adenovirus 40/41 Norovirus Rotavirus	*Cryptosporidium* *Entamoeba histolytica* *Giardia*

multiple target.[41] Although a patient may have multiple GI illnesses concurrently, more likely scenarios are asymptomatic colonization or viral shedding owing to past exposure. False-positive results have been reported for low incidence targets *Vibrio cholera* and *Entamoeba histolytica*.[47] Another major downside is the inclusion of *Clostridioides difficile* in some panels. *C difficile* colonizes the GI tract of 5% to 10% of asymptomatic adults,[48] and more than one-half of children under 1 year of age. Detection of *C difficile* toxin does not differentiate between infection and colonization, so it is essential that testing only be performed in the appropriate clinical context. There are many instances of testing for other GI pathogens that have led to incidental detection and subsequent treatment of patients colonized with *C difficile*. In hospitalized patients, the identification of *C difficile* in any context risks being classified as a hospital-acquired infection, which affects Centers for Medicare and Medicaid Services reimbursement. For this reason, many laboratories have elected not to report syndromic panel *C difficile* results at all or have selected panels that do not include a *C difficile* target.

There are few outcome data surrounding GI syndromic panel testing. The majority of the targets do not have an associated antimicrobial treatment. Even for those targets with treatments, most GI infections are self-limited and treatment is not recommended. A retrospective study by Beal and colleagues[46] showed that the number of days on antibiotics, imaging studies, hospital length of stay, and cost of hospitalization were modestly decreased with GI syndromic panel testing compared with traditional testing methods. Another study of nearly 10,000 patients found that GI syndromic panel testing resulted in fewer endoscopies, fewer abdominal radiographs, and a decrease in antibiotic prescriptions.[49] Although these studies are promising, more studies are needed to capture the full impact of syndromic GI testing on patient care and hospital finances.

DIAGNOSTIC AND LABORATORY STEWARDSHIP

Every single in vitro diagnostic test offered in the clinical laboratories requires clinical correlation. This caveat has become more evident in the era of syndromic testing where the simplicity and ease of ordering and testing have led to an urgency and a "need to know" mindset that can be detrimental to patient care. For example, in the absence of respiratory symptoms, it would be inconceivable for viral cultures to be ordered; yet the same asymptomatic patients are tested for multiple respiratory viral and atypical bacterial targets by syndromic panel. Thus, the exhaustive overuse overshadows and hinders the true benefits of syndromic testing.

Messacar and colleagues[50] eloquently defined the goal of diagnostic stewardship as "to select the right test for the right patient, generating accurate, clinically relevant results at the right time to optimally influence clinical care and to conserve health care resources." The laboratory is at the forefront of this mission, functioning as stewards to maximize clinical excellence. Independent of the actual performance of the syndromic panels, clinical microbiology laboratory directors must determine the added value of the panel compared with existing standard of care tests. Will the test provide highly accurate, actionable results that can improve patient outcomes? Does the test potentially improve the workload in the clinical laboratory by replacing a laborious test? Suffice to say, this decision is often made in collaboration with our infectious disease colleagues and/or antimicrobial stewardship team. Further, costs and reimbursements concerns play a significant role in the equation. It is imperative that a thorough assessment is pursued for every new diagnostic test to ensure that we are not viewing the tests with rose-colored glasses.

Once implemented, strict scrutiny must be applied to establish the most clinically relevant population to test and to optimize how the results are being communicated to the provider. Applications of laboratory stewardship include defining who to test, how often the same patient should be tested, and what targets should be reported is paramount. For instance, stewardship surrounding multiplex upper respiratory panels is a topic of discussion in most clinical microbiology laboratories. How can we identify patients that would benefit clinically from large multiplex syndromic panels to justify the increased cost? How can we identify patients for whom limited testing such as influenza and/or RSV is sufficient? Some laboratories have adopted a practice of testing all specimens for influenza with or without RSV first, and reflexing to the broad respiratory panel only if initial targets are not detected. Other stewardship measures include limiting certain syndromic upper respiratory panels to hospitalized, critically ill, or specialty clinics such as pulmonary and prohibiting repeat testing within a set period of time as retesting within a 20-day window have demonstrated minimal changes in test results.[51] Clinicians should also refrain from testing asymptomatic patients, performing repeat testing owing to low assurance of the initial result, or for test of cure because it can significantly contribute to overuse without any benefit to patient care. Last, for some testing, preauthorization by the clinical microbiology laboratory director or infectious disease team may be a potential solution. Expensive and complex testing, such as metagenomic next-generation sequencing, should only be done in conjunction with an infectious disease consultation and with clinical microbiology laboratory director oversight for clinical review, testing approval, and results interpretation.

Communication between clinical microbiologists and health care providers is absolutely essential to maximize the benefit of test results in the context of the patient. This point is particularly important as tests become increasingly complex and often detect multiple organisms, some of which may not be the cause of the patient's infection. Inclusion of consult notes and recommendations to help guide the provider appropriately interpret these molecular results can be extremely valuable and may help mitigate potential harms that arise owing to limitations associated with a test such as low clinical sensitivity or specificity.

It is near impossible nor sustainable for microbiologists to advocate for appropriate use of syndromic panels at the preanalytical level in the absence of automated gatekeeping through the electronic medical record. The development of support tools range from soft stops, which function as a warning for providers to reconsider whether or not the test should be ordered, to hard stops, which require providers to actively seek approval from the laboratory director.[52] A prime example is restricting orders on patients previously positive or negative for *C difficile* toxin within a 7- to 14-day period. However, sufficient information technology resources, information technology personnel with a clear understanding of microbiology, and the support of hospital and medical group administration is compulsory in the development of these tools. Nonetheless, these tools must be paired with continued provider education and establishment of key indicators of quality metrics to maximize their success.

SUMMARY

Syndromic panels have allowed clinical microbiology laboratories to rapidly identify bacteria, viruses, fungi, and parasites with high sensitivity and specificity to aid physicians in the diagnosis of many infectious clinical syndromes. These panels are now fully integrated into many clinical laboratories' standard testing practices. Thus, laboratories must implement strict measures to ensure that syndromic panels are being used responsibly through optimal clinician ordering practices, prohibiting repeat testing, and continuous education of clinicians on assay usefulness and limitations. Thoughtful reporting of results with interpretative comments and/or consultation with the clinical microbiology laboratory director is needed to aid provider interpretation. Diagnostic stewardship is our best hope to maximize the benefits of syndromic panels.

DISCLOSURE

J.D. Bard is a consultant for BioFire Diagnostics and Accelerate Diagnostics and is involved in clinical trials activities with BioFire Diagnostics, Luminex Corporation, DiaSorin Molecular, Applied BioCode. E. McElvania receives speaking fees, consulting fees, and research support from BD.

REFERENCES

1. Kumar A, Roberts D, Wood KE, et al. Duration of hypotension before initiation of effective antimicrobial therapy is the critical determinant of survival in human septic shock. Crit Care Med 2006;34:1589–96.
2. She RC, Bender JM. Advances in rapid molecular blood culture diagnostics: healthcare impact, laboratory implications, and multiplex technologies. J Appl Lab Med 2019;3:617–30.
3. Pancholi P, Carroll KC, Buchan BW, et al. Multicenter evaluation of the accelerate PhenoTest BC Kit for rapid identification and phenotypic antimicrobial susceptibility testing using morphokinetic cellular analysis. J Clin Microbiol 2018;56(4): e01329-17.
4. MacVane SH, Nolte FS. Benefits of adding a rapid PCR-based blood culture identification panel to an established antimicrobial stewardship program. J Clin Microbiol 2016;54:2455–63.
5. Perez KK, Olsen RJ, Musick WL, et al. Integrating rapid diagnostics and antimicrobial stewardship improves outcomes in patients with antibiotic-resistant Gram-negative bacteremia. J Infect 2014;69:216–25.
6. Sango A, McCarter YS, Johnson D, et al. Stewardship approach for optimizing antimicrobial therapy through use of a rapid microarray assay on blood cultures positive for Enterococcus species. J Clin Microbiol 2013;51:4008–11.
7. Walker T, Dumadag S, Lee CJ, et al. Clinical impact of laboratory implementation of Verigene BC-GN microarray-based assay for detection of gram-negative bacteria in positive blood cultures. J Clin Microbiol 2016;54:1789–96.
8. Patel TS, Kaakeh R, Nagel JL, et al. Cost analysis of implementing matrix-assisted laser desorption ionization-time of flight mass spectrometry plus real-time antimicrobial stewardship intervention for bloodstream infections. J Clin Microbiol 2017;55:60–7.
9. Perez KK, Olsen RJ, Musick WL, et al. Integrating rapid pathogen identification and antimicrobial stewardship significantly decreases hospital costs. Arch Pathol Lab Med 2013;137:1247–54.
10. Banerjee R, Teng CB, Cunningham SA, et al. Randomized trial of rapid multiplex polymerase chain reaction-based blood culture identification and susceptibility testing. Clin Infect Dis 2015;61:1071–80.
11. Juttukonda LJ, Katz S, Gillon J, et al. Impact of a rapid blood culture diagnostic test in a children's hospital depends on Gram-positive versus Gram-negative organism and day versus night shift. J Clin Microbiol 2020;58(4):e01400–19.

12. Pliakos EE, Andreatos N, Shehadeh F, et al. The cost-effectiveness of rapid diagnostic testing for the diagnosis of bloodstream infections with or without antimicrobial stewardship. Clin Microbiol Rev 2018;31(3):e00095-17.
13. Blauwkamp TA, Thair S, Rosen MJ, et al. Analytical and clinical validation of a microbial cell-free DNA sequencing test for infectious disease. Nat Microbiol 2019; 4:663–74.
14. Hogan CA, Yang S, Garner OB, et al. Clinical impact of metagenomic next-generation sequencing of plasma cell-free DNA for the diagnosis of infectious diseases: a multicenter retrospective cohort study. Clin Infect Dis 2020;ciaa035.
15. Hagen A, Eichinger A, Meyer-Buehn M, et al. Comparison of antibiotic and acyclovir usage before and after the implementation of an on-site FilmArray meningitis/encephalitis panel in an academic tertiary pediatric hospital: a retrospective observational study. BMC Pediatr 2020;20:56.
16. Van TT, Mongkolrattanothai K, Arevalo M, et al. Impact of a rapid herpes simplex virus PCR assay on duration of acyclovir therapy. J Clin Microbiol 2017;55: 1557–65.
17. Blaschke AJ, Holmberg KM, Daly JA, et al. Retrospective evaluation of infants aged 1 to 60 days with residual cerebrospinal fluid (CSF) tested using the FilmArray Meningitis/Encephalitis (ME) panel. J Clin Microbiol 2018;56(7):e00277-18.
18. Cailleaux M, Pilmis B, Mizrahi A, et al. Impact of a multiplex PCR assay (FilmArray(R)) on the management of patients with suspected central nervous system infections. Eur J Clin Microbiol Infect Dis 2020;39:293–7.
19. Nabower AM, Miller S, Biewen B, et al. Association of the FilmArray meningitis/encephalitis panel with clinical management. Hosp Pediatr 2019;9:763–9.
20. Dien Bard J, Alby K. Point-counterpoint: meningitis/encephalitis syndromic testing in the clinical laboratory. J Clin Microbiol 2018;56(4):e00018-18.
21. Leber AL, Everhart K, Balada-Llasat JM, et al. Multicenter evaluation of BioFire FilmArray Meningitis/encephalitis panel for detection of bacteria, viruses, and yeast in cerebrospinal fluid specimens. J Clin Microbiol 2016;54:2251–61.
22. Liesman RM, Strasburg AP, Heitman AK, et al. Evaluation of a commercial multiplex molecular panel for diagnosis of infectious meningitis and encephalitis. J Clin Microbiol 2018;56(4):e01927-17.
23. Messacar K, Breazeale G, Robinson CC, et al. Potential clinical impact of the film array meningitis encephalitis panel in children with suspected central nervous system infections. Diagn Microbiol Infect Dis 2016;86:118–20.
24. Naccache SN, Lustestica M, Fahit M, et al. One year in the life of a rapid syndromic panel for meningitis/encephalitis: a pediatric tertiary care facility's experience. J Clin Microbiol 2018;56(5):e01940-17.
25. Tansarli GS, Chapin KC. Diagnostic test accuracy of the BioFire(R) FilmArray(R) meningitis/encephalitis panel: a systematic review and meta-analysis. Clin Microbiol Infect 2020;26:281–90.
26. Ssebambulidde K, Bangdiwala AS, Kwizera R, et al. Adjunctive sertraline for treatment of HIVaCMT: symptomatic cryptococcal antigenemia presenting as early cryptococcal meningitis with negative cerebral spinal fluid analysis. Clin Infect Dis 2019;68:2094–8.
27. Van TT, Kim TH, Butler-Wu SM. Evaluation of the Biofire FilmArray meningitis/encephalitis assay for the detection of Cryptococcus neoformans/gattii. Clin Microbiol Infect 2020. S1198-743X(20)30031-30038.
28. Green DA, Pereira M, Miko B, et al. Clinical significance of human herpesvirus 6 Positivity on the FilmArray meningitis/encephalitis panel. Clin Infect Dis 2018;67: 1125–8.

29. Pandey U, Greninger AL, Levin GR, et al. Pathogen or bystander: clinical significance of detecting human herpesvirus 6 in pediatric cerebrospinal fluid. J Clin Microbiol 2020;58(5):e00313–20.

30. Agueda S, Campos T, Maia A. Prediction of bacterial meningitis based on cerebrospinal fluid pleocytosis in children. Braz J Infect Dis 2013;17:401–4.

31. Precit MR, Yee R, Pandey U, et al. Cerebrospinal fluid findings are poor predictors of appropriate FilmArray Meningitis/Encephalitis panel utilization in pediatric patients. J Clin Microbiol 2020;58(3):e01592-19.

32. Couturier MR, Bard JD. Direct-from-specimen pathogen identification: evolution of syndromic panels. Clin Lab Med 2019;39:433–51.

33. Sakata KK, Azadeh N, Brighton A, et al. Impact of nasopharyngeal FilmArray respiratory panel results on antimicrobial decisions in hospitalized patients. Can Respir J 2018;2018:9821426.

34. Rappo U, Schuetz AN, Jenkins SG, et al. Impact of early detection of respiratory viruses by multiplex PCR assay on clinical outcomes in adult patients. J Clin Microbiol 2016;54:2096–103.

35. Semret M, Schiller I, Jardin BA, et al. Multiplex respiratory virus testing for antimicrobial stewardship: a prospective assessment of antimicrobial use and clinical outcomes among hospitalized adults. J Infect Dis 2017;216:936–44.

36. Garau J, Baquero F, Perez-Trallero E, et al. Factors impacting on length of stay and mortality of community-acquired pneumonia. Clin Microbiol Infect 2008;14:322–9.

37. Torres A, Lee N, Cilloniz C, et al. Laboratory diagnosis of pneumonia in the molecular age. Eur Respir J 2016;48:1764–78.

38. Jamal W, Al Roomi E, AbdulAziz LR, et al. Evaluation of Curetis Unyvero, a multiplex PCR-based testing system, for rapid detection of bacteria and antibiotic resistance and impact of the assay on management of severe nosocomial pneumonia. J Clin Microbiol 2014;52:2487–92.

39. Lee SH, Ruan SY, Pan SC, et al. Performance of a multiplex PCR pneumonia panel for the identification of respiratory pathogens and the main determinants of resistance from the lower respiratory tract specimens of adult patients in intensive care units. J Microbiol Immunol Infect 2019;52:920–8.

40. Ozongwu C, Personne Y, Platt G, et al. Enne VI: the Unyvero P55 'sample-in, answer-out' pneumonia assay: a performance evaluation. Biomol Detect Quantif 2017;13:1–6.

41. Buss SN, Leber A, Chapin K, et al. Multicenter evaluation of the BioFire FilmArray gastrointestinal panel for etiologic diagnosis of infectious gastroenteritis. J Clin Microbiol 2015;53:915–25.

42. Harrington SM, Buchan BW, Doern C, et al. Multicenter evaluation of the BD max enteric bacterial panel PCR assay for rapid detection of Salmonella spp., Shigella spp., Campylobacter spp. (C. jejuni and C. coli), and Shiga toxin 1 and 2 genes. J Clin Microbiol 2015;53:1639–47.

43. Mengelle C, Mansuy JM, Prere MF, et al. Simultaneous detection of gastrointestinal pathogens with a multiplex Luminex-based molecular assay in stool samples from diarrhoeic patients. Clin Microbiol Infect 2013;19:E458–65.

44. Popowitch EB, O'Neill SS, Miller MB. Comparison of the Biofire FilmArray RP, Genmark eSensor RVP, Luminex xTAG RVPv1, and Luminex xTAG RVP fast multiplex assays for detection of respiratory viruses. J Clin Microbiol 2013;51:1528–33.

45. Bateman AC, Kim YJ, Guaracao AI, et al. Performance and impact of the BioFire FilmArray gastrointestinal panel on a large Cyclospora outbreak in Wisconsin, 2018. J Clin Microbiol 2020;58(2):e01415-9.
46. Beal SG, Tremblay EE, Toffel S, et al. A gastrointestinal PCR panel improves clinical management and lowers health care costs. J Clin Microbiol 2018;56(1): e01457-17.
47. Mhaissen MN, Rodriguez A, Gu Z, et al. Epidemiology of diarrheal illness in pediatric oncology patients. J Pediatric Infect Dis Soc 2017;6:275-80.
48. Loo VG, Bourgault AM, Poirier L, et al. Host and pathogen factors for Clostridium difficile infection and colonization. N Engl J Med 2011;365:1693-703.
49. Axelrad JE, Freedberg DE, Whittier S, et al. Impact of gastrointestinal panel implementation on health care utilization and outcomes. J Clin Microbiol 2019; 57(3):e01775-18.
50. Messacar K, Parker SK, Todd JK, et al. Implementation of rapid molecular infectious disease diagnostics: the role of diagnostic and antimicrobial stewardship. J Clin Microbiol 2017;55:715-23.
51. Mandelia Y, Procop GW, Richter SS, et al. Optimal timing of repeat multiplex molecular testing for respiratory viruses. J Clin Microbiol 2020;58(2):e01203-19.
52. Pritt BS. Optimizing test utilization in the clinical microbiology laboratory: tools and opportunities. J Clin Microbiol 2017;55:3321-3.

Practical Aspects and Considerations When Planning a New Clinical Microbiology Laboratory

Dwight J. Hardy, PhD

KEYWORDS

- Microbiology lab • Lab design • Biosafety • Open floor plan • Shared space
- Flexible space • Lab infrastructure

KEY POINTS

- The scope and success of the new laboratory requires clarity and the combined vision of hospital, departmental, and laboratory leadership.
- You do not have to be an architect or a builder/contractor, but you do need to be able to clearly articulate specific space needs.
- An issue with open floor plans is to ensure that the space is not so cavernous so as to overwhelm our human need for feeling proportionate to and comfortable in the space.
- With the opportunity of new space, plan to locate equipment, instruments, and workstations for greatest efficiency gains depending on workflow and technical assignments.
- Do not assume anything, never be afraid to ask questions and challenge what you believe is incorrect.

So it's finally your turn. After what may have been years of discussions that often seemed to go nowhere, funding for a new a new laboratory for your department has now been approved. You can only hope that the funding will allow for your current and future overall space needs, as well as correct long-standing problems that served to impede workflow and efficiencies. This article is written after more than 30 years of first-hand experience as a laboratory director working most of that time in "old" space with late twentieth century upgrades at best and more recently charged with planning for a new laboratory in an off-campus building undergoing renovations and expansion to accommodate a centralized laboratory for a growing health system. This review is not intended to replace detailed authoritative reviews on the topic of laboratory design and safety, but to put forward an experience-based user-friendly approach to thought processes and important points to remember for a successful new laboratory space.

Clinical Microbiology Laboratories, UR Medicine Labs, Pathology and Laboratory Medicine, University of Rochester Medical Center, Box 710, 601 Elmwood Avenue, Rochester, NY 14642-8710, USA
E-mail address: Dwight_hardy@urmc.rochester.edu

Clin Lab Med 40 (2020) 421–431
https://doi.org/10.1016/j.cll.2020.08.015
0272-2712/20/© 2020 Elsevier Inc. All rights reserved.

labmed.theclinics.com

PREPARATION

The first question a laboratory director or chief supervisor should ask is "what's the scope of the project?" Are you planning a laboratory for a single or multiple hospitals? What menu and volume of testing will the new laboratory be required to perform to support the needs of the various hospitals with different specialty programs? Will the new laboratory support all inpatient and outpatient testing, or outpatient testing only? How many years will elapse between planning and occupying the new laboratory? For how many years to come will the laboratory be expected to serve the needs of the health system? How much annual growth should you expect over the next 5 or 10 or 20 years and are you allowed to plan for such growth? While you can participate in discussions aimed at providing answers to such questions, the combined vision and input of hospital and departmental leadership is mandatory. Likewise, if the centralized laboratory is "off-site" from 1 or more hospitals, it is necessary to have agreement on what testing capabilities will remain at the individual hospitals; distance from hospitals to the new central laboratory and frequency and dependability of courier service will be key factors in determining what testing remains at individual hospitals in the system. Without clarity on these issues, the end product, that is, the new laboratory, will likely not meet present and future needs of the organization.

Armed with answers to at least some of these questions, the next question is "where do I begin?" It's time to prepare yourself for numerous meetings with laboratory administration, hospital space planning, contract space planners, architects, multiple project managers, and so on. While waiting to be introduced to members of the design and planning team identify the major players associated with the project, learn their names and roles and make sure that they come to know you. Plan to attend meetings of the various working groups assigned to plan for your area. If you show little interest in the overall project, decisions that will significantly impact your space and operation for years to come will be made without your input. If not already familiar to you, copies of key references that address important design issues should become part of your daily reading routine.[1–3] Don't be surprised if without consulting you, you are presented with a draft plan for your space and be prepared to offer rebuttal or alternate proposals; the quicker you are with your response to draft proposals the more seriously your proposals will be considered and the more willing planners may be to walk back from proposals that have already begun to take shape.

Early in the process of planning for new space, recognize that this is not a 1-person job and assemble your own team of supervisors and technologists who have a knack for identifying space needs, workflow problems, efficiencies, and solutions. Know your current space and what you need from new space, that is, more space, flexible space, better designed space for work efficiency, and so on (no one knows this better than you and your team). A good place to start is to look closely, dispassionately, and objectively at the space you currently occupy with an eye toward determining what's good about it, what is OK but can be improved, and what is really bad and must change. Because you or someone unknown to you will be required to provide current square feet occupied, you should take careful accurate measurements of the space you currently occupy. You should take measurements of current laboratory space including obvious and not so obvious storage space, and areas frequently omitted by space planners, that is, hallways where freezers, refrigerators, and supply cabinets are currently stored, an extra closet space here and there that you may have acquired over the years but is not officially recorded in space surveys held by laboratory or hospital administration. Making this assessment and taking these measurements is not for the purpose of re-creating the space you currently occupy but to give you an idea of overall current space needs. Indeed, in a new space which is better planned, your current and future needs may fit into a space that is smaller than you might predict (don't count on it, but it is within the realm of possibility).

With the opportunity of new space, plan to locate equipment, instruments, and workstations for greatest efficiency gains depending on workflow and technical assignments. Consider each and every bench top and floor-standing instrument and where it should be placed with input from technologists who perform the actual bench work of the laboratory for maximum operational efficiency and minimization of steps. Where possible, plan to colocate low-volume workstations that are the responsibility of a single technologist for enhanced ability to multitask and cross-cover. In times of shortages of licensed medical technologists, consider placing continuous monitoring blood culture instruments in preanalytical areas proximal to nonlicensed staff who may perform non–license-requiring activities, that is, load culture bottles, unload positive culture bottles, and unload negative culture bottles at the end of default incubation times.

ADJUSTING TO AN OPEN FLOOR PLAN

Be prepared to be presented with a vision for your laboratory space that is created by space planners and architects. The vision will likely be that of a large open space with movable work benches that offer flexibility and the ability to quickly respond to changing needs, for example, replace a movable bench with a floor model instrument in a day without requiring major renovations. Open floor plans can also enhance communication and cooperation among various work stations throughout the laboratory. For example, if anaerobic bacterial culture is a separate workstation it should be located near other workstations that have the greatest likelihood of having a companion anaerobic culture. Some disadvantages of large open floor plans, however, include noise and distractions from staff and instrumentation in adjacent areas, noise and distractions created by foot traffic from staff in proximal areas, and a general inability to adjust lighting and room temperature unless the ability for zone control of HVAC and lighting is included in the design to accommodate the comfort level of all staff. Unless you are able to successfully argue for a different approach to space design, a large open floor plan is likely the approach that will be used; after what may be an initial shock from seeing such a plan and the realization of how different it is from current space, consider the advantages of this design and how to mitigate the disadvantages of this design approach. A key issue with large open floor plans is to make sure that the space is not so cavernous so as to have the feel of a warehouse and overwhelm our human need for feeling proportionate to and comfortable in the space. With open floor plans, it is also important to consider the use of materials for walls, floors and ceilings that absorb noise and/or lighting to minimize distractions. In such designs it may also be necessary to implement a plan for traffic flow that minimizes distractions and the potential for laboratory accidents, for example, some areas may be open to all traffic, some areas open to 1-way traffic only and some areas may be "no thru traffic" to limit traffic to staff working in the immediate area only.

BIOSAFETY

In keeping with minimal safety requirements, clinical microbiology laboratories must be designed for working with biosafety level (BSL)-2 level pathogens and require strategically located biological safety cabinets (BSC) for primary specimen setup, conduct of aerosol-generating procedures and recognition of pathogens requiring higher safety level practices. To protect against laboratory-acquired infections and maintain specimen integrity, laboratories should perform all primary specimen setup in a BSC. Separate from standard unidirectional flow of air from corridors into BSL-2 laboratory space (and from BSL-2 into BSL-3 spaces), which is a non-negotiable requirement, a design feature of the laboratory to be introduced to the planning team early in the process is the partitioning of Microbiology space from other laboratory areas.[1] The type of partition and the approach to partitioning depends on desired objectives. If not already part of the design team, Environmental Health and Safety (EH&S) should be a required participant in any and all discussions related to laboratory design and safety; if EH&S has not been invited to participate in such discussion, you should invite them. If the objective is to completely separate Microbiology's space from other laboratory areas in the event of an aerosol-generating laboratory accident, a separate and independent HVAC system is required along with sealed partition walls that cover from floor to deck (ie, the solid impermeable layer above the ceiling tiles). Although a partitioning wall can block airflow and light transmission between areas, glass or other light-permitting materials can not only prevent aerosol movements but can also allow for an open feel to the space and ameliorate a feeling of being "boxed in." It is noteworthy that a separate air handling system with walls from floor to deck adds significant cost to the overall project. If, however, the objective of a partitioning wall is to provide "some" protection against infectious aerosol movements from one space to another, a partitioning wall from floor to ceiling tile with an HVAC system that has easily accessible controls for shutting down airflow from the Microbiology Laboratory can be incorporated into the space design; this design can allow for a quick laboratory evacuation and may be a practical compromise for laboratories in which the likelihood of such accidents is extremely low.

Throughout BSL-2 laboratory areas include space for the placement of BSCs proximal to appropriate work areas, for example, specimen setup; for maximum worker safety, all specimens should be setup in a BSC with separate BSC for setup of sterile site specimens and nonsterile site specimens. Include a BSC for workup of positive blood cultures proximal to blood culture instruments (if inside the partitioned microbiology space) and instruments for molecular identification of organisms in positive culture bottles. For maximum worker safety, include BSCs throughout the laboratory for the examination and workup of cultures potentially growing agents of high-risk for laboratory-acquired infections and/or environmental contamination (eg, *Legionella pneumophila*, *Neisseria meningitidis*, *Brucella*, *Francisella*, *Burkholderia mallei/pseudomallei*, unsuspected molds, severe acute respiratory syndrome coronavirus 2 [SARS-CoV-2]) or handling of specimens requiring procedures with potential for aerosol generation. Although laboratory procedures have largely transitioned away from potentially toxic chemicals such as formalin and formaldehyde for safety reasons, any new laboratory should still have at least 1 chemical fume hood for current procedures as well as procedures that might be used in the future.

SPECIMEN RECEIVING

Within the brick and mortar of the clinical laboratory space, specimen receiving is where it all begins. Whether specimens are received by pneumatic tube systems, internal transporters, or external couriers, ample space is required for the registration and accessioning of specimens upon arrival in the laboratory. With regard to specimen receiving and accessioning for microbiological specimens, a distinct space for Microbiology Specimen Receiving (MSR) should be maintained recognizing that this function is a specialty area requiring dedicated and experienced staff. MSR can be safely located outside of the partitioned space defining Microbiology because specimens remain in sealed containers preferably in individual zip-lock bags during log-in and accessioning activities. It is important for MSR to be proximal to or adjacent to where all specimens are delivered by couriers or pneumatic tube systems. Proximity to specimen receiving for other laboratory specimens and other preanalytical areas is also ideal when it comes to sharing clinical specimens, including but not limited to urine, body fluids and blood, and for sendouts to reference laboratories. Proximity to these receiving areas can be helpful for patient registrations that are required even before specimens for microbiology can be accessioned. When planning for MSR in laboratories, consideration should be given to locating automated blood culture systems in that area to allow preanalytical staff to load blood culture bottles immediately after receipt in the laboratory; culture bottles can be unloaded by preanalytical staff from the automated system when instrument-flagged positive and transferred to adjacent areas for workup by medical technologists.

SPECIMEN TRIAGE AND STAT TESTING

The next logical step for specimens from the MSR area is a triage workstation located within the partitioned microbiology laboratory space that should be immediately adjacent to MSR. Ample space for unopened specimen triage is important to directing specimens to a nearby STAT station or other routine processing stations deeper into the laboratory. A STAT workstation near specimen receiving with BSC(s) allows for rapid turnaround for procedures such as Gram stain, lateral flow immunochromatographic tests (ie, for detection of human immunodeficiency virus, malaria, *Legionella, Streptococcus pneumoniae, Clostridium difficile*), and molecular instrumentation for detection of a variety of infectious agents, including but not limited to influenza virus, respiratory syncytial virus, SARS-CoV-2, methicillin-resistant *Staphylococcus aureus, C difficile* toxin, and Group A Streptococcus.

SPECIMEN SETUP: BACTERIOLOGY AND MYCOLOGY

It may be efficient to perform manual setup of bacterial and fungal cultures in the STAT area with incubation of inoculated media in the same area or transfer of inoculated media to the inner laboratory for incubation. All specimen setup should be performed within BSCs and consideration should be given to providing separate BSCs for setup of sterile site specimens versus nonsterile specimens. If design of new space presents opportunity for installation of a total automated system for culture setup, incubation, and workup, complete specifications of the automated system should be given to space planners at the earliest possible time. Furthermore, vendor experts should be in personal communication with space planners to ensure that the space is appropriate to precisely accommodate large and expensive equipment with fixed and very specific power and information technology (IT) needs to avoid costly design missteps.

VIROLOGY AND MOLECULAR MICROBIOLOGY

Over the course of a few short years, testing for viruses has transitioned from a tissue culture–based laboratory with dedicated technologists highly trained in the specifics of tissue culture and cytopathic effects to a largely molecular operation. This includes manual "open" laboratory-developed molecular tests requiring expertise in nucleic acid extraction, amplification and detection to commercially available "closed" molecular test platforms that require general but little specific knowledge of targeted viral agents. Instrumentation performing molecular testing for many viruses is not specific to virology and is often placed the STAT area of the microbiology laboratory for rapid testing on a 24/7 basis. Routine molecular testing for other viruses, such as those causing gastrointestinal disease, is also included in test platforms not specific to virology, that is, platforms that detect bacterial, parasitic and viral agents, that can be placed in areas of the microbiology laboratory convenient for cross-coverage by technologists from other subdisciplines of microbiology. When locating test platforms for any infectious agent recall that the maximum promise of molecular technology is achieved only when these platforms are not powered down and locked up at the end of the day shift, which means such test platforms should be convenient to evening and night shift personnel.

Other high-volume molecular tests such as for the detection of agents of sexually transmitted diseases can be located in areas of the laboratory that serve best advantage for efficiencies, cross-coverage, and testing on different shifts. Molecular tests for viruses that are performed on platforms used only for the detection of viral agents can be colocated in areas of the laboratory where there is advantage for cross-coverage and other efficiencies. These examples serve to illustrate that with the introduction of commercially available "closed" molecular amplification test systems, testing for some infectious agents can be located in discipline-neutral areas of the microbiology laboratory as long as content experts are readily accessible and supportive equipment, for example, BSC, is conveniently located and provided in quantities necessary to meet the test volume need. It is also important to emphasize that per current Centers for Disease Control and Prevention guidelines and recommendations, the processing of specimens for routine SARS-CoV-2 diagnostic testing can be safely performed in BSC within a BSL-2 laboratory by staff trained in sterile technique and practices requiring careful and nimble manipulations. Although molecular test platforms may be located in different areas of the clinical laboratory, the example of SARS-CoV-2 underscores the importance of locating molecular tests for diagnosis of infectious diseases with the content experts in clinical microbiology.

The introduction of commercially available Food and Drug Administration (FDA)-cleared products and test platforms for molecular amplification of an ever-growing list of infectious agents has reduced the need for "PCR suites" in clinical microbiology laboratories with 1-way traffic and separate rooms dedicated to reagent preparation, extraction, amplification and amplicon detection which are all part of open laboratory-developed tests. The experience of Coronavirus Disease 2019 (COVID-19), however, reminds us that the availability of such space is one factor that allows for the rapid creation and implementation of laboratory-developed tests where commercially available FDA-cleared tests do not exist. Not all laboratories may need such space, but, larger regional laboratories and academic-based laboratories should consider including such space in planning for new facilities.

MYCOLOGY AND MYCOBACTERIOLOGY (SECTIONS WITH BIOSAFETY LEVEL-3 CONSIDERATIONS)

From what might be described as a central or core BSL-2 laboratory space, an adjacent space or suite for separate BLS-3 laboratories for mycology and mycobacteriology can make for good workflow patterns. A single anteroom off of the core BSL-2 laboratory with separate entry into separate laboratories for mycology and mycobacteriology can save space. The need for separate spaces for these specialty areas depends on the type of laboratory and patient populations served by the laboratory. Laboratories that only culture yeasts may not need BSL-3 mycology space, whereas laboratories that culture specimens from severely immunocompromised patients at risk for spore-forming molds such as *Histoplasma* and *Coccidioides* and workup such cultures require BSL-3 space. Similarly, laboratories that serve severely immunocompromised patients at risk for mycobacterial infections, including *Mycobacterium tuberculosis*, require BSL-3 level space. The design of BSL-3 space should strictly adhere to efficient workflow and recommendations for required square footage per person so as to prevent crowding, which may lead to laboratory accidents.[1] Include space for as many BSCs as required to safely perform work and keep "dirty" procedures, for example, processing and decontamination of specimens, from "clean" procedures, for example, culture workup. Positioning these 2 laboratories in adjacent spaces allows for cross-coverage of those laboratories and can also make for the efficient location of separate double-door autoclaves in each laboratory that empty into a common discharge area.

SEROLOGY

Serologic testing for antibodies/antigens of infectious agents and for markers of autoimmune diseases use bench top test platforms or large floor model instruments. Bench top platforms using enzyme-linked immunosorbent assay technology require places for microplate setup, plate washers, plate readers, and other standard small equipment, such as vortexers, water baths, centrifuges, and PC work station, which when taken in totality can require more than 6 feet of linear bench. If possible, equipment common to such workstations should be placed between or proximal to test setup for different assays to share the equipment and avoid duplication of equipment (although some redundancy in equipment is desired). Larger floor model platforms should be placed such that equipment has sufficient "breathing" space and can also be accessed from sides and back for maintenance and repairs; these large high-volume instruments should be directly connected to distilled/deionized water as needed and be proximal to floor drains for waste drainage. When positioning any of these platforms, consideration should be given to cross-coverage by technologists for maximum efficiencies. Storage space for liter or larger qualities of buffers and reagents for these platforms should be nearby.

Serologic testing follows the same testing guidelines for all BSL-2 activities. Splash/spray of specimens when uncapping specimen tubes is a major concern for avoiding laboratory-acquired infections. Providing ample bench space with fixed or movable splash guards or BSC (as deemed necessary) and centrifuges with containment for specimen preparation and test execution is sufficient per current safety recommendations. After specimen centrifugation in closed containers, testing with large floor model instruments provides containment for actual testing and has the advantage of waste drains that empty directly into floor drains for minimizing contact with potentially infectious material.

After years of performing fluorescent or dark-field microscopy in sub-standard inadequate space be sure to plan for a room to house fluorescent microscopes within the BSL-2 laboratory space. For efficient use of space, include microscopes to examine fluorochrome stains for mycobacteria, calcofluor stains for fungi, immunofluorescent stains for viruses, and immunofluorescent stains for markers of autoimmune diseases (eg, antinuclear antibody, antineutrophil cytoplasmic antibody). Locating microscopes for these various stains in the same room can succeed if different work groups can "play well together" and schedule nonconflicting times during the workday for use of the room.

SHARED SPACES

A feature frequently incorporated into new laboratory design is that of "shared" space. If you're told that freezers that will not require daily or frequent access will be stored in a shared "freezer farm," be sure to make your space and electrical needs known and argue for the location of such shared space to be proximal to the laboratory. Similarly, if you're told that shared storage space for dry goods and items, including test kits, which can be stored at room temperature is incorporated into the new design, be sure to make your needs known and argue for location of such shared space to be proximal to the major laboratory sections. For refrigerated items, the strategic placement of floor model refrigerators throughout the laboratory for storage of small items near point-of-use is certainly advantageous. Be prepared, however, to argue that individual floor model refrigerators do not substitute for walk-in cold rooms. Refrigerated storage of commercially prepared media used in high volumes and large boxes/cartons of test kits do not fit efficiently into floor model refrigerator units. Involve individuals from Supply Chain in this discussion because they will likely be responsible for stocking, inventory management, and transport of supplies from cold rooms, which should be immediately accessible to point-of-use areas within the laboratory. If Supply Chain or Inventory Management is not involved in the laboratory design process from the outset, be sure to bring them into the discussion and invite them to meetings early in the process to ensure adequate and proximal storage space; it's unfortunate, but architects and planners may be more likely to listen to Supply Chain than to you when planning for storage space. The experience of COVID-19 and its impact on supply chain disruptions documents the failure of just-in-time delivery for basic laboratory products and the need for ample space to store routine and esoteric items necessary for operation of laboratories in "normal" times and in times of epidemic/pandemic outbreaks. Shared space can also include space for waste storage, which is often overlooked and underestimated; left to nonmicrobiologists, space for waste storage will likely be insufficient for weekends and holiday weekends when waste pickup is less frequent. Another aspect of shared space can also include space for record retention and storage.

TEACHING AND TELEMEDICINE

Designing and building a new laboratory provides an opportunity to include adequate and appropriate space for teaching. The kind, amount, and design of teaching space required by an individual laboratory depends on several factors, including the different categories of students and/or trainees, the number of students in each category and the nature of the teaching required to satisfy the learning experience for each category. For example, space needs for teaching students of medical technology may require a classroom for the delivery of didactic lectures and a space to perform microscopy and wet laboratory exercises, which is separate from the space where routine clinical work is performed. Another example of teaching by a clinical laboratory in terms of space needs includes "shadowing" of experienced technologists by newly hired technologists or residents from different specialties in which the required educational experience can be achieved by observation; such teaching may be accommodated at existing work benches in the clinical laboratory or may require an additional "teaching bench" within the footprint of the clinical laboratory, but does not require a classroom or separate wet teaching laboratory. Although different from in-person teaching, recent experience with COVID-19 has demonstrated that the clinical laboratory must also provide a learning experience to off-site participants including students, attendees of clinical rounds and medical conferences, and staff of affiliate laboratories by remote transmission (eg, Zoom) of lectures, case presentations, and plate rounds with still or real-time high-resolution macroscopic and microscopic images[4]; such technology can also be used by affiliate laboratories to transmit images to a core laboratory for review by more experienced central laboratory based technologists.[5] The IT needs for remote teaching from the clinical laboratory may be met by software on personal computers available in an office or conference room. Similarly, the clinical laboratory should have a sufficient number of small and large conference rooms that can be shared by all laboratory disciplines and that can accommodate the receiving of remote seminars, clinical rounds, and conferences for the educational experience of laboratory faculty and technologists.

GENERAL CONSIDERATIONS

When planning for a new laboratory, it is important to consider the number of required work benches and what constitutes appropriate space per bench. It is not unreasonable to plan for a minimum of 6 linear feet of bench top per designated workstation with 1 or 2 shelves of similar length above the bench and shelf/drawer unit below the bench for storage of protocol binders and materials required for that workstation; locate benchtop equipment such as centrifuges and microscopes on 6-foot benches proximal to where needed. Also include separate and dedicated bench/desk areas for the performance of quality control (QC) activities required for new lots and shipments of media and test reagents/kits, quality assurance activities, special projects; if need in the area of QC, including media assessment and preparation, is sufficiently large a separate room adjacent to the core laboratory may be warranted. As you plan for the workspace, make sure to include sufficient number of electrical outlets for required equipment and ancillary devices (eg, computer/keyboard/barcode scanner; monitor; computer printer; label printers for Laboratory Information System (LIS), antimicrobial susceptibility testing (AST), and total laboratory automation (TLA) systems; bench top lamp; electric incinerators for sterilizing loops; heat block; vortex; slide warmer;) because each workstation can have 5 to 10 devices requiring electricity; request that electrical outlets be placed to the left and to the right side of the bench to avoid long electrical cords or use of extension cords spanning across the work bench. Similarly, include sufficient number of IT ports for each workstation (eg, computer, printer, label printers, other ancillary devices) and instrument remote access. Don't forget to include IT connection for phone at each workstation requiring a phone. Does your laboratory use natural gas for sterile flaming? Does your laboratory operation require in-house vacuum and/or in-house deionized or distilled water connections? Remember that the cost to install electrical outlets and IT ports for computer, telephones, printers, ancillary devices, as well as natural gas jets, vacuum jests, deionized or distilled water connections is significantly less (a fraction of the cost) when installed at the time of construction versus after construction is complete. Indeed, it may not be possible due to infrastructure challenges or cost to install new or additional electrical outlets, IT drops, water or gas connections, and/or plumbing drains after construction is complete.

When planning for equipment, instruments, and people, remember to consider temperature requirements for optimal operation and function (and this includes people). Where practical and possible attempt to incorporate independent temperature zones for individual comfort and instrument/equipment performance. Computerized and distant temperature monitoring of spaces and instruments relieves laboratory staff from manually monitoring and recording of such information and is a desired feature in any new space.

Be sure to include strategically located clean and dirty sinks throughout the laboratory, as well, as hand-washing sinks near exits to encourage frequent hand washing and overall good and safe hygiene practices. For instruments that require distilled or deionized water for reagent mixing, have water lines placed proximally. For maximum flexibility, have floor drains placed proximal to the planned placement of instruments that have waste drains to avoid having to lift and empty large carboys of waste water/reagents/specimens into dirty sinks causing splashing and injured backs; for greatest flexibility have additional floor drains placed throughout the laboratory in the event space needs change and equipment needs to be moved.

Planning for new laboratory space may allow for the incorporation of long sought after instruments and platforms that current space was unable to accommodate. Don't forget to plan for these needs because the opportunity for additional space may not come around again anytime soon. For something as large and complex as a total automated platform for setup, incubation, reading, and workup of cultures be sure to bring together the system manufacturer with building project management and electrical consultants to hear first-hand of specific needs and requirements; don't leave the placement and infrastructure support of such a large, complex, and expensive system to "middle men" communicating to content experts via e-mail.

Be prepared to provide copies of electrical and IT specifications/requirements for each instrument in the laboratory. Although generally obvious that differences between 110 V versus 220 V must be taken into account, differences between plug configurations on each instrument must also be taken into account. Keep copies of all information you provide to planners, architects, and project managers because you will likely be requested to send the same information to other individuals or requested to re-send the same information to the same individuals. All new construction should include provision of normal electrical power, as well as emergency backup power. It would be simple and easy to say that all laboratory equipment, instruments, and workstations require emergency electrical backup power. Because that approach may be cost prohibitive to some projects, consider each instrument, each workstation, and each piece of equipment to determine whether it is imperative for the real-time delivery of patient care and employee safety. In brief, all instruments and systems absolutely required for patient care and employee safety should be on emergency electrical backup, for example, all continuous monitoring blood culture incubators/cabinets and controllers, instrumentation required for delivery of STAT testing for inpatients and emergency department patients (think influenza virus testing), all BSCs and all fans responsible for maintaining negative pressure in laboratory spaces. In addition, a significant number of PCs with ancillary devices connecting to LIS (but not necessarily all) should be on emergency electrical back, where duplicate instrumentation exists for high-volume non-STAT testing (think sexually transmitted disease testing) 1 of 2 or more instruments should be considered for backup power, whereas pencil sharpeners do not require such backup. Each laboratory needs to develop a conscious plan that takes into account every piece of equipment and balances needs versus cost. Some new construction also includes electrical line conditioning for the entire building, which combined with facility-provided emergency power backup, can obviate the need for an individual Uninterruptible Power Supply (UPS) connected to each large instrument in the laboratory. Consult with the project managers and electrical consultants to determine the precise specifications of what your facility will provide. If the building provides dependable instantaneous electrical backup and continuous line conditioning, why clutter floor space with unnecessary UPS that will just attract and trap dust bunnies?

Last, office space for directors, supervisors, and support staff specific to clinical microbiology should be immediately adjacent to the laboratory to make for easy first-hand observations and communication with technologists. Locating offices in nonadjacent areas will result in delayed or lost opportunities for positively impacting patient care. In addition, locating offices immediately adjacent to the laboratory allows for directors and supervisors to be visible, available, and accessible to technologists and assists in improving overall staff satisfaction and performance.

DISCLOSURE

The author has nothing to disclose.

REFERENCES

1. Miller JM, Astles R, Baszler T, et al. Guidelines for safe work practices in human and animal medical diagnostic laboratories. Recommendations of a CDC-convened, Biosafety Blue Ribbon Panel. MMWR Suppl 2012;61(01):1–101.
2. Doern CD, Holfelder M. Automation and design of the clinical microbiology laboratory. In: Manual of clinical microbiology. Washington, DC: ASM Press; 2015.
3. CLSI. Laboratory design. In: CLSI standard QMSO4. 3rd edition. Wayne (PA): Clinical and Laboratory Standards Institute; 2016.
4. Pentella M, Weinstein MP, Beckmann SE, et al. Impact of changes in clinical microbiology laboratory location and ownership of the practice of infectious diseases. J Clin Micobiol 2019. https://doi.org/10.1128/JCM.01508-19.
5. Martinez RM. Remote technical review of blood culture gram stains at a large integrated healthcare network. J Appl Lab Med 2019;3(4):733–4.

Update on Susceptibility Testing
Genotypic and Phenotypic Methods

Romney M. Humphries, PhD, D(ABMM)

KEYWORDS

- Antimicrobial susceptibility testing • Antimicrobial resistance • Bacteriology

KEY POINTS

- Two primary methods are used for antimicrobial susceptibility testing: phenotypic methods and genotypic methods.
- Global standards for antimicrobial susceptibility testing (AST) are defined by the Clinical and Laboratory Standards Institute and the European Committee on Antimicrobial Susceptibility Testing.
- Several new technologies in development seek to reduce the time to results for phenotypic testing, applying a variety of novel detection methods.
- Genomic testing using machine learning holds potential to provide quantitative AST data

INTRODUCTION

The continued emergence of antimicrobial-resistant bacteria has brought the value of antimicrobial susceptibility testing (AST) to the forefront of clinical medicine. In simple terms, AST should provide a prediction of the likelihood for clinical success for an antimicrobial. At a higher level, AST allows monitoring of the emergence and spread of resistant microorganisms. Both these feats are challenged by both the ever-evolving nature of antimicrobial resistance (AMR) and the AST methods used by a majority of clinical laboratories (**Box 1**).

AMR challenges are pervasive. The US Centers for Disease Control and Prevention (CDC) 2019 AMR threats list includes common bacteria isolated daily in clinical laboratories (ie, Enterobacterales, *Pseudomonas aeruginosa*, *Acinetobacter baumannii*, *Staphylococcus aureus*, enterococci, and *Streptococcus pneumoniae*).[1] Determination of whether these bacteria are resistant to commonly prescribed antimicrobials, or meet CDC criteria as AMR threats, relies on AST. Two primary approaches are used for AST: phenotypic and genotypic.[2] The former evaluates the response of a

Pathology, Microbiology and Immunology, Vanderbilt University Medical Center, 1161 21st Avenue South C-3322 MCN, Nashville, TN 37232-2561, USA
E-mail address: romney.humphries@vumc.org
Twitter: @romneyinla (R.M.H.)

Clin Lab Med 40 (2020) 433–446
https://doi.org/10.1016/j.cll.2020.08.002
0272-2712/20/© 2020 Elsevier Inc. All rights reserved.

Box 1
Challenges associated with antimicrobial susceptibility testing in the twenty-first century

Increased prevalence of bacterial resistant to empirical therapy choices
- Time to results should be as short as possible, to ensure rapid therapy optimization for serious infections (eg, sepsis).
- Traditional MIC testing methods require 2 days to 3 days post–specimen collection to yield a result.

Emergence and rapid dissemination of novel resistance mechanisms
- Laboratories and test developers must ensure current technologies can accurately detect resistance mechanism

Development of novel antimicrobial agents
- Laboratories must adopt several new agents annually to test menu.
- Few reference laboratories are available to test new agents.
- Some new agents (eg, antivirulence agents) are not amenable to standard AST methods.

Increased emphasis on quantitative AST methods
- As the number of antimicrobials with activity dwindle, alternative dosing regimens may be used to treat low-level resistance.
- Precision of AST test is ±1 dilution, which is not amenable to PK/PD calculations, which use the MIC as the denominator.

Continual updates by CLSI and EUCAST to AST standards (breakpoints) to address emerging resistance, new PK/PD data
- Interpretations require update by laboratories and commercial manufacturers, including regulatory review, if applicable
- In the United States, many laboratories are not up to date with these standards, making tracking of resistance a challenge.[35,36]

---

microorganism in the presence of an antimicrobial and the latter seeks resistance markers that predict resistance. Each approach has its own advantages and limitations (**Table 1**) and a hybrid approach is used by most laboratories.

ANTIMICROBIAL RESISTANCE AND INTERPRETATION

Bacteria become resistant to antimicrobial agents via acquired and/or mutational mechanisms (**Fig. 1**). Testing for these is complicated by the fact that AMR often results from the actions of greater than 1 mechanism in concert. For example, the *Klebsiella pneumoniae* carbapenemase (KPC) gene, bla_{KPC}, is a widespread and important carbapenem resistance marker among Enterobacterales.[3] Expression of bla_{KPC} alone leads to only modest increases in meropenem minimum inhibitory concentration (MIC) (approximately 4 µg/mL) and alterations to outer membrane porins are needed for a full resistance phenotype (MIC >256 µg/mL). Similarly, isolates with extended spectrum β-lactamases can result in a carbapenem-resistant phenotype if coupled with permeability barriers, even though these enzymes have poor inherent carbapenem hydrolytic activity.[4,5] The gene copy number and expression level of the KPC also have a significant impact on MIC.[6]

For these reasons, there is an increased emphasis on the quantitative nature of AMR, which is expressed in terms of the MIC. MICs are physiologically meaningful, because they indicate the level of resistance that must be overcome by antimicrobial dosing. MIC determinations can aid the practitioner to determine if low-level resistance can be overcome with alternative dosing of the antimicrobial, a practice that

Table 1
Genotypic and phenotypic antimicrobial susceptibility testing methods compared

Parameter	Phenotypic	Genotypic
Detection of resistance	Detection of a phenotypic response (typically growth) in the presence of an antimicrobial that indicates AMR	Detection of 1 or more genes that are known to confer resistance to an antimicrobial and predict AMR
Detection of susceptibility	Inferred by inhibition of growth in the presence of a concentration of antimicrobial that is clinically attainable	Inferred by the absence of gene(s) that are known to confer resistance to an antimicrobial
Inoculum	Typically performed on isolated colonies, but newer technologies enable direct-from-specimen testing	Can be performed direct-from-specimen or on isolated colonies
Required concentration of microorganism	Traditionally 10^5 CFU/mL, although biosensor technology enables lower limits of detection	Limited by lower limit of detection for the technology, but typically 10^3–10^4 CFU/mL, but may be much lower
Minimum time to results	<4 h	<1 h
Ability to detect novel resistance?	Yes	Not at present
Readout	Quantitative (ie, MIC) and qualitative (Susceptible vs. resistant)	Qualitative to date

is most needed to treat infections caused by bacteria resistant to all other antimicrobials.[7]

More typically, MICs are interpreted using breakpoints that categorize MICs as indicating susceptibility versus resistance. Breakpoints are defined through the evaluation of 3 data sets: MIC distributions, pharmacokinetics/pharmacodynamics (PK/PD), and

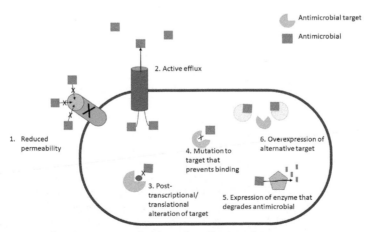

Fig. 1. Summary of major AMR mechanisms described to date.

clinical outcomes.[8] Two organizations establish clinical breakpoint: the Clinical and Laboratory Standards Institute (CLSI)[8] and the European Committee on Antimicrobial Susceptibility Testing (EUCAST). Both organizations are used globally, but in the United States, commercial manufacturers must adhere to Food and Drug Administration (FDA)-recognized interpretive criteria, which are published on the FDA Susceptibility Testing Interpretive Criteria Web site. CLSI is a recognized standards organization for the FDA but not all CLSI standards have been adopted by the agency.[9,10]

Scientific uncertainty often exists in 1 or more data sets used to establish a breakpoint. There often is a dearth of clinical outcome studies, especially for older antimicrobials. Trade-offs, such as the risk of lowering a breakpoint so far that it effectively eliminates the antimicrobial from clinical practice versus the risk of PK/PD-predicted treatment failures, commonly need to be made. It is not infrequent that CLSI and EUCAST independently arrive at different breakpoint decisions and, as a result, global harmonization of breakpoints has remained elusive.[8]

One area of recent schism between CLSI and EUCAST is regarding the intermediate interpretive category.[11] Both agree that antimicrobial dose, frequency, and mode of administration can be modulated to treat infections caused by isolates with low-level resistance—an important concept toward personalized antimicrobial therapy. This possibility is indicated by the intermediate category: that is, possibility of treatment success with dosing regimens that lead to increased antimicrobial exposure. The intermediate category also serves as a buffer zone for AST imprecision between the susceptible and resistant categories and defines the possibility of treating an infection confined to an anatomic location where an antimicrobial concentrates, such in the bladder for cystitis.[12] These complex concepts are not delineated on the patient report, leading clinicians and laboratorians to view intermediate as tantamount to resistant.

Both organizations in 2019 introduced measures to help resolve confusion associated with a catch-all definition for the intermediate category. CLSI adopted a susceptible, dose-dependent category for select breakpoints where increased-exposure dosing was clinically feasible and helped resolve scenarios where MIC distribution and PK/PD data pointed to disparate breakpoints (ie, Enterobacterales with cefepime, Enterococcus faecium with daptomycin, and S aureus with ceftaroline).[13] Intermediate continues to be used by CLSI for other breakpoints, and the possibility of increased exposure is now indicated through a footnote.[11,12] In contrast, EUCAST redefined intermediate to indicate susceptible, increased exposure. A new category, called the area of technical uncertainty, was introduced to account for AST imprecision.[11] Furthering their emphasis on appropriate antimicrobial dosing, in 2020, EUCAST lowered the susceptible MIC and disk diffusion breakpoints for many organism-antimicrobial combinations such that the only interpretation would be susceptible, increased exposure.[11] Continued refinement to these approaches by both organizations should be expected, because AST interpretation rarely is straightforward.

PHENOTYPIC TESTING METHODS

Observation of phenotypic responses has long been the standard method for AST. Alexander Fleming[14] first applied this technique with his discovery of penicillin, evaluating the MIC of bacteria in a 2-fold dilution series of penicillin in broth (a scheme selected to mimic the 2-fold dilution scheme immunoserology testing used). This method, with some adaptations, remains the global standard AST technique of 2020,[15] approximately a century later.

Traditional phenotypic testing has several limitations:
- Requirement of pure culture of bacterium
- 10^5 colony-forming units (CFU)/mL starting concentration of bacterium
- Extensive (approximately 16+ hours) incubation in the presence of antimicrobial to observe the phenotype

Together, these premises have limited the ability of direct-from-specimen, rapid testing. Furthermore, due to small, uncontrolled factors, the reproducibility of phenotypic testing is within a $\log_2$ MIC.[16] It is becoming increasingly apparent that for some isolates and/or antimicrobials, variability of MICs may be even greater.[17] Together, these factors and others (see **Box 1**) have led to significant desire—and progress toward—an improved phenotypic susceptibility test, which is quicker, requires a lower inoculum, and ideally is more precise.[18]

Rapid Disk Diffusion Methods

At a basic level, traditional AST methods can be adapted to yield a more rapid result. For instance, shortcuts, such as testing positive blood culture broth directly or reading disk diffusion zones after short incubations, have been used in laboratories for decades.[19] Standardization of these approaches has been undertaken by EUCAST. The rapid AST method published by EUCAST includes a methodology and early-read breakpoints for some organisms and antimicrobials at 4 hours, 6 hours, and 8 hours incubation.[20] CLSI has evaluated a similar method with plans to publish early-read breakpoints.[21] The availability of a standardized method will make implementation (or reimplementation) by laboratories easier, because results can be compared between laboratories and against quality control standards.

Total laboratory automation (TLA) is another development that may bring early-read disk diffusion testing into the mainstream. TLA instrumentation allows automated setup and reading of disk diffusion zones, providing increased consistency. Furthermore, incubation temperature and atmosphere of these instruments is highly regulated, enabling more rapid growth, and possibly even earlier reading.[22]

Adaption of Matrix-Assisted Laser Desorption Ionization/Time-of-Flight/Mass Spectrometry

Matrix-assisted laser desorption ionization/time-of-flight/mass spectrometry (MALDI-TOF-MS) is a technique that now is widely adopted by clinical laboratories for microorganism identification. The literature is rife with methods by which to adapt this technology to AST, including detection of resistance markers, strain typing predictive of AST profiles, evaluation of protein changes postexposure to antimicrobials, and evaluation of antimicrobial alteration (eg, products from hydrolysis resistance mechanisms, such as β-lactamases).[23,24] It At this time, none of these techniques is amenable to clinical laboratory workflows, requiring laborious specimen preparation and/or modification of MALDI-TOF-MS spectra.

Novel Technologies

Several novel technologies either have recently become commercially available or are in late-phase development, seeking to increase the speed and perhaps precision of phenotypic testing (**Fig. 2, Table 2**). All these technologies are based on the premise that exposure to antimicrobials induces a morphologic and/or physiologic response that can be measured earlier in the course of exposure than the traditional 16 hours to 20 hours. Examples of responses include changes to cell size, mass, membrane integrity, metabolism, and DNA transcription. Methods that have been evaluated to

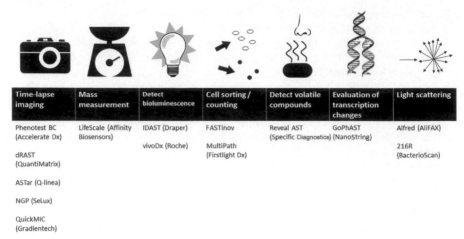

Time-lapse imaging	Mass measurement	Detect bioluminescence	Cell sorting / counting	Detect volatile compounds	Evaluation of transcription changes	Light scattering
Phenotest BC (Accelerate Dx)	LifeScale (Affinity Biosensors)	IDAST (Draper)	FASTinov	Reveal AST (Specific Diagnostics)	GoPhAST (NanoString)	Alfred (AliFAX)
		vivoDx (Roche)	MultiPath (Firstlight Dx)			
dRAST (QuantiMatrix)						216R (BacterioScan)
ASTar (Q-linea)						
NGP (SeLux)						
QuickMIC (Gradientech)						

Fig. 2. Summary of detection modalities applied by novel rapid phenotypic AST methods.

measure these responses include real-time microscopy, microcalorimetry, flow cytometry, microcantilever weighing, high-frequency electromagnet sensors, pH sensors, mass spectrometry, capacitance sensors, nuclear magnetic resonance, microsound detection, Raman spectroscopy, semiconductor quantum wells, and fluorescence detection and are discussed in an excellent review by Behera and colleagues[25] (see **Fig. 2**).

GENOTYPIC ANTIMICROBIAL SUSCEPTIBILITY TESTING

The application of genotypic techniques to AST has been used to both help improve the time to results and, in some cases, the accuracy of AST. To date, however, molecular testing has been able to provide only a qualitative, not a quantitative, readout of resistance. With a few exceptions (described later), molecular methods have only been used to rule out, not rule in, therapy options. The absence of a resistance gene does not always indicate a susceptible result, because AMR is multifactorial for most bacteria (see **Fig. 1**). Conversely, the presence of a resistance gene does not always indicate likely treatment failure because it may confer only low-level resistance or may not be expressed.

Genotypic methods have been subclassified into genetic (detection and/or sequencing of an individual gene) and genomic (sequencing of the entire genome of a microorganism, with bioinformatic analysis of the readout).

Genetic Methods

Many assays based on the detection of 1 or more AMR genes present in an isolate, positive blood culture or specimen are available commercially and used routinely in the clinical laboratory. Most of these are based on polymerase chain reaction technology and several take a syndromic approach to detecting a broad array of both microorganisms and resistance genes directly from clinical specimens. The typical genes queried, and their prediction of susceptibility and resistance, are shown in **Table 3**. Many of these tests also are useful for epidemiologic (surveillance) testing.

Broadly, genetic tests have not supplanted the need for phenotypic testing. Genetic tests cannot assign a detected resistance gene to a specific bacterium in a polymicrobial specimen, which may result in overcalling resistance. For example, *mecA*

Table 2
Rapid phenotypic antimicrobial susceptibility testing methods on market or in late development[a]

Test	Specimen	Antimicrobial Susceptibility Testing Technology	Identification Technology	TTR	Regulatory Status
PhenoTest BC (Accelerate Diagnostics)[37]	PBC	Time lapse imaging of bacterial cells under darkfield microscopy. Morphologic and kinetic changes analyzed.	FISH	7 h	US-IVD (2017) CE-IVD (2017)
dRAST (QuantaMatrix)[38]	PBC	Time-lapse microscopic imaging of bacterial cells immobilized in a gel matrix, on micropatterned plastic microchips.	None	6 h	CE-IVD
Reveal AST (Specific Diagnostics)	PBC, colonies	Sensor array measures volatile organic compounds emitted during microorganism growth.	None	4.5 h	CE-IVD In clinical trials
ASTar (Q-linea)	PBC, colonies	Time-lapse imaging of bacterial growth in broth that quantifies accumulated bacterial biomass.	None	3-6 h	CE-IVD
MultiPath (First Light Diagnostics)	PBC	FISH-based enumeration using nonmagnified digital imaging.	Yes	4 h	Under development
IDAST Lumiphage (Draper)	PBC	Bacteriophage-based luminescence assay that allows determination of cell viability.	Yes	6 h	Under development
vivoDx MRSA (Roche)	Nares swabs	Bioparticle-delivered luciferase gene that is expressed by viable cells.	Yes	2 h for MRSA	FDA IVD for MRSA
NGP (SeLux)[33]	PBC, colonies	Measurement of antibiotic-induced bacterial growth changes using a bacterial surface-binding fluorescent amplifier.	None	5 h	In development

(continued on next page)

Table 2
(continued)

Test	Specimen	Antimicrobial Susceptibility Testing Technology	Identification Technology	TTR	Regulatory Status
Droplet-based AST (Pattern Bioscience)		Neural networks that recognize unique biometric fingerprint produced by different bacterial species that are encapsulated within microfluidic droplets.	Yes	4 h	In development
FASTinov	PBC, colonies	Flow cytometry applying fluorescent dyes that reveal cell damage during treatment	No	80 min	CE-IVD 2017
LifeScale (Affinity Biosensors)	PBC, colony	Mass measurement using a microcantilever	No	4 h	CE-IVD 2018 In trials for US
QuickMIC (Gradientech)[40]	PBC	Real-time monitoring of bacterial growth in antibiotic gradients within a microfluidic system.	No	2h	In development
Alfred (AliFAX)[41]	PBC and colonies	Light scattering to detect bacterial growth in liquid culture broth.	No	3–5 h	CE-IVD
GoPhAST (NanoString)[42]	In development	Evaluation of antibiotic-induced transcriptional changes and simultaneous detection of resistance genes	ND	<4 h	In development
216R (BacterioScan)[43]	Urine, colonies	Laser light scattering to detect growth	No	2.5 h	In development

Abbreviation: CE-IVD, conformite european in vitro diagnostic; FISH, fluorescent in situ hybridization; IVD, in vitro diagnostic; MRSA, methicillin resistant Staphylococcus aureus; PBC, positive blood culture; TTR, time to results; US-IVD, United States FDA cleared in vitro diagnostic.
[a] This is not an all-inclusive list due to the dynamic nature of this field.

Table 3
Common resistance determinants queried by commercially available genetic tests[12]

Gene	Organism(s)	Prediction of Resistance	Prediction of Susceptibility	Limitation
mecA and mecC	Staphylococci	Confers resistance to all β-lactams except ceftaroline	Absence of these genes predicts susceptibility to penicillinase stable penicillins with high sensitivity.	Some rare isolates are resistant to β-lactams by other mechanisms (eg, hyperexpression of blaZ).
vanA and vanB	Enterococcus faecium Enterococcus faecalis	Confers resistance to vancomycin	Absence of these genes generally indicates vancomycin susceptibility for these species of Enterococcus.	vanB is found in many commensal anaerobes, limiting test from specimens where anaerobes are prevalent. Other van genes are present in other enterococci. Susceptibility for agents to treat vancomycin resistant enterococci is not universal (eg, linezolid and daptomycin) and phenotypic testing for these is needed.
blaCTX-M	Enterobacterales	Confers resistance to most cephalosporins	Negative result does not confer susceptibility but may be associated with high predictive values[44] Other resistance mechanisms prevalent, dependent on geography[45]	Different CTX-M enzymes confer differing levels of resistance to the various cephalosporins; confirmatory testing by phenotypic methods highly recommended.
blaKPC	Enterobacterales P aeruginosa	Confers resistance to β-lactams, except newer agents like cefiderocol, ceftazidime-avibactam, meropenem vaborbactam, imipenem-relebactam Often present on plasmid with multiple other resistance	Negative result does not confer susceptibility. Other resistance mechanisms prevalent, dependent on geography[45] Presence of KPC does not necessarily infer susceptibility to ceftazidime-avibactam.[46]	

(continued on next page)

Table 3
(continued)

Gene	Organism(s)	Prediction of Resistance	Prediction of Susceptibility	Limitation
		markers, leading to multidrug-resistant phenotype		
*bla*IMP	Enterobacterales *P aeruginosa*	Confers resistance to β-lactams except cefiderocol.	Negative result does not confer susceptibility. Other resistance mechanisms prevalent, dependent on geography	Often associated with low-level resistance Uncommon in the US
*bla*OXA-48	Enterobacterales *P aeruginosa*	Confers resistance to β-lactams, except newer agents like cefiderocol, ceftazidime-avibactam, imipenem-relebactam	Negative result does not confer susceptibility. Other resistance mechanisms prevalent, dependent on geography	Often associated with low-level resistance
*bla*VIM	Enterobacterales *P aeruginosa*	Confers resistance to β-lactams, except cefiderocol	Negative result does not confer susceptibility. Other resistance mechanisms prevalent, dependent on geography	Often associated with low-level resistance Uncommon in the US
*bla*NDM	Enterobacterales *P aeruginosa*	Confers resistance to β-lactams except aztreonam and cefiderocol Often present on plasmid with multiple other resistance markers, leading to multidrug-resistant phenotype	Negative result does not confer susceptibility. Other resistance mechanisms prevalent, dependent on geography	Often associated with low-level resistance Uncommon in the US

detection in a specimen harboring both S aureus and S epidermidis could lead to incorrect assigning of this gene to the pathogen and not the contaminant. Furthermore, new mutations and resistance mechanisms are continually evolving, which may limit the ability of certain genetic tests to predict resistance, particularly if a mutation occurs in primer complementary regions.[26]

Genomic Methods

Application of whole-genome sequencing (WGS) to the challenge of AMR enables not only excellent epidemiologic tracking but also the possibility of predicting antimicrobial susceptibility from an organism's genomic content. Currently there are no plug-and-play commercial methods for such testing, but some companies are working on this challenge.[2] Laboratory-developed tests are challenged by unstandardized bioinformatic pipelines and databases, which can lead to divergent interpretation of results from the same isolate/specimen tested.[27] Traditional evaluation of genomes using these pipelines may incorrectly assign antimicrobial function to paralogous non-AMR genes or fail to identify mutations in intergenic regions, such as regulatory and promoter sequencing. Machine learning has the potential to correct these deficiencies and further predict MICs based on WGS data. Examples of such technology include application of short, WGS-derived, nucleotide k-mers and traditional MICs as features of AMR in training sets for machine learning algorithms, leading to generation of MIC-level data from genomic sequences.[28,29]

CLINICAL IMPACT OF ANTIMICROBIAL SUSCEPTIBILITY TESTING

Implementation of all new AST technologies is undoubtedly at increased cost to the laboratory over existing methods, and demonstration of clinical value is paramount. Recently, data from the MERINO trial demonstrated an increased mortality rate for patients treated with piperacillin-tazobactam over meropenem for infections caused by ceftriaxone resistant Escherichia coli and K pneumoniae.[30] Post hoc analysis of this trial revealed that false-susceptible results for piperacillin-tazobactam were association with outcome,[31] underscoring the value of an accurate AST result in traditional timeframes. No studies to date, however, have been sufficiently powered to determine the impact on mortality or length of hospitalization associated with a more rapid (and accurate) AST method.

Performing outcome studies for AST devices is challenging because diagnostic test results are several degrees removed from the patient—relying on 1 (or several) intermediaries to take action on results. Blunt endpoints like mortality or length of hospitalization are exceedingly difficult to measure in the context of this noise. Some investigators have proposed evaluation of process-based changes, such as earlier adjustment of therapy with a rapid AST result, which then can be inferred to result in better overall patient care and therefore outcomes.[32] Demonstrating no harm done with earlier de-escalation informed by rapid AST results also may help support use cases. Two randomized controlled trials and a plethora of quasiexperimental pre/poststudies have demonstrated that both genetic and phenotypic rapid ASTs, when implemented in tandem with antimicrobial stewardship activities, can result in significant differences in patient management.[33,34] Translation of these data into stories that are meaningful to hospital C-suites, payers, and professional societies alike will be the task of clinical microbiologists in the coming years, to ensure continued development of novel technologies for AST.

SUMMARY

The AST technology space has become active in the past 5 years, with several companies and researchers developing novel technologies aimed at increasing the accuracy, time to results, and standardization of AST methods. The ultimate goal is to change the antimicrobial treatment paradigm from upfront broad, empirical therapy that is optimized only several days later upon receipt of laboratory results to an upfront, rapid test that informs optimal therapy from the get-go. This is a lofty goal, but the AST development field is a dynamic and fast-moving one. It is not difficult to envision this new paradigm soon becoming reality.

DISCLOSURE

R.M. Humphries is a past employee of Accelerate Diagnostics and a current shareholder.

REFERENCES

1. CDC. Antibiotic resistance threats in the United States, 2019. Atlanta (GA): Centers for Disease Control and Prevention; 2019.
2. van Belkum A, Burnham CD, Rossen JWA, et al. Innovative and rapid antimicrobial susceptibility testing systems. Nat Rev Microbiol 2020;18(5):299–311.
3. Porreca AM, Sullivan KV, Gallagher JC. The epidemiology, evolution, and treatment of KPC-producing organisms. Curr Infect Dis Rep 2018;20(6):13.
4. Martinez-Martinez L. Extended-spectrum beta-lactamases and the permeability barrier. Clin Microbiol Infect 2008;14(Suppl 1):82–9.
5. Jacoby GA, Mills DM, Chow N. Role of beta-lactamases and porins in resistance to ertapenem and other beta-lactams in Klebsiella pneumoniae. Antimicrob Agents Chemother 2004;48(8):3203–6.
6. Cheruvanky A, Stoesser N, Sheppard AE, et al. Enhanced Klebsiella pneumoniae carbapenemase expression from a novel Tn4401 deletion. Antimicrob Agents Chemother 2017;61(6). e00025-17.
7. Heffernan AJ, Sime FB, Lipman J, et al. Individualising therapy to minimize bacterial multidrug resistance. Drugs 2018;78(6):621–41.
8. Weinstein MP, Lewis JS 2nd. The clinical and laboratory standards institute subcommittee on antimicrobial susceptibility testing: background, organization, functions, and processes. J Clin Microbiol 2020;58(3). e01864-19.
9. Humphries RM, Ferraro MJ, Hindler JA. Impact of 21st century cures act on breakpoints and commercial antimicrobial susceptibility test systems: progress and pitfalls. J Clin Microbiol 2018;56(5). e00139-18.
10. Humphries RM, Hindler J, Jane Ferraro M, et al. Twenty-first century cures act and antimicrobial susceptibility testing: clinical implications in the era of multidrug resistance. Clin Infect Dis 2018;67(7):1132–8.
11. Kahlmeter G, Giske CG, Kirn TJ, et al. Point-counterpoint: differences between the european committee on antimicrobial susceptibility testing and clinical and laboratory standards institute recommendations for reporting antimicrobial susceptibility results. J Clin Microbiol 2019;57(9). e01129-19.
12. CLSI. Performance standards for antimicrobial susceptibility testing. *M100*. 30th edition. Wayne (PA): Clinical and Laboratory Standards Institute; 2020.
13. Humphries RM, Abbott AN, Hindler JA. Understanding and Addressing CLSI breakpoint revisions: a primer for clinical laboratories. J Clin Microbiol 2019; 57(6). e00203-19.

14. Fleming A. In-vitro tests of penicillin potency. Lancet 1942;239(6199):732–3.

15. ISO. ISO 20776: clinical laboratory testing and in vitro diagnostic systems - susceptibility testing of infectious agents and evaluation of performance of antimicrobial susceptibility test devices. Part 1: reference method for testing the in vitro activity of antimicrobial agents against rapidly growing aerobic baceria involved in infectious diseases. Geneva (Switzerland): International Organization for Standardization; 2019.

16. CLSI. Development of in vitro susceptibility testing criteria and quality control parameters, M23. 5th edition. Wayne (PA): Clinical and laboratory standards institute; 2018.

17. Campeau SA, Schuetz AN, Kohner P, et al. Variability of Daptomycin MIC values for enterococcus faecium when measured by reference broth microdilution and gradient diffusion tests. Antimicrob Agents Chemother 2018;62(9). e00745-18.

18. van Belkum A, Bachmann TT, Ludke G, et al. Developmental roadmap for antimicrobial susceptibility testing systems. Nat Rev Microbiol 2019;17(1):51–62.

19. Barry AL, Joyce LJ, Adams AP, et al. Rapid determination of antimicrobial susceptibility for urgent clinical situations. Am J Clin Pathol 1973;59(5):693–9.

20. Jonasson E, Matuschek E, Kahlmeter G. The EUCAST rapid disc diffusion method for antimicrobial susceptibility testing directly from positive blood culture bottles. J Antimicrob Chemother 2020;75(4):968–78.

21. Chandrasekaran S, Abbott A, Campeau S, et al. Direct-from-Blood-Culture disk diffusion to determine antimicrobial susceptibility of gram-negative bacteria: preliminary report from the clinical and laboratory standards institute methods development and standardization working group. J Clin Microbiol 2018;56(3). e01678-17.

22. Dauwalder O, Vandenesch F. Disc diffusion AST automation: one of the last pieces missing for full microbiology laboratory automation. Clin Microbiol Infect 2020;26(5):539–41.

23. Oviano M, Bou G. Matrix-assisted laser desorption ionization-time of flight mass spectrometry for the rapid detection of antimicrobial resistance mechanisms and beyond. Clin Microbiol Rev 2019;32(1). e00037-18.

24. Burckhardt I, Zimmermann S. Susceptibility testing of bacteria using Maldi-tof mass spectrometry. Front Microbiol 2018;9:1744.

25. Behera B, Anil Vishnu GK, Chatterjee S, et al. Emerging technologies for antibiotic susceptibility testing. Biosens Bioelectron 2019;142:111552.

26. Hemarajata P, Yang S, Hindler JA, et al. Development of a novel real-time PCR assay with high-resolution melt analysis to detect and differentiate OXA-48-Like beta-lactamases in carbapenem-resistant Enterobacteriaceae. Antimicrob Agents Chemother 2015;59(9):5574–80.

27. Couto N, Schuele L, Raangs EC, et al. Critical steps in clinical shotgun metagenomics for the concomitant detection and typing of microbial pathogens. Sci Rep 2018;8(1):13767.

28. Nguyen M, Brettin T, Long SW, et al. Developing an in silico minimum inhibitory concentration panel test for Klebsiella pneumoniae. Sci Rep 2018;8(1):421.

29. Eyre DW, De Silva D, Cole K, et al. WGS to predict antibiotic MICs for Neisseria gonorrhoeae. J Antimicrob Chemother 2017;72(7):1937–47.

30. Harris PNA, Tambyah PA, Lye DC, et al. Effect of piperacillin-tazobactam vs meropenem on 30-day mortality for patients with E coli or Klebsiella pneumoniae bloodstream infection and ceftriaxone resistance: a randomized clinical trial. JAMA 2018;320(10):984–94.

31. Henderson A, Humphries R. Building a better test for piperacillin-tazobactam susceptibility testing: would that it were so simple (it's complicated). J Clin Microbiol 2020;58(2). e01649-19.
32. Miller MB, Atrzadeh F, Burnham CA, et al. Clinical utility of advanced microbiology testing tools. J Clin Microbiol 2019;57(9). e00495-19.
33. Banerjee R, Teng CB, Cunningham SA, et al. Randomized trial of rapid multiplex polymerase chain reaction-based blood culture identification and susceptibility testing. Clin Infect Dis 2015;61(7):1071–80.
34. Banerjee R, Komarow L, Virk A, et al. Randomized trial evaluating clinical impact of RAPid IDentification and Susceptibility testing for Gram Negative bacteremia (RAPIDS-GN). Clin Infect Dis 2020. https://doi.org/10.1093/cid/ciaa528.
35. Viau RA, Hujer AM, Marshall SH, et al. Silent" dissemination of Klebsiella pneumoniae isolates bearing K. pneumoniae carbapenemase in a long-term care facility for children and young adults in Northeast Ohio. Clin Infect Dis 2012;54(9): 1314–21.
36. Humphries RM, Hindler JA, Epson E, et al. Carbapenem-resistant enterobacteriaceae detection practices in California: what are we missing? Clin Infect Dis 2018;66(7):1061–7.
37. Pancholi P, Carroll KC, Buchan BW, et al. Multicenter Evaluation of the Accelerate PhenoTest BC kit for rapid identification and phenotypic antimicrobial susceptibility testing using morphokinetic cellular analysis. J Clin Microbiol 2018;56(4). e01329-17.
38. Choi J, Jeong HY, Lee GY, et al. Direct, rapid antimicrobial susceptibility test from positive blood cultures based on microscopic imaging analysis. Sci Rep 2017; 7(1):1148.
39. Flentie K, Spears BR, Chen F, et al. Microplate-based surface area assay for rapid phenotypic antibiotic susceptibility testing. Sci Rep 2019;9(1):237.
40. Malmberg C, Yuen P, Spaak J, et al. A novel microfluidic assay for rapid phenotypic antibiotic susceptibility testing of bacteria detected in clinical blood cultures. PLoS One 2016;11(12):e0167356.
41. Anton-Vazquez V, Adjepong S, Suarez C, et al. Evaluation of a new rapid antimicrobial susceptibility system for gram-negative and gram-positive bloodstream infections: speed and accuracy of Alfred 60AST. BMC Microbiol 2019;19(1):268.
42. Bhattacharyya RP, Bandyopadhyay N, Ma P, et al. Simultaneous detection of genotype and phenotype enables rapid and accurate antibiotic susceptibility determination. Nat Med 2019;25(12):1858–64.
43. Idelevich EA, Hoy M, Gorlich D, et al. Rapid phenotypic detection of microbial resistance in gram-positive bacteria by a real-time laser scattering method. Front Microbiol 2017;8:1064.
44. Pogue JM, Heil EL, Lephart P, et al. An antibiotic stewardship program blueprint for optimizing verigene BC-GN within an institution: a tale of two cities. Antimicrob Agents Chemother 2018;62(5). e02538-17.
45. Spafford K, MacVane S, Humphries R. Evaluation of empiric beta-lactam susceptibility prediction among enterobacteriaceae by molecular beta-lactamase gene testing. J Clin Microbiol 2019;57(10). e00674-19.
46. Shields RK, Nguyen MH, Press EG, et al. Emergence of ceftazidime-avibactam resistance and restoration of carbapenem susceptibility in klebsiella pneumoniae carbapenemase-producing k pneumoniae: a case report and review of literature. Open Forum Infect Dis 2017;4(3):ofx101.

Clinical Pathogen Genomics

Andrew Cameron, PhD[a,1], Jessica L. Bohrhunter, PhD[a,1],
Samantha Taffner, MS[a], Adel Malek, PhD[b], Nicole D. Pecora, MD, PhD[a,*]

KEYWORDS

- Pathogen whole-genome sequencing • Clinical pathogen genomics
- Clinical metagenomics • Next-generation sequencing

KEY POINTS

- Next-generation sequencing performed on cultured isolates of bacteria and fungi can assist with pathogen identification and assessment of susceptibility to antibiotics.
- Whole-genome sequence-level discrimination of potential outbreaks and surveillance isolates can inform infection prevention strategies by establishing clonal relatedness and the local pathogen genomic landscape.
- Metagenomic next-generation sequencing of primary specimens provides a universal test capable of pan-taxonomic identification (including viruses, bacteria, fungi, and parasites).
- Metagenomic approaches can be unbiased or targeted toward pathogens using enrichment strategies.
- Challenges of in-house pathogen genomic programs include considerations of cost, infrastructure, validation, and reporting.

INTRODUCTION

Over the past 10 years, clinical pathogen genomics has gone from a cutting-edge research method for investigating organism relatedness to being the gold-standard for assessing potential outbreaks.[1] Although pathogen clonality is often the main question, next-generation sequencing (NGS) provides a rich trove of information to diagnose, assess antimicrobial resistance genes (ARGs) and virulence factors, monitor for high-risk clones, and understand the local genomic landscape. Additional benefits include the characterization of emerging and/or unusual pathogens.

Whole-genome sequencing (WGS) of cultured isolates has become commonplace in research programs, and mainstream in public health laboratories, particularly for bacterial pathogens.[2,3] Genomic assessment of fungal pathogens is an active but still developing field.[4–6] The introduction and application of microbial genomics in clinical

[a] Department of Pathology and Laboratory Medicine, UR Medicine Central Laboratory, West Henrietta, NY 14586, USA; [b] Faculty of Laboratory Medicine, Memorial University, St John's, Newfoundland and Labrador, Canada
[1] A. Cameron and J.L. Bohrhunter contributed equally to this work.
* Corresponding author.
E-mail address: nicole_pecora@urmc.rochester.edu

Clin Lab Med 40 (2020) 447–458
https://doi.org/10.1016/j.cll.2020.08.003
0272-2712/20/© 2020 Elsevier Inc. All rights reserved.

laboratories remains uneven: the necessary instrumentation is often not available and the lack of assays cleared by the US Food and Drug Administration makes clinical-level validations onerous.[7] Although these challenges are real, there are clear advantages of local (in-house) expertise and WGS data.

There have been several reviews discussing the use of pathogen NGS for clinical care.[8–10] Commercial solutions for the sequencing of cultured isolates are now available through many reference laboratories and increasingly for sequencing from primary specimens as well.[11,12] In this article, we provide an update on the current benefits and challenges of bringing this technology in-house for clinical microbiology laboratories. The focus is not on sequencing technologies, which have been extensively covered elsewhere, but rather on current practical uses and how they may develop in the future.[13] We will discuss the use of NGS pathogen genomics for both cultured isolates and primary specimens, for which this diagnostic modality is truly pan-phylogenetic. Metagenomic-based NGS (mNGS) approaches are increasingly at the forefront because they also provide coverage of viral pathogens, which are rarely cultured in the modern clinical laboratory, and not detectable using universal targets common among bacteria (eg, 16S) and fungi (eg, internal transcribed spacer). Logistical and infrastructural considerations for bringing this technology into a diagnostic microbiology laboratory are also discussed.

WHOLE-GENOME SEQUENCING OF CULTURED ISOLATES

For a clinical laboratory, the essential goals of WGS performed on cultured isolates of bacteria and fungi (**Fig. 1**) are:

- Pathogen identification, focusing on cultured bacteria and fungi.
- Assessment of susceptibility to antibiotics.
- Infection prevention, specifically for outbreak investigations and pathogen/antimicrobial resistance surveillance.

Pathogen Identification

Standard clinical techniques—that is, culture, microscopy, biochemical characterization, nucleic acid tests (NATs), matrix-assisted laser desorption ionization - time of flight mass spectrometry—provide sufficient identification for the majority of frequently encountered pathogens. Occasionally, additional resolution is needed, either for accurate speciation or when subspecies information is required. This can be achieved through multilocus sequence typing, but typing schemes are tailored to a particular microbial species. And although sequencing multiple genetic loci by traditional Sanger methods is possible, scalability is a limitation of Sanger-based approaches, and costs can rapidly outstrip those of WGS if multiple targets are sequenced.

Bacterial pathogens

In some circumstances a WGS-based approach is advantageous because it can provide clinically-actionable information. This can include:

- Distinguishing between members of a clonal complex. For example, the NAP1 or ST1 group of *Clostridiodes difficile* is a clinically relevant and high-risk clone easily identified by WGS.[14]
- Identifying high-risk clones and detection of virulence genes. Combined with WGS, the detection of *rmpA* and *iucA* virulence genes in *Klebsiella pneumoniae*

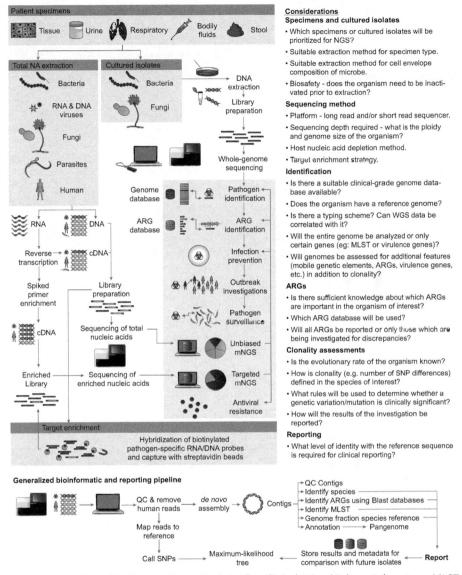

Fig. 1. Integration of Pathogen Genomics into the Clinical Microbiology Laboratory. MLST, multilocus sequence typing; QC, quality control; SNP, single nucleotide polymorphism.

are often markers of a hypervirulent phenotype associated with severe invasive infections.[15]

Fungal pathogens

Although curated databases for the identification of fungi using internal transcribed spacer sequencing are available,[16,17] many fungal taxa cannot be speciated by internal transcribed spacer sequencing alone.[17] Databases available for the identification of fungal pathogens have been reviewed recently[18] and their limitations highlight the need for WGS approaches. Other considerations for fungal WGS include the following.

- Many fungal species do not have reference genomes.[19]
- Large genome size and ploidy variation necessitates specialized bioinformatics tools.[19,20]
- Clinical-grade WGS databases for fungal pathogens do not exist.

Assessment of Susceptibility to Antibiotics: Detection of Antimicrobial Resistance Genes

Phenotypic antibiotic susceptibility testing is inexpensive, robust, and usually agnostic to the mechanism of antibiotic resistance. Antibiotic susceptibility testing methods are commonly augmented by rapid molecular assays or NATs, which detect high-risk and high-probability ARGs. For these reasons, phenotypic antibiotic susceptibility testing is unlikely to be replaced by WGS. However, there are instances where WGS can provide important information about susceptibility. For example:

- The identification of rare ARGs, chromosomal mutations, and variant alleles not detected by NATs.
- Resolution of discrepancies between phenotypic and NAT results, for example, a phenotypically susceptible organism with an ARG detected by NAT.
- Risk assessment by identifying genes involved in ARG mobilization and horizontal transfer (ie, transposons, insertion sequences, integrons, plasmids).

Infection Prevention

Infection prevention is a major application of WGS of cultured isolates and facilitates both outbreak investigation and prospective surveillance (see **Fig. 1**).

Outbreak investigation
The most common use of WGS in clinical laboratories is outbreak investigation. WGS of isolates from a suspected outbreak allows for determination of clonality, correlation with regional and national data, and establishment of transmission timelines.[21–24] Although other methods exist for determining isolate clonality (eg, pulsed-field gel electrophoresis), only WGS also identifies ARGs and virulence genes, and finely resolves degrees of relatedness.[23,25,26] WGS is also the preferred method for fungal genotyping in outbreak investigations, because many of these pathogens lack a pre-existing typing scheme.[19,27] Although there are unique challenges for WGS-based fungal outbreak investigations, it has been successfully used in this context.[19,28,29]

Surveillance
WGS is a powerful tool for prospective genomic surveillance and allows for the detection of cryptic outbreaks[30] and for monitoring the introduction of high-risk clones and ARGs into the hospital environment.[22,25,31,32] Prospective surveillance by WGS also allows each facility to put outbreaks into the context of the local genomic landscape of circulating clones. This process can help to indicate whether potential outbreak strains are newly introduced or known clones circulating in the hospital or local community. Consistent sampling over a long period of time provides better data than sporadic collections of archived strains.

CLINICAL METAGENOMIC NEXT-GENERATION SEQUENCING OF PRIMARY SPECIMENS

Total nucleic acid sequencing (mNGS directly from primary specimens) as a universal diagnostic test has been reviewed thoroughly in recent years.[33–35] Traditional clinical laboratory methods can fail to establish a causative agent, even in patients with features strongly suggestive of infectious disease. Although the ongoing development of multiplex syndromic NAT panels is a partial solution to this problem, mNGS offers a more comprehensive approach. This is because multiplex syndromic NAT panels have limited inclusivity, generally targeting a select range of the most probable syndromic etiologies, and expansion drives up costs.[36] Unlike mNGS, established syndromic NAT panels may be incapable of detecting new or emerging strains. This challenge was evident in the coronavirus disease-19 pandemic where the severe acute respiratory syndrome coronavirus-2 was not detectable by respiratory panels otherwise capable of detecting human coronaviruses (HCoV-229E, HCoV-HKU1, HCoV-NL63, and HCoV-OC43).[37]

Applications of Clinical Pathogen Metagenomic-Based Next-Generation Sequencing

The power of mNGS for infectious disease diagnostics is the provision of unbiased pan-taxonomic identification by total nucleic acid sequencing of primary specimens. Other applications include:

- Identification of DNA and RNA viruses.
- Identification of unculturable or fastidious pathogens, including cases complicated by antibiotic exposure.[38]
- Taxonomic profiling of polymicrobial infections.[39,40]
- ARG screening in complex, polymicrobial matrices.
- Assessment of antiviral resistance.
- Outbreak and infection prevention surveillance.

Unbiased Metagenomic-Based Next-Generation Sequencing and Targeted Metagenomic-Based Next-Generation Sequencing Approaches

Unbiased metagenomic-based next-generation sequencing approach

An unbiased mNGS approach refers to en masse shotgun sequencing of all microbial and host NA present in a patient specimen (see **Fig. 1**). Because it does not rely on prior culture, enrichment, or amplification, mNGS is considered to be unbiased, and is capable of the simultaneous detection of major pathogens from different domains (eg, virus, bacteria, fungi, and parasites). Pathogen detection relies on computational analysis of the resulting sequences to identify those aligning with known pathogen sequences. Depending on the method of library preparation, detection may be limited to DNA or may include both RNA and DNA.

Targeted metagenomic-based next-generation sequencing approach

Several modifications can be made to mNGS workflows to selectively profile target organisms or improve recovery of pathogen-specific nucleic acids. These include amplicon sequencing and target enrichment (see **Fig. 1**). A targeted mNGS sequencing based on sequencing amplicons (polymerase chain reaction-amplified conserved sequences) provides little beyond phylogenetic information and relative abundance (**Table 1**). Furthermore, amplicon sequencing does not allow for extended sequence-based characterization of detected pathogens, although it may be more sensitive owing to polymerase chain reaction amplification. Target enrichment through hybridization capture (panels of pathogen-specific RNA/DNA probes) can enrich for select pathogens while providing WGS level information about each of them, but practical limitations means that the extent of genome coverage is often inversely related to the number of organisms the panel can detect.

Table 1	
Advantages and disadvantages of unbiased and targeted mNGS approaches	
Advantages	Disadvantages
Unbiased mNGS	

Unbiased testing of patient specimen
Discovery of novel organisms or traits
Characterization of
  polymicrobial infections
Extended pathogen characterization
	Host background (human/microbial)
	More costly than targeted amplicon
	  sequencing
	Sequencing depth must be sufficient
	Easily contaminated with environmental
	  nucleic acid
	More challenging computational analysis

Targeted/amplicon mNGS	

More sensitive for organism detection
Less costly than an unbiased approach
	Often requires amplification using
	  primers that may be suboptimal for
	  the pathogen
	Only a small fragment of the genome
	  may be sequenced
	  (ie, 16s amplicon profiling)
	Easily contaminated with environmental
	  nucleic acid

CLINICAL MICROBIOLOGY NEXT-GENERATION SEQUENCING WORKFLOWS

The implementation of a preanalytical clinical microbiology genomics workflow for infectious disease diagnosis requires consideration of specimen storage, nucleic acid extraction techniques, and sequence library preparation.[41] The mNGS assays require additional considerations, owing to an increased risk of contamination and bias.[42]

Unbiased recovery of nucleic acids from a cultured isolate or primary specimen and successful NGS without the introduction of contaminants necessitates consideration of the following:

- Specimen collection, storage, and handling (for both WGS and mNGS).
  - Aseptic technique.
  - Transport and storage conditions.
  - Freeze–thaw cycles.
  - Specimen and nucleic acid preservation methods.
- Nucleic acid extraction (for both WGS and mNGS).
  - Commonly used methods include mechanical (bead beating, cryofracturing), and enzymatic.
  - Optimal lysis methods need to be determined for each specimen type.
  - Extraction method can bias microbial community profiles.
- Host nucleic acid depletion (for mNGS).
  - Host nucleic acid depletion aims to increase the ratio of microbial to host nucleic acid.[43]
  - Technically challenging, expensive, and time consuming, that is, the removal of CpG-methylated host DNA or the selective lysis and degradation of host cells and DNA before extraction.[43]
  - Can introduce additional bias into the workflow.
- Target enrichment by capture hybridization- and amplification-based technologies (for mNGS).
  - Spiked primer enrichment during reverse transcription can amplify specific sequences and simultaneously retain sensitivity for other pathogens.[44]

o Probe-and-capture strategies can selectively enrich relevant nucleic acid sequences though may require large probe sets.[45]
o Target enrichment can preclude identification of novel pathogens.

ADVANTAGES OF IN-HOUSE PATHOGEN NEXT-GENERATION SEQUENCING

Although many of the applications described elsewhere in this article can be done through reference laboratories, there are distinct advantages to developing a pathogen NGS program within the clinical diagnostic laboratory. In-house testing provides a faster turnaround time to resolve questions of identification and the detection of resistance genes pertinent to patient care.[46] With respect to surveillance and outbreak questions, in-house testing additionally allows each institution to query databases of their local genomic landscape. Other benefits, particularly in academic institutions, include the development of familiarity with the technology and analytical literacy of NGS among staff and trainees, which can nurture expansion of NGS into more diverse applications.

CHALLENGES OF IN-HOUSE PATHOGEN NEXT-GENERATION SEQUENCING: COSTS, INFRASTRUCTURE, VALIDATION, AND REPORTING

Bringing pathogen NGS in-house presents challenges, not least of which are the costs and logistics associated with building the technical and analytical infrastructure. Other considerations include the need for a clinical-grade validation, quality control measures, a proficiency testing program, and the development of a reporting structure, both for patient care and hospital infection prevention programs.

Costs and Infrastructure

It is still uncommon for instrumentation capable of NGS to be housed directly in a clinical microbiology laboratory. Pathogen NGS is often developed in collaboration with molecular diagnostic laboratories; however, this practice may change as costs of NGS platforms continue to decrease. For example, nanopore long read technology is approachable for most clinical laboratories, and there is growing interest in its application toward clinical questions.[47]

Commercial analysis platforms are becoming available that can answer many outbreak and typing questions without requiring the skills of a professional bioinformatician. Examples include SeqSphere (Ridom, Munster, Germany) and Bionumerics (Applied Maths, Austin, TX). Other commercial solutions can help with more specific questions, including pathogen identification and viral genotyping/resistance assessment (IDbyDNA, Salt Lake City, UT; SmartGene, Lausanne, Switzerland; etc). Several public agencies have also developed analytical resources to address questions of pathogen identification, antimicrobial resistance, and clonality.[48]

Less standardized questions, such as plasmid and transposon analysis in bacteria or viral typing, may require in-house bioinformatics personnel and customized analysis pipelines (see **Fig. 1**). A high-performance computing cluster is required; the amount of computing power required depends on the number of samples, expected turnaround times, and specific tools chosen within a pipeline. Furthermore, a large amount of data storage is necessary for archival purposes.

The design of a clinical pathogen genomics bioinformatics pipeline should focus on scalability and robustness. Running tasks in parallel greatly increases computational efficiency. A modular design allows for easier testing, validation, and upgrades. Generally, a pipeline includes 3 phases:

1. Read quality control.
2. Either de novo assembly into contigs or read alignment to a reference genome.
3. Genotyping, identifying resistance and virulence factors, single nucleotide polymorphism discovery, and phylogenetic tree building.

Clinical bioinformatics pipelines also need to be adaptable and relevant to any species. Pipelines should contain vetted references and regularly updated databases of strain types and ARGs, while also allowing for custom BLAST databases.

Validation

Validation and proficiency testing requirements associated with a pathogen NGS program vary considerably between WGS tests for cultured isolates and mNGS assays. Several authors have described development of pathogen WGS validation, including the use of test panels, appropriate controls, sequence quality control, and proficiency testing.[49–51] Additional guidance is available from state and national organizations.[52,53] Validation of mNGS assays is less established, but has been described in several publications.[35,54–56]

Reporting

Distilling information from pathogen NGS into an approachable report is challenging.[57] For surveillance and outbreak reporting to infection prevention teams, the report should include an introduction, a list of isolates/patients, and a description of the question at hand. For questions of antibiotic resistance, a table of pertinent ARGs and their connection to phenotypic susceptibility should be included. For questions of clonality (ie, a potential outbreak), a phylogenetic tree and single nucleotide polymorphism distance matrix are appropriate. As with any clinical report, a description of technical and analytical methods must be included. Reporting of clinical metagenomics is more straightforward and has been discussed elsewhere.[34,35,56]

SUMMARY

NGS-based diagnostics for infectious disease is poised to enter routine clinical practice for a variety of applications. Here we have summarized its usefulness for assays based on cultured isolates and primary specimens.

Improved turnaround times, the ability to compile a comprehensive database of local pathogens and clones, enhanced literacy among trainees and laboratory directors, and the ability to develop applications for the unique needs of individual medical centers all number among the benefits of in-house NGS testing. Toward this, a well thought out reporting structure and ongoing dialogue with clinicians is critical for making pathogen NGS data actionable.

The challenges of in-house pathogen NGS include financial, technical, and validation/quality control issues. The need to batch tests for efficiency of scale may necessitate a strategy for bringing pathogen NGS in-house on multiple fronts. For example, although the sequencing of cultured bacterial isolates is a good founder test, planning for other applications should follow closely behind.

The future may bring microbiome-based diagnostics and other paradigm-shifting mNGS assays. For example, although host reads are an obstacle to pathogen detection, host transcriptional profiling (ie, RNA-based sequencing) could provide clinically relevant information about the immune response. An mNGS understanding of host response to infection may also help distinguish colonization from infectious disease (analogous to the enumeration of host polymorphonuclear neutrophils in smears prepared from sterile site specimens).[58,59] As the price of NGS comes down, and literacy and comfort levels go up, it will be exciting to see how these platforms and technologies enter into routine practice.

DISCLOSURE

No author has commercial or financial conflicts of interest. N.D. Pecora is supported by funds available from the Department of Pathology and Laboratory Medicine, University of Rochester Medical Center.

REFERENCES

1. Quainoo S, Coolen JPM, van Hijum S, et al. Whole-genome sequencing of bacterial pathogens: the future of nosocomial outbreak analysis. Clin Microbiol Rev 2017;30(4):1015–63.
2. Allard MW, Bell R, Ferreira CM, et al. Genomics of foodborne pathogens for microbial food safety. Curr Opin Biotechnol 2018;49:224–9.
3. Koser CU, Ellington MJ, Cartwright EJ, et al. Routine use of microbial whole genome sequencing in diagnostic and public health microbiology. PLoS Pathog 2012;8(8):e1002824.
4. Spatafora JW, Aime MC, Grigoriev IV, et al. The fungal tree of life: from molecular systematics to genome-scale phylogenies. Microbiol Spectr 2017;5(5). https://doi.org/10.1128/microbiolspec.FUNK-0053-2016.
5. Cuomo CA. Harnessing whole genome sequencing in medical mycology. Curr Fungal Infect Rep 2017;11(2):52–9.
6. Kidd SE, Chen SC, Meyer W, et al. A new age in molecular diagnostics for invasive fungal disease: are we ready? Front Microbiol 2019;10:2903.
7. Fricke WF, Rasko DA. Bacterial genome sequencing in the clinic: bioinformatic challenges and solutions. Nat Rev Genet 2014;15(1):49–55.
8. Goldberg B, Sichtig H, Geyer C, et al. Making the leap from research laboratory to clinic: challenges and opportunities for next-generation sequencing in infectious disease diagnostics. mBio 2015;6(6). e01888-01815.
9. Mitchell SL, Simner PJ. Next-generation sequencing in clinical microbiology: are we there yet? Clin Lab Med 2019;39(3):405–18.
10. Boers SA, Jansen R, Hays JP. Understanding and overcoming the pitfalls and biases of next-generation sequencing (NGS) methods for use in the routine clinical microbiological diagnostic laboratory. Eur J Clin Microbiol Infect Dis 2019; 38(6):1059–70.
11. Blauwkamp TA, Thair S, Rosen MJ, et al. Analytical and clinical validation of a microbial cell-free DNA sequencing test for infectious disease. Nat Microbiol 2019; 4(4):663–74.
12. Martin RM, Burke K, Verma D, et al. Contact transmission of vaccinia to an infant diagnosed by viral culture and metagenomic sequencing. Open Forum Infect Dis 2020;7(4).
13. Levy SE, Myers RM. Advancements in next-generation sequencing. Annu Rev Genomics Hum Genet 2016;17:95–115.
14. McDonald LC, Killgore GE, Thompson A, et al. An epidemic, toxin gene-variant strain of Clostridium difficile. N Engl J Med 2005;353(23):2433–41.
15. Russo TA, Marr CM. Hypervirulent Klebsiella pneumoniae. Clin Microbiol Rev 2019;32(3).
16. Ratnasingham S, Hebert PDN. bold: the Barcode of Life Data System (http://www.barcodinglife.org/). Mol Ecol Notes 2007;7(3):355–64.

17. Irinyi L, Serena C, Garcia-Hermoso D, et al. International Society of Human and Animal Mycology (ISHAM)-ITS reference DNA barcoding database–the quality controlled standard tool for routine identification of human and animal pathogenic fungi. Med Mycol 2015;53(4):313–37.

18. Prakash PY, Irinyi L, Halliday C, et al. Online databases for taxonomy and identification of pathogenic fungi and proposal for a cloud-based dynamic data network platform. J Clin Microbiol 2017;55(4):1011–24.

19. Bougnoux M-E, Brun S, Zahar J-R. Healthcare-associated fungal outbreaks: new and uncommon species, New molecular tools for investigation and prevention. Antimicrob Resist Infect Control 2018;7(1):45.

20. Litvintseva AP, Brandt ME, Mody RK, et al. Investigating fungal outbreaks in the 21st century. PLoS Pathog 2015;11(5):e1004804.

21. Wendel AF, Malecki M, Otchwemah R, et al. One-year molecular surveillance of carbapenem-susceptible A. baumannii on a German intensive care unit: diversity or clonality. Antimicrob Resist Infect Control 2018;7:145.

22. Ugolotti E, Larghero P, Vanni I, et al. Whole-genome sequencing as standard practice for the analysis of clonality in outbreaks of methicillin-resistant Staphylococcus aureus in a paediatric setting. J Hosp Infect 2016;93(4):375–81.

23. Martineau C, Li X, Lalancette C, et al. Serratia marcescens outbreak in a neonatal intensive care unit: new insights from next-generation sequencing applications. J Clin Microbiol 2018;56(9). e00235-18.

24. Shenoy ES, Pierce VM, Sater MRA, et al. Community-acquired in name only: a cluster of carbapenem-resistant Acinetobacter baumannii in a burn intensive care unit and beyond. Infect Control Hosp Epidemiol 2020;41(5):531–8.

25. Malek A, McGlynn K, Taffner S, et al. Next-generation-sequencing-based hospital outbreak investigation yields insight into klebsiella aerogenes population structure and determinants of carbapenem resistance and pathogenicity. Antimicrob Agents Chemother 2019;63(6). e02577-18.

26. Nakanishi N, Yonezawa T, Tanaka S, et al. Assessment of the local clonal spread of Streptococcus pneumoniae serotype 12F caused invasive pneumococcal diseases among children and adults. J Infect Public Health 2019;12(6):867–72.

27. Alanio A, Desnos-Ollivier M, Garcia-Hermoso D, et al. Investigating clinical issues by genotyping of medically important fungi: why and how? Clin Microbiol Rev 2017;30(3):671–707.

28. Meyer W, Irinyi L, Hoang MTV, et al. Database establishment for the secondary fungal DNA barcode translational elongation factor 1alpha (TEF1alpha) (1). Genome 2019;62(3):160–9.

29. Garcia-Hermoso D, Criscuolo A, Lee SC, et al. Outbreak of invasive wound mucormycosis in a burn unit due to multiple strains of Mucor circinelloides resolved by whole-genome sequencing. mBio 2018;9(2). e00573-00518.

30. Park KH, Greenwood-Quaintance KE, Uhl JR, et al. Molecular epidemiology of Staphylococcus aureus bacteremia in a single large Minnesota medical center in 2015 as assessed using MLST, core genome MLST and spa typing. PLoS One 2017;12(6):e0179003.

31. Roach DJ, Burton JN, Lee C, et al. A year of infection in the intensive care unit: prospective whole genome sequencing of bacterial clinical isolates reveals cryptic transmissions and novel microbiota. PLoS Genet 2015;11(7):e1005413.

32. Leong KWC, Cooley LA, Anderson TL, et al. Emergence of vancomycin-resistant enterococcus faecium at an Australian hospital: a whole genome sequencing analysis. Sci Rep 2018;8(1):6274.

33. Han D, Li Z, Li R, et al. mNGS in clinical microbiology laboratories: on the road to maturity. Crit Rev Microbiol 2019;45(5–6):668–85.
34. Chiu CY, Miller SA. Clinical metagenomics. Nat Rev Genet 2019;20(6):341–55.
35. Gu W, Miller S, Chiu CY. Clinical metagenomic next-generation sequencing for pathogen detection. Annu Rev Pathol 2019;14:319–38.
36. Relich RF, Abbott AN. Syndromic and point-of-care molecular testing. Adv Mol Pathol 2018;1(1):97.
37. Phan T. Novel coronavirus: from discovery to clinical diagnostics. Infect Genet Evol 2020;79:104211.
38. Miao Q, Ma Y, Wang Q, et al. Microbiological diagnostic performance of metagenomic next-generation sequencing when applied to clinical practice. Clin Infect Dis 2018;67(suppl_2):S231–40.
39. Chen M-F, Chang C-H, Chiang-Ni C, et al. Rapid analysis of bacterial composition in prosthetic joint infection by 16S rRNA metagenomic sequencing. Bone Joint Res 2019;8(8):367–77.
40. Ruppé E, Lazarevic V, Girard M, et al. Clinical metagenomics of bone and joint infections: a proof of concept study. Sci Rep 2017;7(1):1–12.
41. Bachmann NL, Rockett RJ, Timms VJ, et al. Advances in clinical sample preparation for identification and characterization of bacterial pathogens using metagenomics. Front Public Health 2018;6:363.
42. McLaren MR, Willis AD, Callahan BJ. Consistent and correctable bias in metagenomic sequencing experiments. Elife 2019;8:e46923.
43. Thoendel M, Jeraldo PR, Greenwood-Quaintance KE, et al. Comparison of microbial DNA enrichment tools for metagenomic whole genome sequencing. J Microbiol Methods 2016;127:141–5.
44. Deng X, Achari A, Federman S, et al. Metagenomic sequencing with spiked primer enrichment for viral diagnostics and genomic surveillance. Nat Microbiol 2020;5(3):443–54.
45. Guitor AK, Raphenya AR, Klunk J, et al. Capturing the Resistome: a targeted capture method to reveal antibiotic resistance determinants in metagenomes. Antimicrob Agents Chemother 2019;64(1). e01324-19.
46. McGann P, Bunin JL, Snesrud E, et al. Real time application of whole genome sequencing for outbreak investigation - what is an achievable turnaround time? Diagn Microbiol Infect Dis 2016;85(3):277–82.
47. Petersen LM, Martin IW, Moschetti WE, et al. Third-generation sequencing in the clinical laboratory: exploring the advantages and challenges of nanopore sequencing. J Clin Microbiol 2019;58(1). e01315-19.
48. Sichtig H, Minogue T, Yan Y, et al. FDA-ARGOS is a database with public quality-controlled reference genomes for diagnostic use and regulatory science. Nat Commun 2019;10(1):3313.
49. Arnold C, Edwards K, Desai M, et al. Setup, validation, and quality control of a centralized whole-genome-sequencing laboratory: lessons learned. J Clin Microbiol 2018;56(8):e00261-18.
50. Kozyreva VK, Truong CL, Greninger AL, et al. Validation and implementation of clinical laboratory improvements act-compliant whole-genome sequencing in the public health microbiology laboratory. J Clin Microbiol 2017;55(8):2502–20.
51. Timme RE, Rand H, Sanchez Leon M, et al. GenomeTrakr proficiency testing for foodborne pathogen surveillance: an exercise from 2015. Microb Genom 2018;4(7):e000185.

52. Lefterova MI, Suarez CJ, Banaei N, et al. Next-generation sequencing for infectious disease diagnosis and management: a report of the association for molecular pathology. J Mol Diagn 2015;17(6):623–34.
53. Aziz N, Zhao Q, Bry L, et al. College of American Pathologists' laboratory standards for next-generation sequencing clinical tests. Arch Pathol Lab Med 2015;139(4):481–93.
54. Miller S, Naccache SN, Samayoa E, et al. Laboratory validation of a clinical metagenomic sequencing assay for pathogen detection in cerebrospinal fluid. Genome Res 2019;29(5):831–42.
55. Brinkmann A, Andrusch A, Belka A, et al. Proficiency testing of virus diagnostics based on bioinformatics analysis of simulated in silico high-throughput sequencing data sets. J Clin Microbiol 2019;57(8). e00466-19.
56. Schlaberg R, Chiu CY, Miller S, et al. Validation of metagenomic next-generation sequencing tests for universal pathogen detection. Arch Pathol Lab Med 2017; 141(6):776–86.
57. Crisan A, McKee G, Munzner T, et al. Evidence-based design and evaluation of a whole genome sequencing clinical report for the reference microbiology laboratory. PeerJ 2018;6:e4218.
58. Cheng AP, Burnham P, Lee JR, et al. A cell-free DNA metagenomic sequencing assay that integrates the host injury response to infection. Proc Natl Acad Sci U S A 2019;116(37):18738–44.
59. Peña-Gonzalez A, Soto-Girón MJ, Smith S, et al. Metagenomic signatures of gut infections caused by different Escherichia coli pathotypes. Appl Environ Microbiol 2019;85(24). e01820-19.

Coronavirus Detection in the Clinical Microbiology Laboratory

Are We Ready for Identifying and Diagnosing a Novel Virus?

Katharine Uhteg, MS, Karen C. Carroll, MD,
Heba H. Mostafa, MD, PhD, D(ABMM)*

KEYWORDS

- Coronaviruses • SARS • MERS • COVID-19 • SARS-CoV-2 (2019-nCoV)
- Sequencing • Molecular diagnosis

KEY POINTS

- Human coronaviruses are differentiated into endemic types, which cause largely self-limiting respiratory infections, and highly pathogenic types with high case fatality rates.
- Specific primers for diagnosing the endemic strains are routinely included in the most commonly used extended molecular respiratory panels.
- Highly pathogenic strains were first identified by molecular assays that include amplification with pancoronavirus primers and amplicon sequencing, and most recently with metagenomic next-generation sequencing.
- Specific molecular assays for the diagnosis of highly pathogenic coronaviruses were developed and are usually only available at public health laboratories and the US Centers for Disease Control and Prevention, but public health as well as clinical laboratories should harbor this diagnostic capacity in order to nimbly respond to an outbreak.
- Metagenomic whole-genome sequencing is a promising tool for the quick detection and epidemiologic characterization of novel coronaviruses.

INTRODUCTION

Coronaviruses were first described as viruses of animals, causing a wide spectrum of diseases that include gastroenteritis of pigs (transmissible gastroenteritis virus and porcine epidemic diarrhea virus), encephalitis in pigs (porcine hemagglutinating encephalomyelitis virus), lethal peritonitis in cats (feline infectious peritonitis virus),

Division of Medical Microbiology, Department of Pathology, Johns Hopkins University School of Medicine, Meyer B 121F, 600 North Wolfe Street, Baltimore, MD 21287-7093, USA
* Corresponding author.
E-mail address: hmostaf2@jhmi.edu

Clin Lab Med 40 (2020) 459–472
https://doi.org/10.1016/j.cll.2020.08.004
labmed.theclinics.com

and bronchitis in chickens (infectious bronchitis virus).[1] However, their potential to cause disease in humans was not described until the 1960s.[2] Seven human coronaviruses (HCoVs) were identified, the first 2 of which, HCoV-OC43 and HCoV-229E, were isolated from patients with respiratory tract infections.[3,4] Since then, these 2 coronaviruses were established as endemic strains associated with mild disease, and it was not until 2003 that a third HCoV was identified as a cause of severe acute respiratory syndrome (SARS).[5,6] Two additional HCoVs were discovered in 2004 (HCoV-NL63)[7] and 2005 (HCoV-HKU1),[8] followed by the Middle East respiratory syndrome (MERS)–CoV, which emerged in 2012.[9] Recently (December of 2019), the seventh HCoV (SARS-CoV-2) emerged in Wuhan, China, causing millions of confirmed cases with high mortality (the World Health Organization [WHO] has named the disease coronavirus disease 2019 [COVID-19]).[10]

Coronaviruses belong to the family *Coronaviridae* order *Nidovirales*. Two subfamilies make up the *Coronaviridae* family: *Letovirinae* and *Orthocoronavirinae*. *Orthocoronavirinae* has 4 genera: *Alphacoronavirus*, *Betacoronavirus*, *Gammacoronavirus*, and *Deltacoronavirus*. Coronaviruses that infect mammals belong to the *Alphacoronavirus* and *Betacoronavirus* genera[11] (**Fig. 1**).

ENDEMIC VERSUS HIGHLY PATHOGENIC CORONAVIRUSES

Four human coronaviruses have been established as endemic: HCoV-NL63, HCoV-229E, HCoV-OC43, and HCoV-HKU1. These endemic strains have been identified as significant causes of acute respiratory infection and the common cold, causing 15% to 30% of respiratory tract infections each year.[1,12–17] Infection with endemic coronaviruses can be severe, and the first isolation of HCoV-NL63 and HCoV-HKU1 were from cases of bronchiolitis and pneumonia.[3,8] Although these endemic coronaviruses have the potential to cause severe disease, which is largely associated with immunocompromising conditions or young age,[18–20] these viruses received scant attention because of their association with milder disease in immunocompetent individuals. The outbreak of SARS in China in 2002 to 2003 highlighted the potential of these and/or related viruses to cause outbreaks of severe disease, because more than 8000 cases were diagnosed with close to a 10% case fatality rate.[21] This highly pathogenic strain that is thought to be transmitted to humans by direct contact with market civets[22] was controlled after the 2003 outbreak with no additional cases reported since 2004. In 2012, another highly pathogenic coronavirus, MERS-CoV, was isolated from a patient with fatal pneumonia in Saudi Arabia.[9] This virus was traced to dromedary camels. Apparently, frequent transmission events of this virus to this Middle East species of camel have occurred.[23,24] This virus has affected 2494 individuals, with new cases being diagnosed every month, mainly from Saudi Arabia (WHO-MERS-CoV), with a case fatality rate higher than SARS-CoV (~35%).[2] In December 2019, a novel coronavirus (SARS-CoV-2) was first isolated from the city of Wuhan, China, and rapidly millions of cases were reported from almost every country in the world. This most novel coronavirus was characterized by extensive spread and apparently higher infectivity or more efficient human-to-human transmission. At the time of this submission (July 1, 2020), 511,860 deaths were associated with COVID-19 of a total of 10,501,482 confirmed global cases (https://coronavirus.jhu.edu/map.html).

Most of the animal and human coronaviruses are thought to originate from bats. Next-genome sequencing (NGS) of the bat virome revealed that 35% are coronaviruses, more than 200 of which were novel species.[25] SARS-like CoV was isolated from the Chinese horseshoe bat years after the SARS-CoV outbreak, and MERS-CoV was found to be

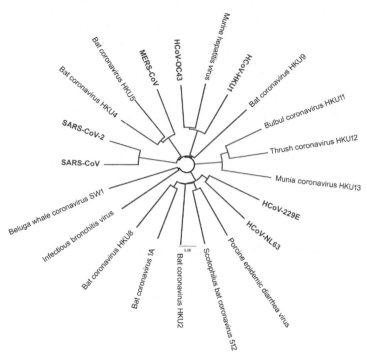

Fig. 1. Phylogenetic relationship of human coronaviruses. Viruses in the subfamily group into 4 genera that include *Alphacoronavirus* (*blue arms*), *Betacoronavirus* (*pink*), *Gammacoronavirus* (*purple*), and *Deltacoronavirus* (*green*). The human coronaviruses belong to *Alphacoronavirus* and *Betacoronavirus* genera and are highlighted in red. The tree was created by Geneious version 2020.0 created by Biomatters. Available from https://www.geneious.com. Accession numbers for selected whole genomes are as follows: AY291315.1, MN908947.3, EF065505.1, EF065509.1, KF186564.1, AY391777.1, AY700211.1, AY597011.2, EF065513.1, FJ376619.2, FJ376621.1, FJ376622.1, AF304460.1, AY567487.2, AF353511.1, NC_009657.1, EF203064.1, NC_010437.1, NC_010438.1, AY514485.1, and EU111742.1.

related to viruses isolated from various bat species of the *Vespertilionidae* family.[26] In addition, sequences similar to HCoV-NL63 and HCoV-229E have been identified in other species of bats.[25] Because human coronaviruses all have zoonotic origin, it is essential to understand the determinants of spillover from bats or other natural reservoirs to humans. Surveillance studies with thorough genomic characterization are vital to predict the next novel highly pathogenic coronavirus epidemic.

CORONAVIRUS GENOME

The viruses of the *Coronaviridae* family are enveloped with a single-strand, positive-sense RNA genome that has an average size of 30 Kb.[1] The name corona describes the crown-shaped projections of the surface when visualized with electron microscopy. The genome has a 5′-terminal cap similar to the standard eukaryotic cap structure and a polyadenylated tail at the 3′ end. About two-thirds of the genome encodes for the replicase-transcriptase, which is the only protein that is immediately translated directly from the genome (encoded by open reading frames [ORFs] 1a and 1b, which encode for 16 nonstructural proteins) (**Fig. 2**). Negative-sense genomic and

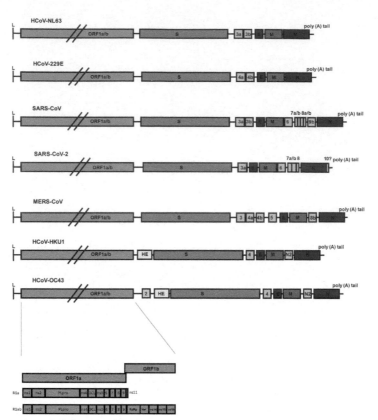

Fig. 2. Genome organization of the 7 human coronaviruses. The genomes range in size from 26 to about 32 kb. The order of the genome is typically 5′-ORF1a-ORF1b-S-E-M-N-3′. ORF1a and ORF1b overlap and occupy the 5′ two-thirds of the genome. Both encode for the components required for replication and transcription. The 3′ one-third of the genome encodes for structural (S-E-M-N) and accessory proteins (*green*). The illustrations and ORFs overlap are not to scale.

subgenomic RNAs are then synthesized with the help of the replicase-transcriptase, which serve as the template for the production of all the downstream ORFs.[27] At least 5 additional ORFs make up the remaining one-third of the genome and encode for structural proteins that include the spike (S), membrane (M), nucleocapsid (N), and envelope (E). Additional accessory genes are dispersed between the structural genes' ORFs downstream of the replicase, which are group specific and required for efficient viral replication (see **Fig. 2**). Transcription regulatory sequences are located between the ORFs that control transcription termination as well as the addition of the leader sequences. The structural protein coding region by sequence alignment of different coronaviruses seems less conserved than the nonstructural protein encoding region; however, both regions show less than 60% identity at the genomic level. Usually, the more conserved *Orf1b* is selected as a target for molecular assay design.[21]

MOLECULAR DIAGNOSIS OF CORONAVIRUSES

Nucleic acid detection methods are more sensitive than traditional methods of diagnosis that include cell culture, and offer higher specificity. In general, there are 3 goals of molecular coronavirus diagnosis in the clinical microbiology and public health laboratories: routine diagnostics of endemic strains, the diagnosis of highly pathogenic strains in endemic areas and during outbreaks, and the detection and characterization of novel unidentified viruses. For coronavirus molecular identification, assays that could generally detect all known human coronaviruses as well as assays that could distinguish the different species were developed. In addition, NGS has advanced the understanding of new coronaviruses and showed a great potential in their identification directly from clinical specimens, although these assays have not yet entered routine practice in the clinical laboratory.

TARGETED CORONAVIRUS MOLECULAR DETECTION

With the wide prevalence of endemic coronaviruses as significant causes of upper respiratory tract infection, implementing methods for routine diagnosis has become a common practice. At present, diagnosing coronaviruses in clinical microbiology laboratories is a part of most of the US Food and Drug Administration (FDA)–cleared respiratory panel assays (**Table 1**). These panels usually are supplemented with oligonucleotides specific for the 4 endemic HCoVs. These assays usually target the N gene; however, several laboratory-developed assays have used primers that target the polymerase, M or S genes, or the 5′ untranslated region. Most of these assays are multiplex or nested real-time polymerase chain reaction (RT-PCR) tests.[28] Because of their species specificity, these assays usually cannot identify novel coronaviruses. The FilmArray respiratory panel (BioFire Diagnostics, Salt Lake City, UT) and the ePlex Respiratory Pathogen Panel (GenMark Diagnostics, Carlsbad, CA) are currently two of the most commonly used extended respiratory panels. In addition to detecting the 4 endemic coronaviruses, the FilmArray Respiratory Panel 2 *plus* and the Pneumonia Panel *plus* have also incorporated specific primers for the detection of MERS-CoV. In addition, the BioFire Respiratory 2.1 (RP2.1) Panel with SARS-CoV-2 received FDA Emergency Use Authorization (EUA) for SARS-CoV-2 diagnosis. The QIAGEN QIAstat-Dx Respiratory SARS-Cov-2 Panel is an extended respiratory panel that also received an EUA for SARS-CoV-2 diagnosis.

Most clinical microbiology laboratories do not offer testing for targeted detection of highly pathogenic HCoVs in house, and, in outbreak situations, suspected specimens are sent out to either local public health laboratories or the US Centers for Disease Control and Prevention (CDC) (see **Table 1**). This work flow is challenging because of hurdles associated with specimen packaging and shipping in addition to prolonged turnaround times and their associated delay in making decisions related to patients' isolation. In response to the recent outbreak of COVID-19, several groups nationally and internationally attempted to develop diagnostic assays that could be available for all clinical laboratories, and multiple diagnostic providers within the United States have been striving to receive EUA from the FDA. This response was secondary to the quick spread of the disease, but it was also largely facilitated by the availability of the virus genomic sequences very quickly early in the pandemic. RT-PCR assays developed by the Chinese National Institute for Viral Disease Control and Prevention, the University of Hong Kong, and the CDC (which received the EUA by FDA on February 4, 2020) were distributed on a large scale, followed by a very quick expansion in the number of the molecular EUA-approved tests. More than 100 assays are currently authorized for SARS-CoV-2 diagnosis, which are largely RT-PCR based. Other technologies have also received FDA authorization, including the CRISPR (clustered regularly interspaced short palindromic repeats)-based assay SHERLOCK (specific

Table 1
Examples of molecular approaches for coronavirus diagnosis, commercially and laboratory developed

Assay	HCoVs Detected	Target	Testing Methodology	Primer Type	Comments
Luminex Respiratory Pathogen Panel NxTAG	HCoV-NL63 HCoV-OC43 HCoV-229E HCoV-HKU1	N gene — Orf1ab	Multiplex RT-PCR and bead array hybridization	Specific	FDA cleared
BioFire FilmArray Respiratory Panel 2 *plus*	HCoV-NL63 HCoV-OC43 HCoV-229E HCoV-HKU1 MERS-CoV	Not disclosed	Multiplex RT-PCR with melt curve analysis	Specific	FDA cleared
BioFire FilmArray Respiratory Panel 2.1	HCoV-NL63 HCoV-OC43 HCoV-229E HCoV-HKU1 SARS-CoV-2				FDA-EUA
GenMark ePlex Respiratory Panel	HCoV-NL63 HCoV-OC43 HCoV-229E HCoV-HKU1	N gene	Digital microfluidics with electrochemical detection	Specific	FDA cleared
Qiagen RespiFinder RG	HCoV-NL63 HCoV-OC43 HCoV-229E HCoV-HKU1	N gene	Multiplex RT-PCR with melt curve analysis	Specific	FDA cleared
QIAGEN Gmbh/Qiastat-Dx Respiratory SARS-Cov-2 Panel	HCoV-NL63 HCoV-OC43 HCoV-229E HCoV-HKU1 SARS-CoV-2				FDA-EUA

CDC[50]	MERS-CoV	UpE and ORF1a	RT-PCR	Specific	UpE: F (5'-GCAACGCGCGATTCAGTT-3') R (5'-GCCTCTACACGGGACCCATA-3') P (5'6- FAM/CTTTCACATAATGCCCCGAGCTCG/3'6-TAMSp) ORF: F (5'- CCACTACTCCCATTTCGTCAG-3') R (5'- CAGTATGTGTAGTGCGCATATAAGCA-3') P (5'6- FAM/TTGCAAATTGGCTTGCCCCACT/3'6-TAMSp)
CDC[51]	SARS-CoV	RNA polymerase, N gene	RT-PCR	Specific	SARS1: F (5'-CATGTGTGGCGGCTCACTATAT-3') R (5'-GACACTATTAGCATAAGCAGTTGTAGCA-3') P (5'-TTAAACCAGGTGGAACATCATCCGGTG-3') SARS2: F (5'-GGAGCCTTGAATACACCCAAAG-3') R (5'-GCACGGTGGCAGCATTG-3') P (5'-CCACATTGGCACCCGCAATCC-3') SARS3: F (5'-CAAACATTGGCCGCAAATT-3') R (5'-CAATGCGTGACATTCCAAAGA-3') P (5'-CACAATTTGCTCCAAGTGCCTCTGCA-3')
CDC	SARS-CoV-2	N gene	RT-PCR	Specific	N1: F (5'-GACCCCAAAATCAGGAAAT-3') R (5'-TCTGGTTACTGCCAGTTGAATCTG-3') P (5'-FAM-ACCCCGCATTACGTTTGGTGGACC-BHQ1-3') N2: F (5'-TTACAAACATTGGCCGCAAA-3') R (5'-GCGCGACATTCCGAAGAA-3') P (5'-FAM-ACAATTTGCCCCAGCGCTTCAG-BHQ1-3')
Zhang, et al,[52] 2018	HCoV-NL63, HCoV-OC43, HCoV-229E, HCoV-HKU1	HCoV-NL63, HCoV-OC43, HCoV-229E ⎱ N gene; HCoV-HKU1 — P gene	Multiplex RT-PCR	Specific	NL63: F (5'-GTTCTTCTGGTACTTCCACTCCT-3') R (5'-TTCCAACGAGGTTTCTTCAA-3') P (5'-FAM-AGCCTCTTTCTCAACCAGGGCTG-BHQ1-3') OC43: F (5'-CCCAAGTAGGCGATGAGGCTA-3') R (5'-AGGAGCAGACCTTCGTGAGC-3') P (5'-FAM-ACTAGGTTTCCGCCTGGCACGGTA-BHQ1-3') 229E: F (5'-CAGAAAACGAAAGATTGCTTCA-3') R (5'-CAAGCAAAGGGCTATAAAGAGA-3') P (5'-VIC-ATGGCTACAGTCAAATGGGCTGATGC-BHQ1-3')

(continued on next page)

Table 1
(continued)

Assay	HCoVs Detected	Target	Testing Methodology	Primer Type	Comments
Gaunt et al,[17] 2010	HCoV-NL63, HCoV-OC43, HCoV-229E, HCoV-HKU1	HCoV-OC43 → M gene; HCoV-229E, HCoV-NL63, HCoV-HKU1 → N gene	One-step multiplex RT-PCR	Specific	HKU1: F (5′-TGAATTTGTTGTTCACATGGT-3′) R (5′-ATAATAGCAACCGCCACACAT-3′) P (5′-VIC-ATCGCCTTGCGAATGAATGTGCTC-BHQ1-3′) NL63: F (5′-GTTCTGATAAGGCACCATATAGG-3′) R (5′-TTTAGGAGGACAAATCAACACAG-3′) OC43: F (5′-CATACYCTGACGGTCACAATAATA-3′) R (5′-ACCTTAGCAACAGTCATATAAGC-3′) 229E: F (5′-CATACTATCAACCATTCAACAAG-3′) R (5′-CACGGCAACTGTCATGTATT-3′) HKU1: F (5′-TCCTACTAYTCAAGAAGCTATCC-3′) R (5′-AATGAACGATTATTGGGTCCAC-3′)
Vijgen et al,[30] 2008	HCoV-NL63, HCoV-OC43, HCoV-229E, HCoV-HKU1, SARS-CoV	RdRp	One-step RT-PCR	Pan	F: (5′-ACWCARHTVAAYYTNAARTAYGC-3′) R: (5′-TCRCAYTTDGGRTARTCCCA-3′)
Canducci et al,[53] 2008	HCoV-NL63, HCoV-OC43, HCoV-229E, HCoV-HKU1, SARS-CoV	RdRp	RT-PCR	Pan	F1: (5′-TTATGGGTYGGGATTATCYAARTGTGAT-3′) R1: (5′-GTACTAGCRTCACCAGAAGTYGTACCACC-3′) F2: (5′-ATGGGATGGGGACTATCCTAAGTGTGATAGAG-3′) R2: (5′-TTGCATCACCACTRCTAGTRCCACCAGGC-3′)

Abbreviations: CDC, US Centers for Disease Control and Prevention; EUA, Emergency Use Authorization; F, forward; M, membrane; N, nucleocapsid; P gene, polyprotein; P, probe; R, reverse; RdRp, RNA-dependent RNA polymerase; RT-PCR, real-time polymerase chain reaction; UpE, upstream E.

high-sensitivity enzymatic reporter unlocking) assay, which combined CRISPR with isothermal amplification as well as the COVIDSeq assay from Illumina (San Diego, CA), a targeted NGS-based assay. Globally, fast implementation of molecular diagnostics in Europe was remarkable,[29] and several international commercial groups have quickly developed assays as well. These assays include a microarray panel developed by Veredus Laboratories (Singapore), which is an amplification-based array method for the quick detection of SARS-CoV, MERS-CoV, and SARS-CoV-2 (Vere-CoV detection kit), in addition to RT-PCR kits that were developed by Amoy Diagnostics (Xiamen, China), Altona Diagnostics (Hamburg, Germany), BGI group (Beijing Genomics Institute, Guangdong, China), among others. A list of all the EUA molecular SARS-CoV-2 assays is available at https://www.fda.gov/medical-devices/coronavirus-disease-2019-covid-19-emergency-use-authorizations-medical-devices/vitro-diagnostics-euas.

One strategy for the detection of all species of coronaviruses requires the use of primers that are capable of recognizing conserved regions in the coronavirus genome. The polymerase gene has been used as a target for these pancoronavirus molecular amplification methods with variable analytical performance.[30,31] In general, these assays are useful for the identification of novel coronaviruses and could be used for an initial screening; however, pancoronavirus detection approaches may suffer from lower sensitivity.[32]

ARE CLINICAL LABORATORIES READY TO IDENTIFY A NOVEL CORONAVIRUS?

Coronaviruses as a cause of seasonal respiratory tract diseases are largely restricted to the 4 endemic human coronaviruses. To date, 3 epidemics have been caused by 3 novel highly pathogenic coronaviruses. The approaches for the initial characterization of these viruses varied. SARS-CoV was first identified by growing the virus in cell culture and using a random amplification polymerase chain reaction (PCR) assay to amplify a 300-nucleotide region. A diagnostic RT-PCR assay was developed based on the obtained sequence.[5] A full genome was available shortly thereafter[6] and multiple specific nucleic acid amplification diagnostic assays were developed.[33] Conventional and molecular approaches were used for the classification of SARS-CoV as a member of *Coronaviridae* about 6 weeks after the Hong Kong outbreak in mid-February 2003.[34] In 2012, the identification of MERS-CoV, which caused severe pneumonia and death of a 60-year-old man, was performed by a pan-CoV PCR assay after cell culture followed by amplicon sequencing.[9] An assay panel was developed for the detection of the N nucleocapsid and the upstream sequence (up) to the E envelope (*upE*) genes, which has become the recommended test for the diagnosis of MERS-CoV by WHO.[35] Eighteen years after the SARS-CoV outbreak, a novel coronavirus was recognized as a cause of another epidemic of severe respiratory infection that started in Wuhan, China. Shortly after the outbreak, clinical specimens were tested both by a pan-CoV PCR assay and NGS. Subsequently, a specific RT-PCR was developed. The SARS-CoV-2 whole genome was available on January 10, almost 1 month after the first report of pneumonia of unknown origin. This process was accelerated compared with SARS-CoV, of which a complete sequence was available in April 2003, a few months after the outbreak started late in 2002. The history of identifying novel epidemic coronaviruses highlights the great impact of using advanced metagenomic NGS (mNGS; discussed later) not only for rapid identification but also for the epidemiologic tracing of the viral reservoir and for elucidating the transmission dynamics.

METAGENOMIC NEXT-GENERATION SEQUENCING FOR CORONAVIRUS DIAGNOSIS

NGS is a high-throughput method that allows massive parallel sequencing of billions of DNA fragments simultaneously. mNGS is an unbiased, untargeted method for sequencing all genomes in a particular specimen.[36] mNGS for viral identification in outbreak situations is very valuable in the absence of prior knowledge of the pathogen and facilitates quick phylogenetic characterization. mNGS has assisted in the characterization of SARS-CoV-2 from respiratory specimens in patients with pneumonia and has provided rapid insight into the genome and its phylogenetic relationship to other coronaviruses. As a response to this outbreak, a metagenomics deep-sequencing method using the MGI DNBSEQ-T7 sequencer (Cambridge, MA) for diagnosing coronaviruses in general was developed. This platform and the metagenomics coronavirus sequencing kit (BGI Group) have received an emergency use approval in China.

On the research side, mNGS was used to propose an evolutionary pathway of the SARS-CoV-2 virus from its origin in bats,[37] for the detection of a cluster of severe lower respiratory tract infections associated with a novel subgenotype of HCoV-NL63,[38] and in identifying an outbreak of health care–associated infections with HCoV-OC43 in hematopoietic stem cell transplant patients,[39] in addition to illuminating a global understanding of the epidemiology of coronaviruses in bats.[40] The applications of mNGS for identification and diagnosis of novel strains of coronaviruses are vast and, when used, initially will provide a quicker and better understanding of the biology and epidemiology of coronaviruses.

THIRD-GENERATION SEQUENCING: A PROMISING TOOL FOR RAPID DIAGNOSIS

A third-generation NGS instrument, the MinION, has become very popular and is a promising tool for developing point-of-care mNGS methods. The MinION is a portable sequencer that uses the innovative Nanopore protein pores for sequencing. Strands of DNA or RNA are directed to the protein pores and a characteristic change in the electric current distinguishes nucleotide bases.[41] Easy-to-prepare libraries and real-time analysis facilitate the use of MinION as a clinical diagnostic tool. Nanopore recently released Flongle, a flow cell designed for individual tests with less cost. This addition will further enhance the potential of the clinical implementation of this technology.

Several studies have shown the great potential of MinION in viral identification[42,43] and confirmed its potential as a point-of-care test, which included the identification of chikungunya, Ebola, and hepatitis C.[43] Recently, diagnosis of influenza virus using MinION directly from respiratory specimens was successful, with excellent sensitivity from specimens with higher viral loads.[44] In addition, a near-complete influenza viral genome was reconstructed by MinION in this study as well as the detection of coinfecting viruses that included coronavirus and human metapneumovirus.[44]

The characterization of the most recent highly pathogenic coronavirus (SARS-CoV-2) was partially performed by MinION sequencing in addition to mNGS.[45] In addition, MinION was used in combination with Sanger-based sequencing for the prospective analysis of specimens from suspected patients in Wuhan in order to characterize the epidemiology of SARS-CoV-2 transmission and to determine the potential for human-to-human transmission.[46]

The use of the MinION as a tool for quick investigation of a novel coronavirus has not only diagnostic potential but also a huge epidemiologic impact. A quick method for direct sequencing of clinical specimens is instrumental for understanding the transmission of the virus, its mutation rate, and polymorphisms associated with disease severity. The ARTIC network was initiated by a group of molecular biologists as a real-time molecular epidemiology response network for processing specimens during viral outbreaks. Based on Nanopore technology, this epidemiologic screening network for viral outbreaks has become feasible in locations with limited resources and is mainly focused on the rapidly evolving RNA viruses. The overall goal is to collect sequencing information in a real-time format to allow the real-time understanding of viral transmission and evolution (https://artic.network/). The ARTIC group has started providing materials and support for sequencing the SARS-CoV-2, which include primers, protocols, and pipelines for data analysis.[47]

Another advantage to using Nanopore sequencing methods is the feasibility of direct RNA sequencing. This approach was used to obtain the whole genome of HCoV-229E and was very successful in identifying not only an accurately built scaffold for the genome but also the several subgenomic-length RNAs.[48] Like other RNA viruses, coronaviruses are characterized by high rates of recombination[49] in addition to the unique replication cycle that results in nested messenger RNAs, largely identical to the original sequence. With the existence of this complex population of variants, long reads sequencing becomes the method of choice. Future research using NGS approaches might give further insight into the biology of replication and polymorphisms of coronaviruses. This method still faces the challenges of high error rate, approaches for maintaining the integrity of RNA samples, and the requirement for high-input RNA.

DISCUSSION

Rapidly emerging viral outbreaks pose a great challenge to clinical laboratories for quickly developing assays with high sensitivity and specificity for diagnosis and infection control. Molecular methods have rapidly replaced traditional methods and assisted the laboratories in real-time epidemiologic surveillance in outbreak situations. The recent outbreak of the novel coronavirus SARS-CoV-2 highlighted a great advance in the molecular diagnosis of evolving viral pathogens. Metagenomics, facilitated by innovative sequencing methodologies, is driving faster pathogen characterization and epidemiologic investigations. Because of the challenges in developing a PCR assay that has the potential for detecting all species of evolving RNA viruses, including coronaviruses, an approach that aims at implementing mNGS directly from clinical specimens along with complementary molecular diagnostic methods is most appropriate for clinically and epidemiologically managing a novel coronavirus outbreak. It is not currently possible to rapidly identify a novel coronavirus, but methodologies are being quickly developed that will change the current workflow in response to an emergent viral strain.

DISCLOSURE

The authors have nothing to disclose.

REFERENCES

1. Fehr AR, Perlman S. Coronaviruses: an overview of their replication and pathogenesis. Methods Mol Biol 2015;1282:1–23.
2. Corman VM, Muth D, Niemeyer D, et al. Hosts and sources of endemic human coronaviruses. Adv Virus Res 2018;100:163–88.
3. Hamre D, Procknow JJ. A new virus isolated from the human respiratory tract. Proc Soc Exp Biol Med 1966;121:190–3.

4. McIntosh K, Dees JH, Becker WB, et al. Recovery in tracheal organ cultures of novel viruses from patients with respiratory disease. Proc Natl Acad Sci U S A 1967;57:933–40.

5. Drosten C, Gunther S, Preiser W, et al. Identification of a novel coronavirus in patients with severe acute respiratory syndrome. N Engl J Med 2003;348:1967–76.

6. Rota PA, Oberste MS, Monroe SS, et al. Characterization of a novel coronavirus associated with severe acute respiratory syndrome. Science 2003;300:1394–9.

7. van der Hoek L, Pyrc K, Jebbink MF, et al. Identification of a new human coronavirus. Nat Med 2004;10:368–73.

8. Woo PC, Lau SK, Chu CM, et al. Characterization and complete genome sequence of a novel coronavirus, coronavirus HKU1, from patients with pneumonia. J Virol 2005;79:884–95.

9. Zaki AM, van Boheemen S, Bestebroer TM, et al. Isolation of a novel coronavirus from a man with pneumonia in Saudi Arabia. N Engl J Med 2012;367:1814–20.

10. Hui DS, Esam IA, Madani TA, et al. The continuing 2019-nCoV epidemic threat of novel coronaviruses to global health - the latest 2019 novel coronavirus outbreak in Wuhan, China. Int J Infect Dis 2020;91:264–6.

11. Woo PC, Huang Y, Lau SK, et al. Coronavirus genomics and bioinformatics analysis. Viruses 2010;2:1804–20.

12. van Elden LJ, van Loon AM, van Alphen F, et al. Frequent detection of human coronaviruses in clinical specimens from patients with respiratory tract infection by use of a novel real-time reverse-transcriptase polymerase chain reaction. J Infect Dis 2004;189:652–7.

13. Owusu M, Annan A, Corman VM, et al. Human coronaviruses associated with upper respiratory tract infections in three rural areas of Ghana. PLoS One 2014;9: e99782.

14. Annan A, Ebach F, Corman VM, et al. Similar virus spectra and seasonality in paediatric patients with acute respiratory disease, Ghana and Germany. Clin Microbiol Infect 2016;22:340–6.

15. Arden KE, Nissen MD, Sloots TP, et al. New human coronavirus, HCoV-NL63, associated with severe lower respiratory tract disease in Australia. J Med Virol 2005;75:455–62.

16. Bastien N, Robinson JL, Tse A, et al. Human coronavirus NL-63 infections in children: a 1-year study. J Clin Microbiol 2005;43:4567–73.

17. Gaunt ER, Hardie A, Claas EC, et al. Epidemiology and clinical presentations of the four human coronaviruses 229E, HKU1, NL63, and OC43 detected over 3 years using a novel multiplex real-time PCR method. J Clin Microbiol 2010;48: 2940–7.

18. Konca C, Korukluoglu G, Tekin M, et al. The first infant death associated with human coronavirus NL63 infection. Pediatr Infect Dis J 2017;36:231–3.

19. Mayer K, Nellessen C, Hahn-Ast C, et al. Fatal outcome of human coronavirus NL63 infection despite successful viral elimination by IFN-alpha in a patient with newly diagnosed ALL. Eur J Haematol 2016;97:208–10.

20. Oosterhof L, Christensen CB, Sengelov H. Fatal lower respiratory tract disease with human corona virus NL63 in an adult haematopoietic cell transplant recipient. Bone Marrow Transplant 2010;45:1115–6.

21. Cheng VC, Lau SK, Woo PC, et al. Severe acute respiratory syndrome coronavirus as an agent of emerging and reemerging infection. Clin Microbiol Rev 2007; 20:660–94.

22. Guan Y, Zheng BJ, He YQ, et al. Isolation and characterization of viruses related to the SARS coronavirus from animals in southern China. Science 2003;302: 276–8.

23. Chu DK, Poon LL, Gomaa MM, et al. MERS coronaviruses in dromedary camels, Egypt. Emerg Infect Dis 2014;20:1049–53.

24. Reusken CB, Haagmans BL, Muller MA, et al. Middle East respiratory syndrome coronavirus neutralising serum antibodies in dromedary camels: a comparative serological study. Lancet Infect Dis 2013;13:859–66.

25. Banerjee A, Kulcsar K, Misra V, et al. Bats and coronaviruses. Viruses 2019;11(1): 41. Available at: https://www.mdpi.com/1999-4915/11/1/41. Accessed January 9, 2019.

26. Anthony SJ, Gilardi K, Menachery VD, et al. Further evidence for bats as the evolutionary source of middle east respiratory syndrome coronavirus. mBio 2017;8. e00373-17.

27. Sawicki SG, Sawicki DL, Siddell SG. A contemporary view of coronavirus transcription. J Virol 2007;81:20–9.

28. Mahony JB, Petrich A, Smieja M. Molecular diagnosis of respiratory virus infections. Crit Rev Clin Lab Sci 2011;48:217–49.

29. Reusken C, Broberg EK, Haagmans B, et al. Laboratory readiness and response for novel coronavirus (2019-nCoV) in expert laboratories in 30 EU/EEA countries, January 2020. Euro Surveill 2020;25:2000082.

30. Vijgen L, Moes E, Keyaerts E, et al. A pancoronavirus RT-PCR assay for detection of all known coronaviruses. Methods Mol Biol 2008;454:3–12.

31. Zlateva KT, Coenjaerts FE, Crusio KM, et al. No novel coronaviruses identified in a large collection of human nasopharyngeal specimens using family-wide CODE-HOP-based primers. Arch Virol 2013;158:251–5.

32. Gerna G, Campanini G, Rovida F, et al. Genetic variability of human coronavirus OC43-, 229E-, and NL63-like strains and their association with lower respiratory tract infections of hospitalized infants and immunocompromised patients. J Med Virol 2006;78:938–49.

33. Mahony JB, Richardson S. Molecular diagnosis of severe acute respiratory syndrome: the state of the art. J Mol Diagn 2005;7:551–9.

34. Chow KY, Hon CC, Hui RK, et al. Molecular advances in severe acute respiratory syndrome-associated coronavirus (SARS-CoV). Genomics Proteomics Bioinformatics 2003;1:247–62.

35. Lu X, Whitaker B, Sakthivel SK, et al. Real-time reverse transcription-PCR assay panel for Middle East respiratory syndrome coronavirus. J Clin Microbiol 2014;52: 67–75.

36. Gu W, Miller S, Chiu CY. Clinical metagenomic next-generation sequencing for pathogen detection. Annu Rev Pathol 2019;14:319–38.

37. Benvenuto D, Giovanetti M, Ciccozzi A, et al. The 2019-new coronavirus epidemic: evidence for virus evolution. J Med Virol 2020. https://doi.org/10.1002/jmv.25688.

38. Wang Y, Li X, Liu W, et al. Discovery of a subgenotype of human coronavirus NL63 associated with severe lower respiratory tract infection in China, 2018. Emerg Microbes Infect 2020;9:246–55.

39. Beury D, Flechon L, Maurier F, et al. Use of whole-genome sequencing in the molecular investigation of care-associated HCoV-OC43 infections in a hematopoietic stem cell transplant unit. J Clin Virol 2020;122:104206.

40. Wong ACP, Li X, Lau SKP, et al. Global epidemiology of bat coronaviruses. Viruses 2019;11:174.

41. Laver T, Harrison J, O'Neill PA, et al. Assessing the performance of the oxford nanopore technologies MinION. Biomol Detect Quantif 2015;3:1–8.
42. Kilianski A, Haas JL, Corriveau EJ, et al. Bacterial and viral identification and differentiation by amplicon sequencing on the MinION nanopore sequencer. Gigascience 2015;4:12.
43. Greninger AL, Naccache SN, Federman S, et al. Rapid metagenomic identification of viral pathogens in clinical samples by real-time nanopore sequencing analysis. Genome Med 2015;7:99.
44. Lewandowski K, Xu Y, Pullan ST, et al. Metagenomic nanopore sequencing of influenza virus direct from clinical respiratory samples. J Clin Microbiol 2019; 58. e00963-19.
45. Zhu N, Zhang D, Wang W, et al. A novel coronavirus from patients with pneumonia in China, 2019. N Engl J Med 2020. https://doi.org/10.1056/NEJMoa2001017.
46. Chan JF, Yuan S, Kok KH, et al. A familial cluster of pneumonia associated with the 2019 novel coronavirus indicating person-to-person transmission: a study of a family cluster. Lancet 2020. https://doi.org/10.1016/S0140-6736(20)30154-9.
47. Itokawa K, Sekizuka T, Hashino M, et al. A proposal of an alternative primer for the ARTIC Network's multiplex PCR to improve coverage of SARS-CoV-2 genome sequencing. bioRxiv 2020. https://doi.org/10.1101/2020.03.10.985150:2020. 2003.2010.985150.
48. Viehweger A, Krautwurst S, Lamkiewicz K, et al. Direct RNA nanopore sequencing of full-length coronavirus genomes provides novel insights into structural variants and enables modification analysis. Genome Res 2019;29:1545–54.
49. Liao CL, Lai MM. RNA recombination in a coronavirus: recombination between viral genomic RNA and transfected RNA fragments. J Virol 1992;66:6117–24.
50. Hemida MG, Chu DK, Poon LL, et al. MERS coronavirus in dromedary camel herd, Saudi Arabia. Emerg Infect Dis 2014;20:1231–4.
51. Emery SL, Erdman DD, Bowen MD, et al. Real-time reverse transcription-polymerase chain reaction assay for SARS-associated coronavirus. Emerg Infect Dis 2004;10:311–6.
52. Zhang D, Mao HY, Lou XY, et al. Clinical evaluation of a panel of multiplex quantitative real-time reverse transcription polymerase chain reaction assays for the detection of 16 respiratory viruses associated with community-acquired pneumonia. Arch Virol 2018;163:2855–60.
53. Canducci F, Debiaggi M, Sampaolo M, et al. Two-year prospective study of single infections and co-infections by respiratory syncytial virus and viruses identified recently in infants with acute respiratory disease. J Med Virol 2008;80:716–23.

Update on Biosafety and Emerging Infections for the Clinical Microbiology Laboratory

Michael A. Pentella, PhD, D(ABMM)[a,b,*]

KEYWORDS

- Biosafety in clinical laboratories • Emerging pathogen • Ebola
- Association of Public Health Laboratories • Biosafety program

KEY POINTS

- This article reviews the current biosafety issues facing the clinical laboratory community.
- It looks at progress in the past 5 years and what has yet to be accomplished.
- It provides a road map for clinical laboratories on building an effective biosafety program.
- It advises on preparation for an emerging threat agent that may appear.

INTRODUCTION

Maintaining a strong biosafety program is a challenge for clinical and public health laboratories. Generally speaking, every specimen that arrives in a clinical microbiology laboratory is an unknown.[1] Samples come from a wide variety of patients who may have traveled from unknown locations. It is rare that a clinical microbiology laboratory hears from the physician that a specific pathogen is suspected.[2] Consequently, the laboratory must be prepared to receive a wide variety of potential pathogens. It is unreasonable to be prepared for every conceivable pathogen; consequently, the laboratory prepares for those pathogens that generally are anticipated based on the geographic demographics where the laboratory provides services. The emergence of new pathogens continues to occur, however, and laboratories must have a strong biosafety program that is flexible and permits a facility to respond to unknown pathogens quickly and effectively. Laboratories not always are located in the facility providing patient care (reference for remote site laboratories).[3] These remote site laboratories have additional concerns of sample transport, communication, and the need to provide rapid results. Most importantly, the laboratory must maintain an awareness

[a] College of Public Health, University of Iowa, Iowa City, IA, USA; [b] State Hygienic Laboratory, University of Iowa, Coralville, IA, USA
* College of Public Health, CPH 433, 145 North Riverside Drive, Room S433 CPHB, Iowa City, IA 52242.
E-mail address: michael-pentella@uiowa.edu

Clin Lab Med 40 (2020) 473–482
https://doi.org/10.1016/j.cll.2020.08.005
0272-2712/20/© 2020 Elsevier Inc. All rights reserved.

labmed.theclinics.com

of the importance of biosafety in the laboratory, which can be difficult to do because, over time, laboratorians may become complacent and accustomed to the risk.

Prior practices, such as mouth pipetting, eating and drinking in the laboratory, and application of lip balm, for example, that previously placed laboratorians at risk of laboratory-acquired infections, now mostly are part of history. There are new risks, however, such as (1) use of mobile phones in laboratories that can pose the risk of infection[4,5] and (2) the ever-present risk of emerging pathogens.

Checklists are the driving force behind biosafety programs in clinical laboratories, and laboratories rely on a prescriptive approach to requirements. Generally, the checklists of the College of American Pathologists (CAP) are soundly based on the Occupational Safety and Health Administration requirements with additional items added. Admirably, CAP's concern for laboratory safety was demonstrated in the first checklist, in 1965, that asked if safety precautions were adequate. CAP addresses blood-borne pathogens and other infectious hazards as well. CAP checklists require use of personal protective equipment (PPE), training, and hand-washing. CAP also requires policies and procedures for recognition of biothreat agents, safe handling of potential agents, and the use of a biological safety cabinet (BSC) when biothreat agents suspected. The Clinical Laboratory Improvement Amendments (CLIA) program checklists are less prescriptive and rely on the director to ensure that the testing environment is safe and states that safety procedures must be established.

In 2014, when the first case of a patient infected with Ebola virus was detected in Dallas, Texas, most laboratories would not have included Ebola virus as a pathogen to reasonably expect. Because of the strong biosafety program at the facility (B. Dickson, personal communication;2015), however, there were no infections among laboratory workers in the facility. Facing the spread of an emerging pathogen for which there was no treatment and a high fatality rate,[6] other facilities in the United States made the decision to not test patients suspected to be infected with Ebola virus until the infection had been ruled out. This had a tragic outcome for at least 2 patients who had their testing delayed and subsequently tested negative for Ebola. These 2 patients later died of malaria.[7] Based on this experience, it became apparent that many laboratories were unfamiliar with the risk assessment process and had not adopted biosafety competencies. Importantly, clinical laboratories often only consider pathogens a threat in the microbiology laboratory section, hence, only considering the risk of emerging infectious agent in the microbiology laboratory section, not chemistry, hematology, or anatomic pathology. In February 2020, when severe acute respiratory syndrome coronavirus 2 (SARS-CoV-2) cases appeared in the United States, some clinical laboratories began to review facility-specific biosafety practices and performed risk assessments. As an emerging pathogen, there was scarce information about SARS-CoV-2; fortunately, both the Centers for Disease Control and Prevention (CDC) and the World Health Organization provided interim guidelines for specimen handling and testing.[8,9]

Another concern is that some in the clinical laboratory community lack a clear understanding of the terms, *risk* and *hazard*.[10] In the laboratory, a hazard is the ability of a pathogen to cause an adverse effect to an exposed person whereas the risk considers the probability and the consequence of an exposure. This confusion may lead the uninformed laboratory staff to refuse to work with some potential hazards. Many of the specimens handled in the laboratory contain hazards; the purpose of the risk assessment is to determine the necessary steps to reduce the likelihood and consequence of an exposure. For example, the hazard is working with *Neisseria meningitidis* on the open bench. By performing a risk assessment, it is determined that working in a biosafety cabinet reduces the likelihood of exposure and providing vaccination reduces the consequence of exposure.

During the Ebola outbreak, some instrument manufacturers refused to service instruments used to test patients' specimens under investigation for Ebola infection. This led to the recognition that biosafety issues, cleaning and disinfecting instruments, were not a top priority for the instrument manufacturers. This can extend to other new instruments that are brought into the laboratory, for example, the use of matrix assisted laser desorption ionization time-of-flight mass spectrometry.[11]

CURRENT PRACTICES

In order to determine the biosafety practices and needs in clinical laboratories, the Association of Public Health Laboratories (APHL), launched a comprehensive survey. The estimated size of the target audience was 5000 laboratories that met the definition of a sentinel clinical laboratory.[12] From that audience, 489 responses were received. Respondents came from 47 states. Some states, Georgia and New York, had high response rates, of 11%, with 54 responding facilities in each of those states. At the other end of the spectrum, 7 states had only 1 responding facility. When asked if the institution had a biosafety plan in place, 91.4% responded affirmatively. Because performance of a risk assessment is identified as a critical first step in developing the biosafety program,[13] it is significant that 37.4% had completed at least 1 risk assessment for an infectious agent between May 2015 and May 2018; 19% had completed at least 2 risk assessments.

The survey attempts to determine if there is a staff member in the facility who is responsible for biosafety; 91 (18.6%) indicated that they had at least 1 full-time staff member dedicated to biosafety. Yet only 15.9% of the respondents indicated that the person responsible for biosafety was an "experienced biosafety professional." The most common response was that 54.4% indicated that there was not a full-time staff member dedicated to biosafety but that the responsibility is allocated to multiple staff across all institutional laboratories; 85% indicated that they have developed safety-specific competencies for the laboratory staff. Respondents identified sharps hazard, blood-borne pathogens, PPE, spill prevention, and chemical hazards as the top 5 training needs for their staff. Generally, most respondents, 71.6%, indicated that they identified biosafety training needs based on the accreditation certification requirements. This response reaffirms that the checklist mentality is commonplace.

Although the APHL clinical laboratory survey provides a high-level perspective of biosafety programs, it does not delve into specific practices. In order to determine the biosafety culture, Munson and colleagues[1] performed a survey of hospital laboratories in Wisconsin and found deficiencies in basic biosafety practices. For example, only 75.4% of the performing aerosol-generating work in a biosafety cabinet with biosafety level (BSL)-3 practices for high-risk bacterial pathogens. Even more surprising was that only 52.4% are compliant with wearing a laboratory coat when screening cultures.

BEST PRACTICES BIOSAFETY PROGRAM
A Road Map

Building a strong biosafety program takes planning and a dedicated effort long term. The purpose of the road map (**Fig. 1**) is to provide a big picture perspective of what the biosafety program looks like.

Stop 1 is the start, with a risk assessment that serves as the foundation for the rest of the program. The concept of performing a risk assessment should not be that

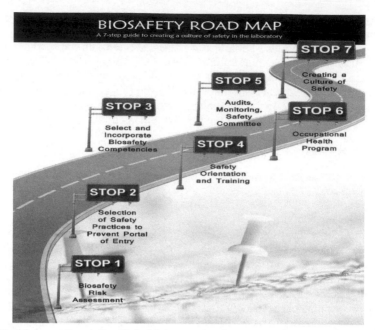

Fig. 1. Biosafety road map for clinical laboratories. (*Courtesy of* Michael A. Pentella, PhD, (D(ABMM), University of Iowa.)

daunting to clinical laboratorians because they perform risk assessments continuously in normal daily activities. Before crossing a street, they look both ways and determine if they can make it across before an oncoming vehicle. The gas gauge is on empty and they determine if there is sufficient fuel to make it to the gas station. In the laboratory, the risk assessment is the process of gathering all available information on a hazardous substance and evaluating it to determine the possible risks associated with exposure.[5,6,13] The clinical laboratorian at this point considers the infectious organisms likely to be encountered in the laboratory, how that organism can be transmitted to the laboratorian, and how the organism causes disease. Performing this activity prior to facing the arrival of the specimen in the laboratory allows for the selection of the mitigation practices to protect the worker. When a new pathogen emerges in the community, a risk assessment is the starting point for the biosafety considerations. The challenge posed by an emerging pathogen is that not all of the information about routes of transmission and infectious dose may be known when performing the risk assessment. In that case, the clinical laboratorian must make the best effort and look to experts, such as the CDC, for guidance.

Additionally, the risk assessment defines processes or activities that present exposure risk, for example, centrifugation, use of needles, and vortexing. It should be recognized that most accidents that lead to an infectious disease exposure in the laboratory are a result of human error and not instrument failures.[14] Therefore, the prevention of laboratory-acquired infections first considers the potential risk for human error.[15]

At stop 2 is the selection of the safety practices to mitigate the risks identified by the risk assessment process. Selection of mitigation practices reduces the risk to the laboratorian by blocking the pathogen's portal of entry into the host. Mitigation selection is a sequential process.[16] Through each step in the process, the risk is reduced but the risk is never reduced to zero. It starts with the most effective mitigation to reduce risk, which is the BSL of the laboratory in which the work is performed. For clinical laboratorians this most often is BSL-2 for most pathogens[15] encountered in the clinical laboratory. A few pathogens, such as *Mycobacterium tuberculosis*, are BSL-3. An emerging pathogen can pose a challenge and it is best to look for expert guidance, for example, from the CDC. The next determination is the engineering controls that should be used to perform the work. For example, when to perform testing inside a biosafety cabinet and which testing can be performed on a bench top? Then, the appropriate PPE is selected. Common in most clinical laboratories today are barrier protective gowns, gloves, and eye protection. There are some instances, such as working with *M tuberculosis*, when a respirator is required. Note that from a mitigation perspective, PPE is not first because it is not the most effective means to mitigate risk. The final mitigation step is to determine the laboratory practices, such as handwashing, restriction of food or drink in the laboratory, and determining disinfection practices. Document the mitigations steps in the safety section of the procedure manual.

Following mitigation stop 3, based on the risk assessment and mitigation strategies, is selecting the appropriate competencies. It should be recognized that the use of competencies is an essential component of the program because the competencies connect the required skill and create the framework of how staff perform regarding biosafety in the organization. Competencies are common practice in clinical laboratories for the performance of tests, and adding biosafety competencies to the existing competency program supports and builds the biosafety culture of the laboratory. There are 2 documents[17,18] that can be used to select applicable competencies for the laboratory. The competency can be written into the safety section of the procedure. Assessment of competencies needs to be determined, using the same assessment processes as that for testing. Review the competencies annually and modify based on changes and identified issues in the laboratory.

With stop 4, the education and training should start with the onboarding process at the beginning of employment and should be ongoing during the duration of employment. This builds a culture of safety in the laboratory and helps bolster individuals whose biosafety vigilance may wane over time. When an emerging pathogen presents itself, it is a good opportunity to provide continuing education to refresh staff biosafety skills. The risk assessments, mitigation plans, and competency assessments can inform the education and training needs. Much biosafety training is now Web based and can be used to document competency. It is important to provide training on the appropriate donning, doffing, and use of PPE because improper use of PPE can lead to exposures. Staff should be trained on the biosafety practices, the pathogens that they might encounter, and the signs and symptoms of the diseases caused by the pathogens worked with in the clinical laboratory. How to report exposures, when to connect with occupational health services, and the postexposure medical surveillance process are critical information for all staff at risk of exposures. Having drills and exercises to practice skills, such as spill cleanup, can be useful training for staff. Training should be tailored to individual laboratory needs. Some facilities can provide training through internal resources; others need to seek external resources or a combination of the 2.

Stop 5 in the process covers the importance of monitoring what is happening in the laboratory through audits and the critical role of the safety committee. The best way to monitor a safety program is for leadership and supervision to observe potential safety issues when in the laboratory. Monitoring staff and equipment performance regularly gives an opportunity for immediate training and correction of potential problems. Audits, both internal audits and external audits by accrediting organizations, are another valuable tool. Linking biosafety to the quality management program in the clinical laboratory helps establish a permanent process to monitor biosafety activities through the internal audit process. Quality management audits then include safety audits. During the audit, make certain that staff are using the appropriate disinfectant and following the manufacturer's directions. Establishing a safety committee with membership consisting of staff and leadership gives everyone ownership of the biosafety responsibility. The safety committee establishes an audit program and provides reports to the laboratory director.

At stop 6, it is essential to point out how important the connection with occupational health is for incidents, exposures, and selection of vaccines. Partnering with an occupational health clinician is a critical component of the biosafety plan. Every laboratory needs a well-described procedure for staff to access the occupational health services in the event of an exposure. When a laboratorian follows the protocol after an exposure and immediately notifies the supervisor, it is far less likely that others will have the same incident occur to them or to cause secondary infections, thus limiting the consequences of the incident.[14] Determining which vaccinations are offered or required is an mitigation determined by the risk assessment process and best determined with input from an occupational health specialist. Staff need to know what signs and symptoms they might exhibit if exposed to pathogens that they work with and the postexposure medical surveillance process. After an exposure event, leadership should review the incident with the occupational health clinician on potential ways to prevent future exposures.

Stop 7 serves to point out how all of the stops collectively establish a strong culture of safety in the laboratory. In a clinical laboratory, staff understand their responsibility to maintain a safe work environment and that exposures are not mistakes on their part but an opportunity for the laboratory to reassess the biosafety program and prevent exposures in the future. Creating a culture of safety is a continual effort; it comes about only when there is strong leadership committed to emphasizing safety despite other priorities. Having an active safety committee that is supported by laboratory leaderships helps maintain the strong culture of safety. Another means of maintaining the culture of safety is to discuss safety topics regularly during staff meetings. Leadership should take every safety issue seriously. Using root cause analysis tools, treat exposures and near-misses as excellent opportunities to review what occurred to improve the biosafety plan. The biosafety program should be reviewed at least annually.

CURRENT EXPOSURES AND THE RISK OF LABORATORY-ACQUIRED INFECTIONS

Unfortunately, neither exposures nor laboratory acquired infections are required reporting. Therefore, there are no data to determine the actual incidence. This lack of data makes studies and recommendations difficult for biosafety professionals and laboratory leaders. There are some data regarding exposures to *Brucella*. From 2008 to 2011, there were 1724 possible *Brucella* exposures reported to CDC.[19,20] Ackelsberg and colleagues[21] reported on 10 *Brucella* exposure incidents from 2015 to 2017 involving 7 clinical laboratories. In none of the incidents was the clinical laboratory alerted to the potential diagnosis of brucellosis. A total of 219 laboratorians were exposed but, fortunately, no laboratory acquired infections occurred. The risk of laboratory acquired infections from *Brucella* is well recognized.[19] Most at risk are laboratorians performing procedures that aerosolize *Brucella*. Because *Brucella* frequently is encountered in the laboratory without prior warning that *Brucella* is part of the differential diagnosis, exposures do occur, especially because *Brucella* initially can stain as gram-positive cocci in broth cultures.[20] Unsuspecting laboratorians then manipulate the cultures on the open bench and are exposed while performing routine procedures. The CDC recommendations[22] guidance includes an exposure risk stratification as high risk, low risk, or minimal risk, depending on proximity to potentially aerosolized *Brucellae*. This is followed by a 3 week, 2-drug postexposure prophylaxis regimen if deemed a high-risk exposure and 24 weeks of symptom and serologic monitoring.

PREPARATION FOR AN EMERGING THREAT AGENT

There always is potential for a new microbial pathogen to emerge anywhere in the world. Clinical laboratory directors pay attention to these issues and receive emails alerting them when an emerging threat agent (ETA) might be encountered. When a director receives notice of a risk, it is time to take action:

1. Learn as much as possible about the suspected routes of transmission of the ETA.
2. Communicate with staff so that they aware of the potential risk.
3. Perform a risk assessment for receiving and handling specimens from patients expected to be infected with the ETA.
4. Based on the risk assessment, use appropriate PPE.
5. Ensure that the BSC certification is current.
6. Ensure all staff who need training on the proper use of a BSC have received it (**Box 1**). The CDC has a free training course, *Fundamentals of Working Safely in a Biological Safety Cabinet*, available at: https://www.cdc.gov/labtraining/training-courses/biological-safety-cabinets.html.
7. Refer to the CDC Web page as to the category of the agent in regards to packaging and shipping of specimens for the ETA. Refresh staff knowledge regarding Category A or Category B packaging and shipping requirements.
8. Determine if the disinfectant commonly used in the facility is able to kill the suspected ETA. Make certain that all staff follow the established disinfection protocols.
9. Remind staff of the importance of proper and regular handwashing.
10. Train staff on the signs and symptoms of the ETA.
11. Contact the state or local public health laboratories for questions or more information.

FUTURE VISION

Future laboratorians need training on biosafety issues and practices at their educational institutions. With some exceptions, this is not happening. An example of the

---

Box 1
Proper use of biosafety cabinet

Training on the proper use of biosafety cabinet should include
1. Review of the written SOP for the BSC
2. Checking the Magnehelic reading and document each day of use
3. Verifying the BSC certification and assuring it is performed annually
4. Checking/cleaning on a regular basis (per SOP), including grills and spill tray
5. Exercising care to ensure that no items are placed over the front intake grills
6. Appropriate PPE that must be worn while working in the BSC
7. Avoidance of passing contaminated materials over uninoculated cultures or clean materials to limit contamination
8. Not using cabinet as a repository for excess laboratory equipment during periods of nonoperation

lack of training is the recent *Salmonella* outbreak that occurred in the academic environment.[23] The curriculum adjustment to build the biosafety competencies needs to occur at a national level. While this is occurring, those currently employed in the field require training in biosafety issues and practices as well so that there is a strong foundation of current staff who are demonstrating best practices.

The field of biosafety in clinical laboratories should align itself with the laboratory quality management system. This change of focus would move the process from checklist-driven requirements to a biorisk management approach.[12] The current approach to biosafety requires policies and rules that enforced by a biosafety officer with administrative support. In the biorisk management system model, everyone in the laboratory has responsibilities and there is reliance on evidence-based decision making. Risk assessments analyze the unique functions in the laboratory. Managers decide on mitigation measures through risk-based decisions not on prescriptive checklists.

What is lacking in the field of biosafety is evidence-based data to support decisions. Data are lacking in 2 areas. First, there is a lack of data on how to prevent errors. Second, there is a lack of data on how mistakes occur. This lack of data, on which to base recommendations, can lead to under-estimating some risks and over-estimating others.[14]

Based on data, it would be extremely useful to develop mathematical models to support further development of knowledge of biosafety, to detect gaps in knowledge, and to support the development and evaluation of new biosafety measures.

SUMMARY

An important question to answer is, Has the Ebola experience resulted in lasting changes in biosafety practices in the clinical laboratories? The answer will be determined only with time and effective studies to determine the change in practices in clinical laboratories. Through CDC and APHL efforts, many more laboratories recognize the importance of biosafety. There is a need to engage academia so that the future workforce has the necessary biosafety skill set to meet the needs. Although the requirements for biosafety in clinical laboratories are limited mostly to the CAP checklists, if the workforce is knowledgeable about biosafety, then a checklist mentality moves to the critical thinking skills necessary to make effective decisions regarding biosafety in a real-time. Important for now is keeping biosafety issues in the forefront of laboratory leadership.

DISCLOSURE

M.A. Pentella is a consultant for Charles River Analytics.

REFERENCES

1. Munson E, Bowles EJ, Dern R, et al. Laboratory Focus on Improving the Culture of biosafety: statewide risk assessment of clinical laboratories that process specimens for microbiologic analysis. J Clin Microbiol 2018;56:1–11.
2. Lagace-Wiens P, Pentella MA. Prevention of laboratory-acquired infections. In: Carroll KC, Pfaller MA, editors. Manual of a clinical microbiology. 12th edition. Washington, DC: ASM Press; 2019. p. 206–23. Chapter 123.
3. Pentella M, Weinstein MP, Beekmann SE, et al. The impact of changes in Clinical Microbiology Laboratory location and ownership on the practice of Infectious Diseases. J Clin Microbiol 2020. https://doi.org/10.1128/JCM.01508-19.

4. Cavari Y, Kaplan O, Zander A, et al. Healthcare workers mobile phone usage: a potential risk for viral contamination. Surveillance pilot study. Infect Dis 2016; 48(6):432–5.

5. Dunn JJ, Sewell DL. In: Garcia L, editor. Laboratory safety. Clinical laboratory management. 2nd edition. Washington, DC: American Society for Microbiology; 2014. Chapter 28:515–536.

6. Chosewood LC, Wilson DE. Biosafety in microbiological and biomedical laboratories. 5th edition. Washington, DC: U.S. Government Printing Office; 2009.

7. Karwowski MP, Meites E, Fullerton KE, et al. Clinical inquiries regarding Ebola virus disease received by CDC–United States, July 9-November 15, 2014. MMWR Morb Mortal Wkly Rep 2014;63:1175–9.

8. Centers for Disease Control and Prevention (CDC). Interim laboratory biosafety guidelines for handling and processing specimens associated with coronavirus disease 2019 (COVID-19). Available at: https://www.cdc.gov/coronavirus/2019-nCoV/lab/lab-biosafety-guidelines.html. Accessed June 14, 2020.

9. World Health Organization. Laboratory biosafety guidance related to the novel coronavirus (2019-nCoV). Available at: https://www.who.int/publications/i/item/laboratory-biosafety-guidance-related-to-coronavirus-disease-(covid-19. Accessed June 14, 2020.

10. Scheer D, Beninghaus C, Beninghaus L, et al. The distinction between risk and hazard, understanding and use in stakeholder communication. Risk Anal 2014; 34(7):1270–85.

11. Dingle TC, Butler-Wu SM, Abbott AN. Accidental exposure to Burkholderia pseudomallei in the laboratory in the era of matrix-assisted laser desorption ionization time of flight mass spectrometry. J Clin Microbiol 2014;52:3490–1.

12. Association of Public Health Laboratories. Biosafety Practices and needs in clinical laboratories survey. Summary data report. 2019. Available at: https://www.aphl.org/programs/preparedness/Biosafety-and-Biosecurity/Documents/Clinical-Lab-Biosafety-Practices-Survey-Data-Report.pdf#search=clinical%20lab%20biosafety%20survey. Accessed February 1, 2020.

13. Salerno RM, Gaudioso J. Laboratory biorisk management: biosafety and biosecurity. Boca Raton, FL: CRC Press; 2015.

14. Ritterson R, Casagrande R. Basic scholarship in in biosafety is critically needed to reduce risk of laboratory accidents. mSphere 2017;2:e00010-17.

15. Miller JM, Astles R, Baszler T, et al. Guidelines for safe work practices in human and animal medical diagnostic laboratories. Recommendations of a CDC-convened, Biosafety Blue Ribbon Panel. MMWR Suppl 2012;61:1–102.

16. Gaudioso J, Boggs S, Griffith NK, et al. Laboratory biorisk management: rethinking mitigation measures. Boca Raton, FL: CRC Press; 2015.

17. Delany JR, Pentella MA, Rodriguez JA, et al. Guidelines for biosafety laboratory competency: CDC and the Association of Public Health Laboratories. MMWR Suppl 2011;60:1–23.

18. Ned-Sykes R, Johnson C, Ridderhof JC, et al. Competency guidelines for public health laboratory professionals: CDC and the Association of Public Health Laboratories. MMWR Suppl 2015;64:1–81.

19. Traxler RM, Lehman MW, Bosserman EA. A literature review of laboratory-acquired brucellosis. J Clin Microbiol 2013;54:3055–62.

20. Yagusky P, Baron EJ. Laboratory exposure to *Brucellae* and implications for bioterrorism. Emerg Infect Dis 2005;11:1180–5.

21. Ackelsberg J, Liddicoat A, Burke T, et al. Brucella exposure risk events in 10 clinical laboratories, New York City, USA, 2015 to 2017. J Clin Microbiol 2020;58. e01096-19.
22. Centers for Disease Control and Prevention. Brucellosis reference guide: exposures, testing, and prevention. 2017. Available at: https://www.cdc.gov/%20brucellosis/pdf/brucellosi-reference-guide.pdf. Accessed February 1, 2020.
23. Centers for Disease Control and Prevention. Human Salmonella Typhimurium infections associated with exposure to clinical and teaching microbiology laboratories (Final Update). 2012. Available at: https://www.cdc.gov/salmonella/2011/lab-exposure-1-17-2012.html. Accessed February 1, 2020.

Point-of-Care Testing in Microbiology

Linoj Samuel, PhD, D(ABMM)

KEYWORDS

- Point of care • Rapid diagnostics • Microbiology

KEY POINTS

- Point-of-care (POC) testing is a rapidly expanding area of growth for infectious diseases due to the consolidation of clinical microbiology laboratories.
- Advances in technology have increased the quality of results available in the POC setting.
- The increasing complexity of the technology involved in POC testing requires oversight by laboratory professionals.

Point-of-care (POC) testing can be defined as testing performed in close proximity to the patient with results available within a timeframe that allows for an intervention to take place while the patient is still in the care of the provider.[1,2] The terms POC and near patient testing may be used interchangeably because they often refer to testing performed using the same systems although the regulatory requirements may vary. The key distinction may be the level of regulatory oversight based on the complexity of testing. POC testing is often used to refer to waived testing under CLIA (Clinical Laboratory Improvement Amendments Act) but could include more complex testing nonwaived testing performed in the near patient setting. Traditional infectious disease–related POC testing typically provides results in 15 to 20 minutes but even results available in <1 hour from the time of specimen receipt are useful in patient management. There are obvious advantages to having results available immediately for patient care:

1. A timely answer can alleviate patient anxiety and improve patient satisfaction.
2. Allows the care provider to initiate appropriate therapy immediately if needed where empiric coverage is adequate, for example, streptococcal pharyngitis and sexually transmitted diseases.
3. Reduces the need for follow-up visits that add to the burden on the patient and the growing cost of health care.
4. Rapid testing results can ensure the optimal use of limited health care resources by determining which patients need to be in isolation due to potential transmissible

Clinical Microbiology, Department of Pathology and Laboratory Medicine, Henry Ford Hospital, 2799 West Grand Boulevard, Detroit, MI 48202, USA
E-mail address: LSAMUEL2@hfhs.org

Clin Lab Med 40 (2020) 483–494
https://doi.org/10.1016/j.cll.2020.08.006
0272-2712/20/© 2020 Elsevier Inc. All rights reserved.

labmed.theclinics.com

pathogens and can play a significant role in interrupting community-based transmission of common pathogens, such as those causing infectious diarrhea or sexually transmitted diseases.

5. POC testing also improves the care of patients who are unlikely to return for subsequent visits. In resource-poor settings where patients have to travel long distances to obtain primary care, it is often unreasonable to expect them to return after laboratory results become available for additional care.

Clinical microbiology diagnostic testing has traditionally centered around the use of time-consuming methods such as viral and bacterial cultures. Bacterial cultures can take anywhere from 1 to 14 days depending on the suspected pathogen. Cultures for specific pathogens such as *Mycobacterium tuberculosis* require an incubation period of 6 to 8 weeks for a negative result. Viral cultures can require 1 to 21 days of incubation but have been mostly replaced by molecular-based methods. The transition from viral cultures to molecular methods has significantly improved the time to result but these assays are often batched and performed at specialized laboratories so that the results are not available in a timely manner.[3] Non–culture-based tests, such as stains for stool-based pathogens, require additional expertise and are not available in the POC setting.

Clinical microbiology laboratories have historically operated on a 9-to-5 schedule with limited services available outside routine working hours and on weekends, but this model has changed over time with increased focus on laboratory utilization and cost-effective strategies that facilitate timely patient care. The manual nature of microbiology testing made it less conducive to automated testing but over the years, improvements in technology have allowed for the implementation of highly automated culture-based platforms. These systems enhance the performance of clinical microbiology laboratories in terms of efficiency, speed, and culture yield.[4] The cost of these automated systems, shortage of trained laboratory personnel, and the constant pressure to reduce health care costs have encouraged the consolidation of microbiology laboratories into core facilities to ensure optimal utilization of these systems. Automated testing still requires prolonged culture incubation, and results are not available during the course of the patient visit. The advantages of this integrated approach to testing include the ability to provide expanded testing services around the clock and improve overall laboratory performance.[5] However, the consolidation of laboratory services into core facilities that are geographically distant from patient care locations and community hospitals within an expanded network can introduce further delays in results due to transport time. The consolidated laboratory model could also lead to batch processing of specimens due to the transport requirements but this may be offset by the extended working hours and the access to automation, advanced expertise, and testing panels.[5] With advances in testing technology, the time spent in transport often represents the largest source of delay for obtaining results.[6]

The transition to diagnosis-based reimbursement in the 1980s was expected to negatively impact centralized laboratory testing but the implementation of the Clinical Laboratory Improvement Amendment 1988 (CLIA 88), discouraged the expansion of laboratory testing into the primary care setting.[6] The recent growth in POC testing coincided with the development of novel technologies and the miniaturization of existing technologies that brought improved assay performance to the near patient setting.

The merger of clinical microbiology laboratories into core facilities coupled with the advances in POC testing system development has led to renewed interest in the role of near patient testing.[1] Some health care institutions have implemented rapid response laboratories with a limited test menu composed of assays that can be performed in less than 3 hours to supplement the capabilities of the core laboratories.[7] These rapid response laboratories provide a limited menu of tests, are typically staffed by qualified laboratory personnel, and provide actionable timely results. This model can range from the traditional concept of POC testing, which is performed by the providers in the patient care setting, to more complex molecular testing and limited processing of positive blood cultures.

The term POC encompasses tests using a broad range of technologies. These include

1. Direct detection of antigen: This relates to the capture of antigen using a specific antibody and the detection of this antigen-antibody complex typically using a lateral flow assay or a variant of this technology, for example, rapid influenza or group A streptococcal antigen testing.
2. Detection of antibody: These are fingerstick assays for the detection of antibody toward specific pathogens, for example, human immunodeficiency virus (HIV).
3. Direct detection of pathogen RNA/DNA: Current nucleic acid amplification technologies (NAAT)-based testing directly detects the presence of pathogen genomic material in the patient sample, for example, polymerase chain reaction (PCR)-based detection of influenza and group A streptococci in respiratory samples.

POC testing has traditionally operated under the premise that speed and ease of use are essential but this is often achieved at the cost of reduced sensitivity and/or specificity. The regulatory framework for POC testing is described later in this document, but for this reason, POC testing has often been limited to settings in which the impact of an errant result is limited or can be mitigated by reflex testing. Clinical microbiologists have tended to question the potential for POC testing because of the inherent performance-related issues. Until recently, a significant proportion of POC testing was limited to lateral flow assays for common respiratory pathogens, such as group A streptococci, influenza, and respiratory syncytial virus (RSV), but performance limitations meant that negative results often had to be confirmed by alternative molecular or culture-based methods. Nevertheless, POC testing can play an important role in the diagnostic algorithm.

- Rapid streptococcal antigen testing allows quick determination and treatment of a common pathogen that can have significant long-term implications for patient health. However, because the sensitivity of the streptococcal antigen tests are only approximately 86%, negative streptococcal antigen results should be confirmed by traditional culture-based or molecular testing, particularly in children.[8,9]
- For the detection of sexually transmitted pathogens, such as *Trichomonas*, provider-performed microscopy was the mainstay of diagnostic testing but the sensitivity of this approach was extremely limited and relied on timely specimen transport and immediate processing as well as expertise in microscopy. The development of *Trichomonas* antigen-based testing allowed for not just significantly improved sensitivity over microscopy-based methods but also reduced the labor and expertise required for testing. In spite of these improvements, POC testing for *Trichomonas* does not rule out infection and negative results need to be confirmed by molecular methods if clinical suspicion persists.[10]
- POC testing for *M tuberculosis* has the potential to significantly impact both patient care and appropriate utilization of institutional resources. In low tuberculosis (TB) incidence countries, 1 to 2 negative TB PCR results can be used to remove

patients from airborne isolation with significant cost savings.[11] In other settings, a rapid TB PCR result can be used to not just to establish a diagnosis but detect the presence of resistance markers in patients who have traveled long distances to obtain care and are unlikely to return for follow-up with traditional methods for diagnosis of M tuberculosis, such as culture, which can take 6 to 8 weeks to obtain a final result.[12] The utility of POC testing in this setting is challenged by the costs and logistical challenges of maintaining expensive PCR-based reagents and equipment in resource-poor settings. In high disease prevalence settings, it may not be cost-effective to rely on expensive molecular-based POC testing.[13]

- Rapid HIV testing has become the mainstay of public health efforts to combat the spread of HIV especially among populations that do not routinely access health care services; these are antibody-based tests that are useful under these circumstances but both positive and negative results should be confirmed in high-risk individuals.[14]

Negative POC antigen-based testing results for most pathogens have limited value in actual patient care due to inadequate sensitivity. Negative results typically represent the vast majority of results and many institutions were routinely confirming negative influenza and RSV antigen results by alternative methods.[15] Recently the Food and Drug Administration (FDA) acknowledged the limitations of POC antigen-based testing for influenza and raised the bar for minimum performance standards for influenza antigen testing.[16] This led to the development of fluorescent immunoassays that detected the antigen using automated readers and fluorescent markers that improved performance.[17] The sensitivity of these improved assays still fell short of being able to rule out infection and it remained common for laboratories to continue to confirm negative results using alternative methods.[17]

Molecular testing or NAAT for infectious disease pathogens offer the advantages of improved sensitivity and specificity over antigen testing. Until recently, technologies such as real-time PCR required the use of significant training and specialized equipment. The challenges associated with use of NAAT include the need for molecular expertise, expensive equipment/reagents, designated testing areas, and the risk of contamination. Testing is often performed in large batches to conserve reagents and reduce costs. Traditional molecular tests were typically not performed in the near patient setting and were not available within a timeframe that allowed for intervention during the patient visit.

REGULATORY FRAMEWORK FOR POINT-OF-CARE TESTING

A number of factors are involved in determination of which tests are appropriate for use in the POC setting.

CLIA 88 governs the classification of testing based on complexity. The level of complexity is determined by the following questions[18]

1. How the test may be used and in which setting?
2. Who can perform the test?
3. What kind of proficiency testing and quality assurance is required?

In addition, the type of testing performed by a laboratory determines the level of regulatory oversight of the performing laboratory.

Three categories of test complexity have been established:

1. Waived
2. Moderate complexity, including provider-performed microscopy (PPM)

3. High complexity.

In the United States, CLIA 88 outlines the different levels of complexity for testing but it is the FDA that issues guidelines on how to interpret CLIA 88 and determines how to categorize a new test in terms of complexity.

Waived tests generally meet the following criteria:

- The technology involved must be simple enough to have an extremely low likelihood of inaccurate results
- Should not require processing of specimens before testing
- Relatively low risk of harm to patients if the test is incorrectly performed

Nonwaived testing refers to moderate or high complexity testing. Laboratories that perform nonwaived testing must hold a CLIA certificate as well as undergo routine inspections and follow a prescribed system of proficiency testing, quality assurance, and personnel requirements. Sites performing waived testing on the other hand only need a CLIA certificate and to follow manufacturer's instructions, although they may be subject to inspections. This makes the use of CLIA-waived testing an attractive prospect to sites that have limited laboratory capability, resources, or access to trained laboratory personnel ,but still want to offer some onsite testing capability for patients with relatively minor health issues. As of March 2020, there were 193,474 sites with CLIA-waived registration.[18] POC testing may be performed under the CLIA waiver by nonlaboratory personnel or by laboratory personnel in near patient settings such as stat laboratories.

TRENDS IN POINT-OF-CARE TESTING

There is also renewed interest in using POC testing in nontraditional settings. The entry of giants in the field of information technology, retail, and pharmacy into the health care space has accelerated the transition in the capability and accessibility of POC testing. Traditional patient care requires the patient to take time out their daily schedule to travel to a dedicated health care facility where they spend a significant amount of time working their way through often inefficient processes to receive care for what are often relatively minor issues or concerns at relatively high costs. These visits are often associated with significant costs and loss of productivity. The entities looking to disrupt this process are seeking to provide patient care outside the confines of traditional health care spaces; the goal being to provide some level of primary care with minimal disruption by bringing care to the patient while they go through their daily routine. Large corporations like Walmart already have the stated goal of bringing low-cost primary care clinics within 15 minutes of 90% of the US population.[19] The effectiveness of these primary care clinics, which are typically staffed by nurse practitioners, hinges on the availability of infectious and noninfectious POC testing.

By integrating care into existing retail and other nontraditional spaces, providers can offer an attractive alternative to patients and achieve efficient delivery of health care. The challenges to this model are the need for trained personnel and the need for a new approach to POC testing. For POC testing to have a meaningful impact, it is necessary for the test to be relatively easy to perform even by a nonlaboratorian and for the results to be accurate enough to be actionable for the care provider without the need for confirmation.

The volume of POC testing is expected to grow 10% to 15% annually.[20] According to the National Community Pharmacists Association (NCPA), "Point-of-care testing provides an excellent opportunity for community pharmacies to enhance revenue by expanding patient care services while improving health at the patient and population levels."[21] According to Deloitte,[22] POC testing is on track to exceed immunizations as a source of revenue for the pharmaceutical retail industry. The top 4 primary opportunities for growth in POC testing as identified by the NCPA are all for infectious disease–related assays including influenza, streptococcal antigen, HIV, and hepatitis C detection assays.[21] The volume of POC testing is growing rapidly globally at with the market expected to be valued at $3 billion annually by 2021.[22]

The provision of care has moved toward telehealth due to the pandemic, but is limited by the lack of access to laboratory test results.[23] The natural progression of POC testing is therefore toward its use in at-home testing. Studies have shown that when given the choice, patients prefer at-home testing.[24] During the SARS-COV-2 outbreak, the FDA authorized the first at-home collection kit for the detection of the virus from saliva.[25] Further advances in technology are required to improve the quality and performance of at-home POC testing with a focus toward reducing the likelihood of errors and automated result interpretation.

It is important to note that the waived classification does not mean that the test is error proof and not all POC testing is able to obtain the waived classification. Early POC testing was limited to lateral flow-based antigen tests with visual detection of the positive signal by the user. These assays suffered from limited performance characteristics with sensitivities ranging from 10%-80% in comparisons with viral culture or real-time PCR.[26] Concerns about the about the poor negative predictive value of antigen-based assays in particular for influenza prompted the FDA to reclassify rapid influenza antigen devices as class II devices with the expectation of improved performance characteristics.[16] These were then replaced by FIA-based antigen detection assays. The performance of these FIA assays for the detection of influenza was significantly improved over traditional antigen-based testing with sensitivity of approximately 80% in multiple studies.[17,27] These assays still fell short of real-time PCR in terms of being able to rule out influenza. In contrast to lateral flow devices, the throughput of these immunofluorescent-based assays was also limited by the number of instruments/readers available with each instrument able to read one patient sample at a time.

Advances in NAAT-based testing allowed for the development of the first CLIA-waived NAAT test for influenza (Abbott ID Now, initially developed as the Alere I).[27] The use of isothermal amplification–based technology eliminated the need for hardware that had the temperature cycling capabilities required for real-time PCR. This development was a revolutionary step forward in being the first time that any molecular amplification–based technology was available to be performed at the level of primary care without the need to follow the CLIA requirements for moderate or high complexity testing. Subsequently additional NAAT-based platforms obtained CLIA waivers for POC testing including (among others) the Roche Liat and the Cepheid GeneXpert, both of which use real-time PCR and are capable of detecting influenza A, B, and RSV as well as group A streptococci using a variety of CLIA-waived assays. The Liat can provide results for influenza A and B as well as RSV from a respiratory sample within 22 minutes. The GeneXpert is able to provide similar results in 30 minutes with minimal sample handling requirements for both platforms. Even more revolutionary was the approval of the Biofire Filmarray Respiratory Panel EZ, which is a multiplex panel for 14 different respiratory pathogens.

IMPACT OF POINT-OF-CARE TESTING

The ability to offer panel-based syndromic testing in the POC setting can appear to be attractive to the clinician, but it is unclear whether there is a significant benefit associated with the detection of viral pathogens in the outpatient setting, especially when there are no interventions associated with some of the positive targets. The value of these syndromic panels has been difficult to demonstrate even in the inpatient setting and the primary care providers might also struggle to interpret panel results that detect multiple targets although in some settings.[28–30] The ResPOC trial evaluated the impact of syndromic panel-based testing in the POC testing and found that the results reduced length of stay (LOS) and improved influenza detection and appropriate antiviral use although it did not reduce antibiotic use.[28] It is possible that similar gains could be achieved using NAAT-based assays targeted at specific pathogens, such as influenza alone. Mercuro and colleagues[29] demonstrated that inhouse testing using syndromic respiratory panels did not have any impact on LOS, duration of therapy, or frequency of drug-related interventions. When appropriately used, NAAT-based POC testing can significantly impact patient care. POC group A streptococcal NAAT-based testing was able to significantly improve appropriate antibiotic use (97.1% vs 87.5%; $P = .0065$) when compared with an antigen-based test.[31] Implementation of an NAAT-based rapid influenza assay reduce in appropriate antiviral use, improved appropriate antibiotic utilization, reduced LOS and also reduced the likelihood of admission when compared with antigen-based testing.[32]

These findings are crucial to the adoption of NAAT-based POC technology because of the significant capital and reagent costs that may be involved with NAAT tests, whereas antigen-based testing does not typically require resources beyond the testing kits and specimen collection materials. It is important for laboratories to demonstrate the direct impact and cost savings in terms of patient care that accrue from the adoption of these technologies. It is also essential to liaison with care providers to improve understanding of assay performance and interpretation of results. This is necessary to ensure that changes in testing platforms translate to changes in patient care. NAAT-based influenza and group A Streptococcal testing can offer greater than 99% sensitivity and specificity allowing the care provider to make decisions on patient care with confidence as compared with antigen tests with limited performance characteristics. There is little doubt that POC and near patient testing is an area of rapid growth. The continued consolidation of laboratories, the challenges with hiring laboratory personnel and the continued development of novel POC platforms and technologies suggests these trends will continue.

OVERSIGHT AND PERFORMANCE OF POINT-OF-CARE TESTING

The performance of NAAT-based platforms represented a significant improvement over the previous iterations of antigen-based tests, both lateral flow and immunofluorescent-based assays.[27] However it does raise concerns about appropriate oversight of testing systems and methods that are far more complex than traditional POC-based testing. Laboratories that perform moderate and high-complexity NAAT testing are required by their accrediting bodies to adhere to rigorous standards and quality control.[33] This includes routine use of control material, monitoring of test statistics and assay performance and environmental sampling to detect potential contamination. The exquisite sensitivity of NAAT-based testing means that failure to adhere to these practices can result in erroneous results and patient harm.[34] Although NAAT-based testing in the POC setting has the potential to significantly impact patient care, there are significant concerns that in the absence of adequate laboratory-based oversight, problems could develop and continue undetected for significant periods of time. In an ideal world, POC testing would be performed by appropriately trained and qualified laboratory personnel but the current shortage of technologists ensures that is not a realistic goal.

A number of questions need to be addressed when moving POC testing using highly complex testing out of the laboratory and into settings in which the users are health care professionals who are not familiar with the challenges of NAAT testing.[35] A colloquium convened by the American Academy of Microbiology recognized the need for near patient and POC infectious disease testing but also strongly recommended that oversight of the quality assurance processes associated with this testing should remain under appropriate laboratory-based personnel.[36]

Examples of situations that demonstrate the need for laboratory oversight of POC and near patient testing systems are not uncommon:

- Invalid results associated with influenza B–positive samples using the Roche Liat system that generated unusual PCR curves that was determined to be related issues with the system software.[37]
- Point mutations in the M gene of influenza that caused false negative results using the Cepheid GeneXpert.[38]
- Engelmann and colleagues[39] suggested there was a need to review PCR curves under specific circumstances when using the Cepheid GeneXpert platform.
- The Abbott ID NOW was demonstrated to have lower sensitivity that other NAAT-based platforms in direct comparison of sensitivity for the detection of influenza due to the dilution effect of transport media.[27]
- Random sampling of the Roche Liat instrument in a testing laboratory determined that target viral RNA could be detected on the surface of and within the instrument testing chamber. Studies eventually demonstrated that the risk of contamination was low even in the presence of environmental contamination with viral genomic material.[40] Nevertheless, these findings reinforce the need for rigorous adherence to protocol and regular monitoring of test results and statistics to rule out contamination.
- False positive *Campylobacter* and *Cryptosporidium* results in Biofire gastrointestinal panel testing of stool samples.[41]
- False positive *Streptococcus pneumoniae* results associated with use of the Biofire ME meningitis panel.[42]

Although the Biofire ME and gastrointestinal panels are not CLIA-waived POC tests, they are often performed in the near patient setting. These quality issues were not limited to NAAT-based testing; false positive results were identified in comparison studies of the Quidel Quickvue Influenza A + B antigen test with NAAT-based testing during the 2009 H1N1 Influenza outbreak.[43]

POINT-OF-CARE TESTING IN THE CORONAVIRUS DISEASE 2019 ERA

During the course of the Coronavirus Disease 2019 (COVID-19) pandemic, the shortage of testing resources and the need for near patient testing became severe enough that the FDA relented and relaxed the rules governing the Emergency Use Authorization (EUA) process to allow for expedited approval of testing platforms.[44] One of the first POC testing platforms to receive approval to operate under a CLIA waiver certificate was the Abbott ID NOW using isothermal amplification.[45] Early results were promising, but as was the case with the Abbott ID Now Influenza assay, issues that could impact the sensitivity of the assay were identified.[46] Subsequently, the FDA also issued a notification that negative results may require confirmation by an alternative NAAT-based assay.[47] Other NAAT-based platforms using real-time PCR that are capable of being used in the POC space are either now available or in development. This includes multiplex and syndromic panels that incorporate SARS-COV-2 detection along with other respiratory viral pathogens. These combinations may prove essential during the flu season when multiple pathogens are circulating in the community and could potentially cause coinfections.[48]

In the antibody testing space, under the EUA authorization, numerous vendors were allowed to market POC antibody detection assays for COVID-19 with the disclaimer that these assays were not intended for diagnostic use.[49] Despite these restrictions, the market was flooded with numerous POC antibody assays with few data on actual performance characteristics. These assays were widely available and being used inappropriately for diagnosis despite the limitations.[50] Responding the reports regarding inappropriate use and substandard performance of the these POC antibody tests, the FDA requested the manufacturers to provide additional information on assay performance characteristics and eventually took action to remove those that did not comply or meet minimum standards.[51]

Despite the performance issues associated with early iterations of POC tests for COVID-19, the need for rapid near patient testing is essential to the management of this outbreak. The pandemic has forced health care providers to consider innovative steps to provide primary care without having potentially infectious patients congregating in close proximity with high-risk individuals. Providers are increasingly relying on telemedicine to continue to provide care to the patient remotely.[52] However, the extent of care is limited by the ability to obtain laboratory test results. The FDA recently approved the first at-home collection kit for testing for COVID-19 in saliva but these assays are not widely available.[53] Subsequent data on the performance of saliva for the detection of COVID-19 has not been consistent and it remains to be determined whether this sample type will be widely adopted. Specimen collection for COVID-19 remains challenging with collection of the preferred specimen type; nasopharyngeal swabs requiring specific training and infection control precautions to minimize risk to the individual collecting specimens. Approval of alternative specimen types such as nasal swabs, sputum, and tracheal aspirates have eased these concerns, although challenges still remain in the availability of swabs and transport media.

SUMMARY

Technological advances have ensured that POC testing can become central to patient care and management. Further studies are necessary to determine the optimal strategies to use these platforms in a partnership between laboratories and care providers. The increasing complexity of these testing systems makes it essential that laboratory personnel are involved in the oversight of POC testing systems and platforms.

DISCLOSURE

L. Samuel is on the Advisory Board of Qvella Diagnostics.

FUNDING SOURCES

Current funding source: Specific Diagnostics.

REFERENCES

1. Drancourt M, Michel-Lepage A, Boyer S, et al. The point-of-care laboratory in clinical microbiology. Clin Microbiol Rev 2016;29(3):429–47.
2. Kozel TR, Burnham-Marusich AR. Point-of-care testing for infectious diseases: past, present, and future. J Clin Microbiol 2017;55(8):2313–20.

3. Leland DS, Ginocchio CC. Role of cell culture for virus detection in the age of technology. Clin Microbiol Rev 2007;20(1):49–78.

4. Yarbrough ML, Lainhart W, McMullen AR, et al. Impact of total laboratory automation on workflow and specimen processing time for culture of urine specimens. Eur J Clin Microbiol Infect Dis 2018;37(12):2405–11.

5. Sautter RL, Thomson RB Jr. Consolidated clinical microbiology laboratories. J Clin Microbiol 2015;53(5):1467–72.

6. Robinson A, Marcon M, Mortensen JE, et al. Controversies affecting the future practice of clinical microbiology. J Clin Microbiol 1999;37(4):883–9.

7. Corrie Simons GC. The pros and cons of centralizing microbiology services. Clinical Laboratory News: AACC 2019. Available at: https://www.aacc.org/cln/articles/2019/julyaug/the-pros-and-cons-of-centralizing-microbiology-services.

8. Shulman ST, Bisno AL, Clegg HW, et al. Clinical practice guideline for the diagnosis and management of group A streptococcal pharyngitis: 2012 update by the Infectious Diseases Society of America. Clin Infect Dis 2012;55(10):1279–82.

9. Cohen JF, Bertille N, Cohen R, et al. Rapid antigen detection test for group A streptococcus in children with pharyngitis. Cochrane Database Syst Rev 2016;(7):CD010502.

10. Campbell L, Woods V, Lloyd T, et al. Evaluation of the OSOM Trichomonas rapid test versus wet preparation examination for detection of Trichomonas vaginalis vaginitis in specimens from women with a low prevalence of infection. J Clin Microbiol 2008;46(10):3467–9.

11. Cowan JF, Chandler AS, Kracen E, et al. Clinical impact and cost-effectiveness of Xpert MTB/RIF testing in hospitalized patients with presumptive pulmonary tuberculosis in the United States. Clin Infect Dis 2017;64(4):482–9.

12. Van Rie A, Page-Shipp L, Scott L, et al. Xpert((R)) MTB/RIF for point-of-care diagnosis of TB in high-HIV burden, resource-limited countries: hype or hope? Expert Rev Mol Diagn 2010;10(7):937–46.

13. Vassall A, Siapka M, Foster N, et al. Cost-effectiveness of Xpert MTB/RIF for tuberculosis diagnosis in South Africa: a real-world cost analysis and economic evaluation. Lancet Glob Health 2017;5(7):e710–9.

14. Hutchinson AB, Ethridge SF, Wesolowski LG, et al. Costs and outcomes of laboratory diagnostic algorithms for the detection of HIV. J Clin Virol 2013;58(Suppl 1):e2–7.

15. Drexler JF, Helmer A, Kirberg H, et al. Poor clinical sensitivity of rapid antigen test for influenza A pandemic (H1N1) 2009 virus. Emerg Infect Dis 2009;15(10):1662–4.

16. FDA. Microbiology devices; reclassification of influenza virus antigen detection test systems intended for use directly with clinical specimens. In. Vol 21 CFR 866. Federalregister.gov 2017:3609-3619.

17. Lewandrowski K, Tamerius J, Menegus M, et al. Detection of influenza A and B viruses with the Sofia analyzer: a novel, rapid immunofluorescence-based in vitro diagnostic device. Am J Clin Pathol 2013;139(5):684–9.

18. CMS. Clinical Laboratory Improvement Amendments (CLIA). Available at: www.cms.gov/clia. Accessed July 1, 2020.

19. Patel N. Walmart Health: A Deep Dive into the $WMT Corporate Strategy in Health Care. 2018; Available at: https://medium.com/@nxpatel/walmart-health-e4e73eebb06c. Accessed July 1, 2020.

20. Wagar E. Point-of-care testing: twenty years' experience. Lab Medicine 2008;39(9):560–2.

21. NCPA. Point-of-Care (POC) Testing. Available at: https://ncpa.org/point-care-poc-testing. Accessed July 1, 2020.

22. Deloitte. Top 10 health care innovations: achieving more for less. Available at: https://www2.deloitte.com/content/dam/Deloitte/global/Documents/Life-Sciences-Health-Care/gx-lshc-top-10-health-care-innovations.pdf2016. Accessed July 1, 2020.

23. FDA. Using telehealth to expand access to essential health services during the COVID-19 pandemic. Available at: https://www.cdc.gov/coronavirus/2019-ncov/hcp/telehealth.html. 2020. Accessed July 10, 2020.

24. Gaydos CA, Jett-Goheen M, Barnes M, et al. Self-testing for *Trichomonas vaginalis* at home using a point-of-care test by women who request kits via the Internet. Sex Health 2016. https://doi.org/10.1071/SH16049.

25. FDA. Coronavirus (COVID-19) update: FDA issues first emergency use authorization for point of care diagnostic. 2020. Available at: https://www.fda.gov/news-events/press-announcements/coronavirus-covid-19-update-fda-issues-first-emergency-use-authorization-point-care-diagnostic. Accessed July 10, 2020.

26. CDC. Guidance for clinicians on the use of rapid influenza diagnostic tests. Available at: https://www.cdc.gov/flu/professionals/diagnosis/clinician_guidance_ridt.htm2020. Accessed July 1, 2020.

27. Nolte FS, Gauld L, Barrett SB. Direct comparison of Alere i and cobas Liat influenza A and B tests for rapid detection of influenza virus infection. J Clin Microbiol 2016;54(11):2763–6.

28. Brendish NJ, Malachira AK, Armstrong L, et al. Routine molecular point-of-care testing for respiratory viruses in adults presenting to hospital with acute respiratory illness (ResPOC): a pragmatic, open-label, randomised controlled trial. Lancet Respir Med 2017;5(5):401–11.

29. Mercuro NJ, Kenney RM, Samuel L, et al. Stewardship opportunities in viral pneumonia: why not the immunocompromised? Transpl Infect Dis 2018;20(2):e12854.

30. Brendish NJ, Malachira AK, Beard KR, et al. Impact of turnaround time on outcome with point-of-care testing for respiratory viruses: a post hoc analysis from a randomised controlled trial. Eur Respir J 2018;52(2):1800555. https://doi.org/10.1183/13993003.00555-2018. Print 2018 Aug.

31. Rao A, Berg B, Quezada T, et al. Diagnosis and antibiotic treatment of group a streptococcal pharyngitis in children in a primary care setting: impact of point-of-care polymerase chain reaction. BMC Pediatr 2019;19(1):24.

32. Mercuro NJ. Impact of rapid influenza molecular testing on diagnosis and patient management. ASM Microbe 2018. San Francisco (CA).

33. CAP. Laboratory Accreditation Program. Available at: https://www.cap.org/laboratory-improvement/accreditation/laboratory-accreditation-program. Accessed July 2, 2020.

34. Mandal S, Tatti KM, Woods-Stout D, et al. Pertussis pseudo-outbreak linked to specimens contaminated by *Bordetella pertussis* DNA from clinic surfaces. Pediatrics 2012;129(2):e424–30.

35. Arboleda VA, Garner OB. Ensuring the quality of point-of-care testing in a large and decentralized ambulatory care setting. Am J Clin Pathol 2017;148(4):336–44.

36. Dolen V, Bahk K, Carroll KC, et al. Changing diagnostic paradigms for microbiology. 2016. Available at: https://pubmed.ncbi.nlm.nih.gov/28796470/

37. Valentin T, Kieslinger P, Stelzl E, et al. Prospective evaluation of three rapid molecular tests for seasonal influenza in patients presenting at an emergency unit. J Clin Virol 2019;111:29–32.

38. Binnicker MJ, Baddour LM, Grys TE, et al. Identification of an influenza A H1N1/ 2009 virus with mutations in the matrix gene causing a negative result by a commercial molecular assay. J Clin Microbiol 2013;51(6):2006–7.

39. Engelmann I, Alidjinou EK, Lazrek M, et al. Necessity to critically review the automatic results of the Xpert Flu assay. Diagn Microbiol Infect Dis 2017;88(1):26–30.

40. Phillips JE, McCune S, Fantz CR, et al. Assay integrity of a PCR influenza point-of-care test remains following artificial system contamination. J Appl Lab Med 2019; 4(3):422–6.

41. FDA. Class 2 device recall FilmArray gastrointestinal (GI) panel. 2019. Available at: https://www.accessdata.fda.gov/scripts/cdrh/cfdocs/cfRES/res.cfm?id=171388. Accessed July 2, 2020.

42. Dien Bard J, Alby K. Point-counterpoint: meningitis/encephalitis syndromic testing in the clinical laboratory. J Clin Microbiol 2018;56(4). e00018-18.

43. Stevenson HL, Loeffelholz MJ. Poor positive accuracy of QuickVue rapid antigen tests during the influenza A (H1N1) 2009 pandemic. J Clin Microbiol 2010;48(10): 3729–31.

44. FDA. COVID-19-related guidance documents for industry, FDA staff, and other stakeholders. 2020. Accessed July 2, 2020.

45. Abbott ID Now EUA authorization [press release]: FDA. Available at: https://www. fda.gov/media/136522/download. Accessed July 1, 2020.

46. Harrington A, Cox B, Snowdon J, et al. Comparison of Abbott ID Now and Abbott m2000 methods for the detection of SARS-CoV-2 from nasopharyngeal and nasal swabs from symptomatic patients. J Clin Microbiol 2020;58(8):e00798-20.

47. FDA. Coronavirus (COVID-19) update: FDA informs public about possible accuracy concerns with Abbott ID NOW point-of-care test. 2020. Available at: https:// www.fda.gov/news-events/press-announcements/coronavirus-covid-19-update-fda-informs-public-about-possible-accuracy-concerns-abbott-id-now-point. Accessed July 2, 2020.

48. Ding Q, Lu P, Fan Y, et al. The clinical characteristics of pneumonia patients co-infected with 2019 novel coronavirus and influenza virus in Wuhan, China. J Med Virol 2020. https://doi.org/10.1002/jmv.25781.

49. Coronavirus (COVID-19) update: serological tests [press release]. Available at: https://www.fda.gov/news-events/press-announcements/coronavirus-covid-19-update-serological-tests2020. Accessed July 1, 2020.

50. Coronavirus (COVID-19) update: FDA issues warning letters to companies inappropriately marketing antibody tests, potentially placing public health at risk [press release]. Available at: https://www.fda.gov/news-events/press-announcements/coronavirus-covid-19-update-fda-issues-warning-letters-companies-inappropriately-marketing-antibody2020. Accessed July 1, 2020.

51. Certain COVID-19 serology/antibody tests should not be used - letter to clinical laboratory staff and health care providers [press release]. Available at: https:// www.fda.gov/medical-devices/letters-health-care-providers/certain-covid-19-serologyantibody-tests-should-not-be-used-letter-clinical-laboratory-staff-and2020. Accessed July 1, 2020.

52. Keesara S, Jonas A, Schulman K. Covid-19 and health care's digital revolution. N Engl J Med 2020;382(23):e82.

53. Coronavirus (COVID-19) update: FDA authorizes first diagnostic test using at-home collection of saliva specimens [press release]. Available at: https://www. fda.gov/news-events/press-announcements/coronavirus-covid-19-update-fda-authorizes-first-diagnostic-test-using-home-collection-saliva2020. Accessed July 1, 2020.

Update in Pediatric Diagnostic Microbiology

James J. Dunn, PhD, D(ABMM)[a,b,*], Paula A. Revell, PhD, D(ABMM)[a,b]

KEYWORDS

- Pediatric microbiology • Measles • Congenital infections • Neonatal infections
- Syphilis • Cytomegalovirus • *Treponema pallidum*

KEY POINTS

- Congenital CMV (cCMV) infection is the most common intrauterine infection in the United States and primary infection in the seronegative mother is associated with the greatest risk of transplacental transmission, which can lead to symptomatic manifestations of the disease in the newborn period.
- Most infants with cCMV are asymptomatic at birth, which makes the diagnosis challenging because universal screening is not mandated. Some states require laboratory testing only on failure of a hearing screen by the infant.
- Prevention of congenital syphilis entails maternal screening with testing at the first prenatal care visit and again at 28 to 32 weeks gestation and at delivery for women at high risk.
- Diagnosis of congenital syphilis is complicated by transplacental transfer of maternal nontreponemal and treponemal IgG antibodies. Infants up to 18 months of age born to mothers with reactive treponemal tests should have serum quantitative nontreponemal testing and be carefully examined for physical signs of congenital syphilis.
- Measles is a highly communicable infectious disease and is one of the leading causes of death among children worldwide despite the availability of a safe and effective vaccine.
- The type of specimen, timing of collection, and vaccination status are important factors to consider in making an accurate diagnosis of measles infection.

INTRODUCTION

The practice of clinical microbiology does not differ significantly between pediatric and adult patient populations. However, infants and young children are uniquely susceptible to potentially severe and long-lasting effects of certain types of infections that in otherwise healthy adults might not have significant clinical manifestations. Children lack the immune and physiologic defenses of older individuals, which makes them more likely to succumb to common illnesses. Despite advances in vaccinology over

---

[a] Medical Microbiology and Virology, Department of Pathology, Texas Children's Hospital, 6621 Fannin Street, Suite AB1195, Houston, TX 77030, USA; [b] Baylor College of Medicine, Houston, TX, USA
* Corresponding author. 6621 Fannin Street, Suite AB1195, Houston, TX 77030.
E-mail address: jjdunn@texaschildrens.org

Clin Lab Med 40 (2020) 495–508
https://doi.org/10.1016/j.cll.2020.08.007
0272-2712/20/© 2020 Elsevier Inc. All rights reserved.

the past 50-plus years, unvaccinated or undervaccinated children remain at risk for acquiring age-old infections or those that have reemerged in recent years (eg, measles). The etiologies and manifestations of infections in pediatric patients are often distinctly different and more severe than those seen in adults. This requires laboratories to implement unique microbiologic methods for rapid and accurate diagnoses in this population. In some instances there are challenges in specimen collection that are unique to pediatrics. For example, the amount of available blood volume for laboratory testing is limited in infants and young children to the extent that iatrogenic anemia becomes an issue in neonatal and pediatric intensive care units. Additionally, serologic diagnosis in neonates and infants is complicated by the presence of maternal antibodies making the type of testing performed crucial to accurate diagnoses. The role of the pediatric microbiology laboratory in providing rapid and accurate results for patient management and public health purposes cannot be understated. This article focuses on two important congenital infections and a disease once nearly eliminated through global vaccination efforts that has reemerged because of the increased prevalence of individuals opting out of the recommended childhood vaccination schedule.

CONGENITAL CYTOMEGALOVIRUS INFECTION

Congenital cytomegalovirus (cCMV) infection is the most common intrauterine infection in the United States. In developed countries the incidence of cCMV is approximately 5 to 7 per 1000 live births, whereas in developing countries the rate is significantly higher at 10 to 30 per 1000 live births.[1,2] Higher rates of cCMV are observed in populations with high seroprevalence, which can vary by geographic area, race, ethnicity, and socioeconomic background.[3]

Primary infection in the seronegative mother is associated with the greatest risk of transplacental transmission (~30%) compared with approximately 1.5% for nonprimary infections and symptomatic infection in newborns occurs most often after primary maternal infection in pregnancy.[4,5] One of the most important risk factors for primary acquisition of CMV during pregnancy is prolonged exposure to young children who secrete the virus in their urine and saliva for several months. Primary infection in pregnancy can occur with increased exposure to these young children and also through sexual activity.[6] Most transplacental transmission events are thought to result from nonprimary maternal infections because of the high seroprevalence and transmission to the fetus is more likely to occur in advanced pregnancy stages because of increased shedding in urine and cervicovaginal secretions as pregnancy progresses. About two-thirds of transmission cases occur in the third trimester and the risk of long-term sequelae to the fetus in this situation is low (~5%). Although transmission in the first trimester occurs less frequently (30%–45%), it is typically associated with a higher rate of long-term sequelae (~25%).[7,8]

Upwards of 90% of infants with cCMV are asymptomatic during the newborn period. Of those with symptoms shortly after birth, the mortality rate is 7% to 12% and most suffer from permanent sequelae, such as sensorineural hearing loss (SNHL), neurodevelopmental delays, retinitis, or cerebral palsy. About 10% to 15% of those asymptomatic in the newborn period develop SNHL and a much smaller percentage develop cognitive impairment or retinitis.[9] The most common signs of cCMV in the neonate are jaundice, petechiae, hepatosplenomegaly, and microcephaly.[10,11] Brain imaging is important to asses for findings of periventricular calcifications, ventricular dilatation, and cysts.[12] These newborns usually have elevated aspartate aminotransferase, hyperbilirubinemia, thrombocytopenia, and elevated cerebrospinal fluid protein.[11]

Prenatal testing for cCMV involves testing of the mother and fetus. Although universal screening in pregnancy is not routinely recommended, cases of suspected primary infection should warrant further testing. Serology provides indirect evidence of recent or prior CMV infection based on changes in antibody titers at different time points. The standard for determining primary infection is CMV seroconversion, detection of CMV IgG in a previously seronegative maternal patient. A CMV IgM-positive result in a pregnant woman may be indicative of primary infection. However, IgM antibodies can persist for several months so it could reflect a recent past infection. The timing of infection is determined by IgG antibody avidity testing in which low avidity represents recent infection and high avidity past remote infection. The combination of IgM-positive with low IgG avidity would be suggestive of recent primary infection.[13] Testing of amniotic fluid is used to demonstrate fetal infection. Amniocentesis should be performed after 21 weeks gestation and 7 weeks after maternal infection because fetal shedding of CMV in the urine occurs at least 5 to 7 weeks after infection. Using the viral load in amniotic fluid to predict outcomes of disease severity in newborns remains a controversial subject because some studies have shown no direct correlation.[14,15]

Postnatal diagnosis involves testing of a newborn's saliva, urine, or blood. Ideally these specimens are collected before 21 days of life to confirm a diagnosis of cCMV. After 3 weeks it is difficult to determine if the infant could have contracted the infection through nursing or by exposure to other individuals shedding the virus. In addition, intrapartum or postnatal acquisition of the virus is not usually associated with long-term sequelae.

CMV is isolated in cell culture from a variety of different specimen types including blood, urine, upper and lower respiratory tract samples, cerebrospinal fluid, saliva, and tissue. Human fibroblast cell lines in either conventional tube or shell vial format support the replication of CMV. In cases of cCMV, the virus is readily recovered in culture from urine and saliva samples collected within the first 21 days of life because of the high concentration of viable virus in those compartments.

Several Food and Drug Administration (FDA)-cleared/approved molecular tests are available for determination of viral load in plasma specimens and several laboratory-developed tests have been used to detect CMV quantitatively and/or qualitatively in a variety of sample types.[16] However, there are currently no FDA-cleared/approved molecular tests for detection of CMV in urine samples. Only one FDA-approved test is commercially available for testing newborn saliva samples (Alethia CMV, Meridian Bioscience, Inc, Cincinnati, OH). In this assay flocked swabs are used to collect saliva from neonates less than 21 days of age and at least 1 hour after nursing. The swabs are placed in a transport tube with or without viral media. The assay uses loop-mediated isothermal amplification chemistry to amplify and detect a conserved region of the CMV genome.[17] Some CLIA–certified reference laboratories test for cCMV in infant dried blood spots using polymerase chain reaction (PCR), although the sensitivity of detection is typically less than that for urine and saliva.[18,19]

Although more than 5000 infants born each year suffer from permanent disability caused by cCMV (**Fig. 1**A), most pregnant women have not heard of CMV infection and its associated sequelae (**Fig. 1**B). Health care providers are also unlikely to have complete information on cCMV and how to prevent CMV infection, and do not routinely provide CMV education or counseling for pregnant women. In the United States, CMV testing is recommended only when there is a clinical suspicion of infection or fetal abnormalities are detected by routine imaging.

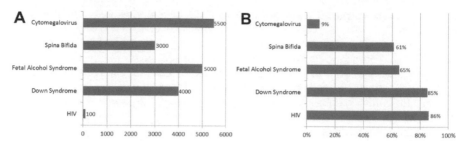

Fig. 1. Number of US children born with or developing long-term medical conditions each year (A). Women's awareness of conditions affecting children (B). HIV, human immunodeficiency virus. (*Data from* www.cdc.gov.)

In 2013, Utah became the first state to implement hearing-targeted CMV screening. If an infant fails a hearing screen within the first 3 weeks of life, testing for CMV must take place, typically PCR of either saliva or urine. The law also directs the Utah Department of Health to create a public education program to inform pregnant women, and women who may become pregnant, about the occurrence of CMV and possible risks to the fetus and neonate. More recently additional states have mandated CMV testing for newborns that fail a hearing screen (Connecticut, Iowa, New York, Virginia, Illinois) and several other states require education of the public and health care professionals about cCMV (**Fig. 2**). These and other measures are important to improve awareness and provide access to reliable diagnostic testing to recognize in a timely manner those infants with cCMV infection and at risk for hearing loss and neurologic disabilities.

Benefits of treatment with antivirals in asymptomatic infants or those with isolated SNHL have not been demonstrated. In infants with symptomatic cCMV, treatment

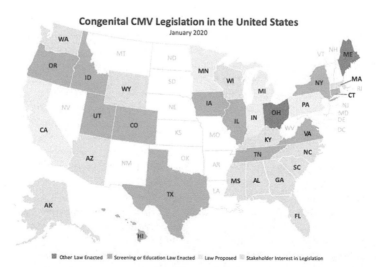

Fig. 2. States with final or proposed legislative mandates for cCMV education and/or testing. (*From* National CMV Foundation. Advocacy. Available at: https://www.nationalcmv.org/about-us/advocacy; with permission.)

with 6 months of valganciclovir therapy has been shown to be beneficial for long-term hearing and neurodevelopmental outcomes.[20]

CONGENITAL SYPHILIS INFECTION

Congenital syphilis (CS) is caused by infection with *Treponema pallidum*. Transmission occurs vertically from mother to fetus, and can occur throughout all stages of pregnancy; however, the likelihood of transmission increases as the stage of pregnancy advances. Transmission can occur through any stage of maternal infection, but the rate of transmission is highest during primary and secondary (P&S) syphilis. Although an ancient disease, syphilis has made a significant resurgence in the United States over the past two decades. In 2000 and 2001, the national rate of reported P&S syphilis cases was 2.1 cases per 100,000 population, the lowest rate since reporting began in 1941. Since 2001 the rate of infection has steadily increased each subsequent year; in 2018 the rate of P&S syphilis cases was 10.8 per 100,000 population. The overall incidence of syphilis infection in all stages has increased from 11.2 to 35.5 cases per 100,000 population in this same time period. This overall trend is reflected in the rate of reported cases of CS because rates of congenital infection coincide with rates of P&S syphilis among women of reproductive age (**Fig. 3**). In 2018, there were 1306 reported cases of CS, with a rate of 33.1 cases per 100,000 live births, the highest rate reported since 1995; rates range from 0.0 to 92.2 cases per 100,000 live births. The highest rates of reported CS cases were observed in the West and South (**Fig. 4**). This increase in 2018 represents a 39.7% more cases relative to 2017 and a 291.0% increase relative to 2012.[21] Untreated syphilis during pregnancy leads to congenital infection, which is associated with significant risk including premature delivery, low birthweight, and fetal and neonatal mortality. Despite the devastating consequences, CS is preventable. In 2007 the World Health Organization (WHO) introduced an initiative to eliminate mother-to-child transmission of syphilis worldwide; in 2015 Cuba was the first country to achieve this goal. Per the WHO initiative, elimination of transmission is defined as a reduction of transmission to such a low level that it no longer constitutes a public health problem. Globally more than 10 countries,

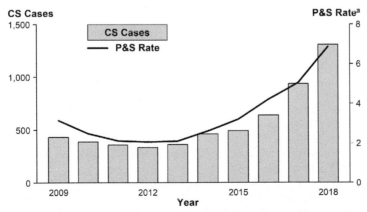

Fig. 3. Congenital syphilis, reported cases by year of birth and rates of reported cases of primary and secondary syphilis among females aged 15 to 44 years, United States, 2009 to 2018. [a] Per 100,000 population. (*From* Centers for Disease Control and Prevention. Sexually transmitted disease surveillance 2018. Atlanta: U.S. Department of Health and Human Services; 2019. https://doi.org/10.15620/cdc.79370.)

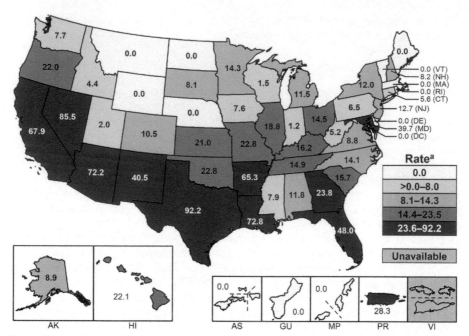

Fig. 4. Congenital syphilis, rates of reported cases by state and territory, United States, 2018. [a] Per 100,000 live births. (*From* Centers for Disease Control and Prevention. Sexually transmitted disease surveillance 2018. Atlanta: U.S. Department of Health and Human Services; 2019. https://doi.org/10.15620/cdc.79370.)

including but not limited to Cuba, Thailand, Armenia, Belarus, and the Republic of Moldova, have eliminated mother-to-child transmission of this devastating disease. Diagnosis and treatment of syphilis infection in pregnant women and their partners are critical to breaking the mother-to-child transmission cycle.[22,23]

Because prevention and identification of CS depends so heavily on careful maternal screening, syphilis testing is recommended at initiation of prenatal care in all women. In 2015 the Centers for Disease Control and Prevention (CDC) published the Sexually Transmitted Disease Treatment Guidelines, which recommend serologic syphilis screening for all women at first prenatal care visit and additional testing at 28 to 32 weeks gestation and at delivery for women at high risk.[24]

Importantly, only select states have mandatory third trimester testing[25] and providers should be aware of geographic prevalence and patient risk factors because the true prevalence of syphilis is not recognized without adequate screening. In New York City a study evaluating factors that contribute to CS infection showed that in approximately one-third of CS cases, the major contributing factor was late initiation of prenatal care, and lack of health care coverage was often cited by patients as a barrier to seeking care.[26]

Aside from issues surrounding access to care, the diagnosis of syphilis has always posed unique challenges; the disease is known as "the great imitator" because of its multiple clinical presentations. Laboratory diagnosis is no less complicated; *T pallidum* cannot be cultivated in vitro or visualized by bright field microscopy. Additionally, no FDA-cleared molecular assays for organism detection are available. Although direct organism visualization with darkfield microscopy can provide presumptive diagnosis early in infection, darkfield microscopy is not widely available and most syphilis cases encountered in clinical practice are asymptomatic. Given these unique challenges, syphilis diagnostics have relied on serologic tests as the mainstay of laboratory diagnosis. Serologic tests for syphilis include detection of non-treponemal antibodies against cardiolipin and treponemal specific antibodies.

Nontreponemal tests (NTTs) include the rapid plasma reagin (RPR) and the venereal disease research laboratory (VDRL) test. These tests detect antibodies against cardiolipins released from host cell damage during infection, and are qualitative or quantitative. Importantly, titers increase with active disease and decrease following adequate therapy. The sensitivities of the NTTs are comparable, and vary depending on the stage of infection. The sensitivity is lowest early and late in infection.[27]

Treponemal tests (TTs) include all assays that detect IgM and IgG antibodies specific to *T. pallidum*. Although these tests can confirm previous *T. pallidum* infection, unlike the NTTs, they cannot differentiate individuals who have been treated from those with current disease. Generally, TTs remain reactive for life following eradication of the infection. Historically the most commonly used TTs were the *T. pallidum* particle agglutination assay (TP-PA) and the fluorescent treponemal antibody absorption (FTA-ABS) assay. Recent advances in the detection of *T. pallidum* antibodies have resulted in several TTs that are highly sensitive and specific and are automated to accommodate high throughput testing. These include enzyme-linked immunosorbent assay, chemiluminescence immunoassay (CIA), and multiplex bead enzyme immunoassay (EIA) formats. The specificity of these assays are comparable to the TP-PA and fluorescent treponemal antibody absorption assay but have better sensitivity for early primary syphilis that is sometimes missed by TP-PA, FTA-ABS, and NTTs.[27]

Because of the limitations of each available laboratory test for syphilis, a diagnostic algorithm composed of multiple tests has historically been used to diagnose syphilis. The algorithm used for decades, referred to as the "traditional algorithm," initiates screening with an NTT screen, such as an RPR, followed by confirmation of reactive specimens with a treponemal-specific test to rule out false-positive results. In 2009 a new algorithm was proposed by a panel of experts, and designated the "reverse algorithm" laboratory diagnostic testing for *T. pallidum*.[28,29] This algorithm initiates screening with a treponemal-specific test (EIA or CIA); reactive samples are tested by quantitative RPR and discrepant samples (those that test RPR nonreactive) are tested by TP-PA to aid in determination of disease and treatment status. If the TP-PA is negative (+EIA/CIA, -RPR, -TP-PA), this typically reflects false-positive EIA/CIA results.

Each of the two algorithms has strengths and weaknesses, and importantly laboratories establish which algorithm best suits the needs of their population. Typically, high-volume laboratories use the reverse algorithm to take advantage of the high sample throughput, automation, and objective test interpretation. In low-volume settings, the traditional algorithm may be more cost-effective despite the requirement for manual operation and subjective interpretation. This recent change in the diagnostic approach to syphilis impacts potential diagnosis of CS, which has long depended on the NTTs. In settings where the reverse algorithm is in place, results of the maternal NTT titer should be available to providers to aid in appropriate evaluation and management of potential congenital infections. In all cases, the same NTT should be performed on the mother and infant so that accurate comparisons are made.

Diagnosis of CS is further complicated by transplacental transfer of maternal nontreponemal and treponemal IgG antibodies to the fetus. The interpretation of reactive serologic tests for syphilis in infants up to 18 months of age must take into account maternal antibody status. Evaluation of neonates with a quantitative NTT should be performed on the neonate's serum, because umbilical cord blood can become contaminated with maternal blood and yield a false-positive result, and Wharton jelly within the umbilical cord can yield a false-negative result.[30] A four-fold higher quantitative NTT titer in an infant relative to the mother is considered definitive for congenital infection; however, in most cases of CS the NTT results show titers that are the same or one to two dilutions lower than the maternal titer. Infants born to mothers with reactive TT results for syphilis should have a serum quantitative NTT performed and be carefully examined for physical signs of CS. In neonates who have a normal physical examination and a serum quantitative NTT titer that is less than four-fold the maternal titer, evaluation and treatment depends on the maternal treatment history. If the mother was not treated or the treatment is undocumented or inadequate, cases are considered possible CS and additional clinical and laboratory evaluation is warranted. In neonates with a normal physical examination and for whom NTT titer is less than four-fold of maternal titer, and if mother was treated greater than 4 weeks before delivery, CS is less likely. These patients are still at risk and as such the CDC recommends a single dose of intramuscular penicillin G.

Overall, laboratories need to be aware of the importance of maternal and neonatal testing for syphilis diagnosis and manage the test availability and reporting accordingly. For example, in laboratories for which the reverse algorithm is the primary serologic approach to diagnosis of syphilis, RPR testing for neonatal serum should also be available because it is critical for assessment of potential congenital infection. Likewise reporting strategies for maternal reverse algorithm results need to always include the quantitative RPR titer rather than reporting only a "positive" or "negative" for the syphilis algorithm result. Laboratories should also provide result interpretation as per the Association of Public Health Laboratories recommendation,[29] and not simply report the individual components of the algorithm. The laboratory remains a critical reservoir for information and interpretation of results that are essential to the cessation of mother-to-child transmission of syphilis.

MEASLES IN CHILDREN

Measles is a highly contagious illness caused by rubeola virus and characterized by fever, cough, coryza, and conjunctivitis followed by exanthem.[31,32] Transmission of measles occurs via person-to-person contact through respiratory droplets, which can remain airborne and infectious on contaminated surfaces for several hours.[31,33] Infection is highly communicable in persons with measles from approximately 4 days before the onset of rash to 4 days after. The occurrence of measles transmission in susceptible close contacts is up to 90%.[31]

Measles remains one of the leading causes of death among young children worldwide, despite the availability of a safe and effective vaccine. In 2017 there were approximately 110,000 deaths globally caused by measles, mostly in children younger than 5 years of age.[34] During the first 6 months of 2019, the WHO reported more than 350,000 measles cases from 182 countries, a greater than 150% increase from the same time period the prior year.[35] In the United States, the incidence of measles declined rapidly after the introduction of the first licensed measles vaccine in 1963 and was officially eliminated in 2000. Since then localized measles outbreaks have occurred sporadically throughout the United States, mainly because of infected international travelers spreading the virus to unvaccinated and undervaccinated populations.[36] In 2019 through October 1 there were 1248 measles cases and 22 measles outbreak in the United States, marking the most cases reported since 1992 **(Table 1)**.[37]

Table 1
Number and vaccination status of measles cases, by age group—United States, January 1, 2019 to October 1, 2019

Age Group	Measles Cases, n (%)	Vaccination Status, n (%)[a]		
		Unvaccinated	Vaccinated	Unknown
0–5 mo	43 (3)	43 (100)	0 (0)	0 (0)
6–11 mo	116 (9)	110 (95)	5 (4)	1 (1)
12–15 mo	118 (9)	106 (90)	12 (10)	0 (0)
16 mo–4 y	274 (22)	238 (87)	33 (12)	3 (1)
5–17 y	339 (27)	295 (87)	26 (8)	18 (5)
18–29 y	144 (12)	49 (34)	41 (28)	54 (38)
30–49 y	160 (13)	25 (16)	22 (14)	113 (71)
≥50 y	55 (4)	6 (11)	3 (5)	46 (84)
Overall	1249	872 (70)	142 (11)	235 (19)

[a] Received greater than 1 dose of measles, mumps, and rubella vaccine.
From Centers for Disease Control and Prevention. National update on measles cases and outbreak – United States, January 1-October 1, 2019. Morb Mortal Wkly Rep 2019;68:893-6.

The incubation period for measles is 7 to 14 days and initial clinical symptoms include fever, cough, coryza, and conjunctivitis. Koplik spots, punctate blue-white spots on the buccal mucosa, can occur shortly before or after the onset of rash and are pathognomonic for measles infection. The maculopapular rash occurs approximately 3 to 5 days after the first clinical symptoms and often begins on the forehead and face and spreads gradually downward to the neck, trunk, and lower limbs. In uncomplicated cases the fever usually decreases when the rash reaches the feet, and then the rash fades out gradually downward. This phase is followed by skin desquamation over a period of up to 2 weeks.

About 20% of measles infections result in complications, such as pneumonia, otitis media, or laryngotracheobronchitis. Diarrhea may sometimes lead to dehydration and ocular complications, such as purulent conjunctivitis, keratitis, and xerophthalmia, may lead to blindness. Neurologic complications, such as severe encephalitis, occur in approximately 1 in 1000 infections. Mortality occurs in less than 1% of cases in otherwise healthy individuals, although the rate may be up to 10% in malnourished children. In pregnant women measles infection can lead to increased risk of prematurity or fetal loss. Subacute sclerosing panencephalitis is a rare complication of measles infection and is characterized by irreversible destruction of brain tissue and death.

Laboratory testing for measles should include collection of serum, respiratory tract specimens, and urine (**Table 2**). Serum for antibody detection should be collected 4 to 5 days after rash onset. Throat and nasopharyngeal swabs for molecular detection and viral isolation should be collected using a flocked synthetic swab and placed in 1 to 3 mL of viral transport medium. Nasopharyngeal aspirates and bronchoalveolar lavage specimens are also acceptable. Ideally, because of the cell-associated nature of the virus, urine (10–50 mL) should be centrifuged at 500 × g for 10 minutes at 4°C and the sediment resuspended in viral transport medium. The timing of respiratory swab and urine collection should occur as soon as possible (at least within 7–10 days) after rash onset to optimize the sensitivity of RNA detection and viral isolation. All samples are maintained at 4°C if testing will occur soon after collection, otherwise

Table 2
Suitability of specimen types for laboratory diagnosis of measles infection

Specimen Type	Utility of Laboratory Method				
	RT-PCR	Culture	IgM Serology	IgG Avidity	Genotyping
Serum (from 4 up to 30 d after rash onset)	+	−	+++	++	+/−
Respiratory (throat/ nasopharyngeal within 7–10 d after rash onset)	+++	++	−	−	++
Urine (10–50 mL, concentrated)	++	+	−	−	++

Abbreviations: RT; reverse transcription.

respiratory and urine specimens are frozen and transported at −20°C or −70°C for molecular detection.[38]

The standard laboratory method for rapid confirmation of measles is detection of virus-specific IgM antibodies in serum by EIA or chemiluminescent immunoassay.[39,40] In most patients, IgM antibodies are detectable approximately 3 days after the onset of rash and levels decline over a time period of up to 6 to 8 weeks. IgG antibodies develop shortly after the appearance of IgM and usually remain detectable for life. Seroconversion is demonstrated using acute and convalescent sera obtained 2 weeks apart and assessed for a greater than or equal to four-fold increase of IgG antibodies. IgG avidity testing is useful in cases, such as suspected vaccine failure.[41] The plaque reduction neutralization test is considered the gold standard to detect neutralizing antibodies but is laborious and time consuming and mostly restricted to specialized reference or public health laboratories.[42]

Nucleic acid amplification tests are used to detect viral RNA in respiratory specimens and urine up to 14 days after rash onset but early sampling is recommended to achieve greater sensitivity.[40] Viremia is typically short-lived in the course of measles infection so RNA may only be detectable using RT-PCR within the first few days after symptom onset.[43] Genotyping of viral RNA is an important part of outbreak investigation and global surveillance and the WHO maintains a sequence database for these purposes.

Virus isolation in cell culture is less commonly used for diagnosis of measles, but like genotyping is important for epidemiologic purposes. Specimens for culture should be collected within 3 days of rash onset to maximize the potential for recovery. Cell culture is performed using Vero/hSLAM cells in which Vero cells have been transfected with a plasmid encoding the gene for human SLAM, a known cellular receptor for rubeola virus. Cell culture confirmation of measles virus isolation is done using either RT-PCR, immunofluorescence, or immunohistochemistry.[43]

Because no specific antiviral therapy for measles is available, treatment consists of supportive care. The WHO recommends administration of once daily vitamin A (200,000 IU) for 2 days to all children 12 months and older with measles and 100,000 IU to children less than 12 months.[44] Susceptible individuals having had contact with a measles case patient within the 4 days before and after rash onset may have been infected and should be monitored by public health authorities for 23 days from last contact with the confirmed case. Unvaccinated contacts greater than or equal to 6 months of age who are eligible for vaccination should be vaccinated within 72 hours of exposure to prevent or reduce the risk of complications following measles infection. For contacts that have contraindications to measles vaccine, human immune globulin may be administered intramuscularly within 6 days of exposure to prevent illness or reduce its severity.[31,45]

The live attenuated measles vaccine are combined with mumps and rubella (MMR vaccine) and also with varicella (MMRV vaccine). The CDC recommends two doses of measles-containing vaccine for all children 12 months of age and older with the second dose given between the ages of 4 and 6 years.[31,46] Standard and airborne precautions should be implemented in anyone with suspected measles.[45,47] Hospitalized patients should be placed in a negative air pressure single room. Airborne transmission precautions are indicated for 4 days after the onset of rash in otherwise healthy children and for the duration of illness in immunocompromised patients. Exposed susceptible patients and health care providers without evidence of measles immunity should be offered the first dose of MMR and placed on airborne precautions from Day 5 after first exposure until 21 days following their last exposure.[45,47]

SUMMARY

Awareness of the unique aspects of diagnostic testing in the pediatric patient population is critical to the health of the individual patient and the community. As is exemplified by diagnostic strategies for detection of cCMV and CS infection, a complete understanding of the requirements for diagnosis in the mother and the fetus or neonate is necessary. Application of approaches that are effective for diagnosis of disease in adult patients can lead to confusion and error when applied to a neonate with maternal antibody present. Likewise rapid and effective diagnosis of measles requires careful consideration of the patient's age and vaccination status. This article articulates the important impact of newer approaches to laboratory diagnosis, such as nucleic acid amplification tests for diagnosis of CMV and measles, and the continued dependence on methods developed decades ago, such as RPR for diagnosis of CS. As testing methodologies change and evolve careful consideration of the unique characteristics of pediatric patients is required to provide best possible care to the littlest among us, and ensure the health of the community as a whole.

DISCLOSURE

The authors have nothing to disclose.

REFERENCES

1. Kenneson A, Cannon MJ. Review and meta-analysis of the epidemiology of congenital cytomegalovirus (CMV) infection. Rev Med Virol 2007;17:253–76.
2. van der Sande MA, Kaye S, Miles DJ, et al. Risk factors for and clinical outcomes of congenital cytomegalovirus infection in a peri-urban West-African birth cohort. PLoS One 2007;2:e492.
3. Manicklal S, Emery VC, Lazzarotto T, et al. The "silent" global burden of congenital cytomegalovirus. Clin Microbiol Rev 2013;26:86–102.
4. Picone O, Vauloup-Fellous C, Cordier AG, et al. A series of 238 cytomegalovirus primary infections during pregnancy: description and outcome. Prenat Diagn 2013;33(8):751–8.

5. Wang C, Zhang X, Bialek S, et al. Attribution of congenital cytomegalovirus infection to primary versus non-primary maternal infection. Clin Infect Dis 2011;52: e11–3.

6. Fowler KB, Boppana SB. Congenital cytomegalovirus infection. Semin Perinatol 2018;42:149–54.

7. Bodeus M, Kabamba-Mukadi B, Zech F, et al. Human cytomegalovirus in utero transmission: follow-up of 524 maternal seroconversions. J Clin Virol 2010;47: 201–2.

8. Pass RF, Fowler KB, Boppana SB, et al. Congenital cytomegalovirus infection following first trimester maternal infection: symptoms at birth and outcome. J Clin Virol 2006;35:216–20.

9. Dollard SC, Grosse SD, Ross DS. New estimates of the prevalence of neurological and sensory sequelae and mortality associated with congenital cytomegalovirus infection. Rev Med Virol 2007;17:355–63.

10. Lanzieri TM, Leung J, Caviness AC, et al. Long-term outcomes of children with symptomatic congenital cytomegalovirus disease. J Perinatol 2017;37:875–80.

11. Dreher AM, Arora N, Fowler KB, et al. Spectrum of disease and outcome in children with symptomatic congenital cytomegalovirus infection. J Pediatr 2014;164: 855–9.

12. Boppana SB, Ross SA, Fowler KB. Congenital cytomegalovirus infection: clinical outcome. Clin Infect Dis 2013;57(Suppl 4):S178–81.

13. Prince HE, Lape-Nixon M. Role of cytomegalovirus (CMV) IgG avidity testing in diagnosing primary CMV infection during pregnancy. Clin Vaccine Immunol 2014;21:1377–84.

14. Ross SA, Novak Z, Pati S, et al. Overview of the diagnosis of cytomegalovirus infection. Infect Disord Drug Targets 2011;11:466–74.

15. Luruez-Ville MSJ, Sellier Y, Guilleminot T, et al. Feasibility of predicting the outcome of fetal infection with cytomegalovirus at the time of prenatal diagnosis. Am J Obstet Gynecol 2016;215:342.e1-9.

16. Razonable RR, Hayden RT. Clinical utility of viral load in management of cytomegalovirus infection after solid organ transplantation. J Clin Microbiol 2013;26: 703–27.

17. Gantt S, Goldfarb DM, Park A, et al. Performance of the Alethia CMV assay for the detection of cytomegalovirus using neonatal saliva swabs. J Clin Microbiol 2020; 58(4):e01951-19.

18. Boppana SB, Ross SA, Novak Z, et al. Dried blood spot real time polymerase chain reaction assays to screen newborns for congenital cytomegalovirus infection. JAMA 2010;303:1375–82.

19. Kharrazi M, Hyde T, Young S, et al. Use of screening dried blood spots for estimation of prevalence, risk factors, and birth outcomes of congenital cytomegalovirus infection. J Pediatr 2010;157:191–7.

20. Kimberlin DW, Jester PM, Sanchez PJ, et al. Valganciclovir for symptomatic congenital cytomegalovirus disease. N Engl J Med 2015;372:933–43.

21. Centers for Disease Control and Prevention. Sexually transmitted disease surveillance 2018. Atlanta (GA): U.S. Department of Health and Human Services; 2019. Available at: https://www.cdc.gov/std/stats18/STDSurveillance2018-full-report.pdf.

22. World Health Organization. New estimates on congenital syphilis. 2020. Available at: https://www.who.int/reproductivehealth/congenital-syphilis-estimates/en/. Accessed January 12, 2020.

23. World Health Organization. WHO validation for the elimination of mother-to-child transmission of HIV and/or syphilis. 2020. Available at: https://www.who.int/reproductivehealth/congenital-syphilis/WHO-validation-EMTCT/en/. Accessed January 12, 2020.
24. Workowski KA, Bolan GA. Sexually transmitted diseases treatment guidelines, 2015. MMWR Morb Mortal Wkly Rep 2015;64:1–137.
25. Hollier LM, Hill J, Sheffield JS, et al. State laws regarding prenatal syphilis screening in the United States. Am J Obstet Gynecol 2003;189:1178–83.
26. Slutsker JS, Hennessy RR, Schillinger JA. Factors contributing to congenital syphilis cases—New York City, 2010-2016. MMWR Morb Mortal Wkly Rep 2018;67:1088–93.
27. Cantor AG, Pappas M, Daeges M, et al. Screening for syphilis: updated evidence report and systematic review for the U.S. Preventive Services Task Force. JAMA 2016;315:2328–37.
28. Centers for Disease Control and Prevention. Discordant results from reverse sequence syphilis screening-five laboratories—United States, 2006-2010. MMWR Morb Mortal Wkly Rep 2011;60:133–7.
29. Association of Public Health Laboratories (APHL). Suggested reporting language for syphilis serology testing. Silver Spring (MD): 2015.
30. Centers for Disease Control and Prevention. 2015 sexually transmitted diseases treatment guidelines 2015. Available at: https://www.cdc.gov/std/tg2015/congenital.htm. Accessed January 12, 2020.
31. Centers for Disease Control and Prevention. Epidemiology and prevention of vaccine-preventable diseases. 13th Edition. Washington, DC: Public Health Foundation; 2015.
32. Moss WJ. Measles. Lancet 2017;390:2490–502.
33. Richardson M, Elliman D, Maguire H, et al. Evidence base of incubation periods, periods of infectiousness and exclusion policies for the control of communicable diseases in schools and preschools. Pediatr Infect Dis J 2001;20:380–91.
34. Dabbagh A, Laws RL, Steulet C, et al. Progress toward regional measles elimination—worldwide, 2000-2017. MMWR Morb Mortal Wkly Rep 2018;67:1323.
35. World Health Organization. Measles. 2019. Available at: https://www.who.int/news-room/fact-sheets/detail/measles. Accessed November 16, 2019.
36. Paules CI, Marston HD, Fauci AS. Measles in 2019—going backward. N Engl J Med 2019;380:2185–7.
37. Patel M, Lee AD, Clemmons NS, et al. National update on measles cases and outbreaks—United States, January 1-October 1, 2019. MMWR Morb Mortal Wkly Rep 2019;68:893–6.
38. Hickman CJ, Icenogle JP. Measles and rubella viruses. In: Carroll KC, Pfaller MA LM, McAdam AJ, et al, editors. Manual of clinical microbiology. 12th edition. Washington, DC: American Society for Microbiology; 2019. p. 1560–75.
39. de Ory F, Minguito T, Balfagon P, et al. Comparison of chemiluminescent immunoassay and ELISA for measles IgG and IgM. APMIS 2015;123:648–51.
40. Hubschen JM, Bork SM, Brown KE, et al. Challenges of measles and rubella laboratory diagnostic in the era of elimination. Clin Microbiol Infect 2017;23:511–5.
41. Hickman CJ, Hyde TB, Sowers SB, et al. Laboratory characterization of measles virus infection in previously vaccinated and unvaccinated individuals. J Infect Dis 2011;204:S549–58.
42. Cohen BJ, Parry RP, Doblas D, et al. Measles immunity testing: comparison of two measles IgG ELISAs with plaque reduction neutralisation assay. J Virol Methods 2006;131:209–12.

43. World Health Organization. Manual for the laboratory diagnosis of measles and rubella virus infection. Geneva, Switzerland: World Health Organization; 2007. Available at: https://apps.who.int/iris/handle/10665/70211. Accessed December 10, 2019.

44. World Health Organization. Vaccine-preventable diseases surveillance standards: measles. 2018. Available at: https://www.who.int/immunization/monitoring_surveillance/burden/vpd/WHO_SurveillanceVaccinePreventable_11_Measles_R2.pdf. Accessed December 10. 2019.

45. American Academy of Pediatrics. Red book: report of the committee on infectious diseases. Measles. In: Kimberlin DW, Brady MT, Jackson MA, editors. Elk Grove Village (IL): American Academy of Pediatrics; 2018. p. 537–50.

46. Centers for Disease Control and Prevention. Prevention of measles, rubella, congenital rubella syndrome, and mumps, 2013: summary recommendations of the Advisory Committee on Immunization Practices (ACIP). MMWR Morb Mortal Wkly Rep 2013;62:1–34.

47. Centers for Disease Control and Prevention. Manual for the surveillance of vaccine-preventable diseases: Measles. 2019. Available at: https://www.cdc.gov/vaccines/pubs/surv-manual/chpt07-measles.html#control. Accessed December 10, 2019.

Antimicrobial Stewardship
What the Clinical Laboratory Needs to Know

Diana Alame, MD[a],*, Bryan Hess, MD[b],
Claudine El-Beyrouty, PharmD, BCPS[c]

KEYWORDS

- Antimicrobial stewardship programs • Antimicrobial misuse
- Antimicrobial resistance • Rapid diagnostics • Antibiogram • Prospective audit
- Prior authorization • Handshake stewardship

KEY POINTS

- Antimicrobial stewardship programs (ASP) promote the appropriate use of antimicrobials in order to optimize patient outcomes and reduce harm, including antimicrobial resistance.
- The Centers for Disease Control and Prevention guidelines define core elements of stewardship programs that are now part of accreditation standards and federal regulations in hospitals participating in Centers for Medicare and Medicaid Services.
- Key ASP members include infectious diseases physicians, pharmacists, clinical microbiologists, nurses, informaticists, and epidemiologists.
- Rapid diagnostics are impactful when combined with ASP in promoting clinical outcomes, and antibiogram data are essential in guiding stewardship interventions.
- ASP interventions may include prospective audit, prior authorization, and handshake stewardship.

INTRODUCTION

The discovery of antimicrobials has been an important driver for unprecedented medical and societal advances. However, evidence suggests that about 30% of all antibiotics prescribed in the US acute care hospitals are either unnecessary or inappropriate,[1,2] and their use can cause side effects and contribute to the development of resistance. Antimicrobial resistance is considered one of the greatest global

[a] Clinical Microbiology, Thomas Jefferson University Hospital, Anatomy and Cell Biology, Sidney Kimmel Medical College at Thomas Jefferson University, 117 South 11th Street, Pavilion Building, Suite 207, Philadelphia, PA 19107-4998, USA; [b] Antimicrobial Stewardship Program, Division of Infectious Diseases, Sidney Kimmel Medical College at Thomas Jefferson University, 1015 Chestnut Street, Suite 1020, Philadelphia, PA 19107, USA; [c] Infectious Diseases, Thomas Jefferson University Hospital, 111 South 11th Street, Suite 2260 Gibbon Building, Philadelphia, PA 19107, USA
* Corresponding author.
E-mail address: DIANA.ALAME@JEFFERSON.EDU

Clin Lab Med 40 (2020) 509–520
https://doi.org/10.1016/j.cll.2020.08.008
0272-2712/20/© 2020 Elsevier Inc. All rights reserved.

health challenges of our time, as it affects health care, food production, and life expectancy. The Centers for Disease Control and Prevention (CDC) estimates that more than 2.8 million antibiotic-resistant infections occur in the United States each year and more than 35,000 people die as a result.[3] Infections with antimicrobial resistant bacteria also have a significant economic impact, as they are often associated with prolonged hospital stays, additional follow-up visits, and treatments with costlier medications.

Although the terminology has evolved since it first appeared in the literature, the accepted definition of antimicrobial stewardship is those efforts related to promoting appropriate use of antimicrobials in order to optimize patient outcomes and reduce harms, including antibiotic resistance.[4] The CDC published "Core Elements" for hospital ASPs, which were later incorporated in Joint Commission accreditation standards. As of 2019, federal regulation requires implementation of ASPs in hospitals and critical access hospitals as a condition of participation in Centers for Medicare and Medicaid Services.[5] As of 2018, the CDC reported 85% of acute care hospitals as meeting all core elements, and this number will undoubtedly continue to grow in light of regulatory efforts.[1]

TEAM ROLES

National guidelines emphasize that ASP teams should be multidisciplinary and include an infectious diseases (ID) specialist, a hospital pharmacist, and a clinical microbiologist.[6] Successful collaboration depends on clear understanding of the skills each team member brings toward stewardship efforts. Key roles are thus summarized in the following section.

Physicians

Physicians are essential team members for any ASP. The ASP physician leader should be well respected in their institution, as they often serve as the "face" of the program.[7] In 2017, the Infectious Diseases Society of America (IDSA), Society for Healthcare Epidemiology of America (SHEA), and Pediatric Infectious Diseases Society released a white paper supporting ID physicians as the ideal leaders or co-leaders of an ASP. They noted that ID physicians are uniquely well equipped to lead ASPs, given their training, clinical expertise, and experience managing multidisciplinary teams as quality leaders.[8] Unfortunately, an estimated 42% of US hospitals lack on-site ID specialists, and alternative staffing models are required.[9] Hospitalists have also proved to be effective physician leaders, especially in smaller hospitals.[1]

Pharmacists

Antimicrobial stewardship is the responsibility of every pharmacist in each practice setting. However, the CDC 2019 core elements recommend that stewardship programs specifically appoint a pharmacist to function as the antibiotic expert and co-leader of the stewardship program.[1] Ideally, pharmacists should be ID trained and/or have experience in antibiotic stewardship. Several formal training and certificate programs exist to allow general clinical pharmacists to gain the necessary skills and knowledge.[6,10] Pharmacists play several roles on the ASP team, including developing antimicrobial guidelines, reviewing individual patient regimens to optimize therapy, educating health care providers on appropriate antimicrobial use, and monitoring/auditing the outcomes of antimicrobial usage.[10]

Clinical Microbiologists

Clinical microbiologists are important participants in the ASP team,[11,12] not only in providing relevant patient-specific and institution-wide data that informs clinical and stewardship policy and activity but also in acting directly in a consultative capacity. The role of microbiologists in stewardship efforts is highlighted by the CDC (**Box 1**).[1]

As clinical breakpoints are periodically updated, clinical microbiologists are essential for interpretation and implementation. Effective collaboration with the ASP, as well as other stakeholders, is critical for communicating the rationale and potential impact of such changes. Decisions on selective reporting of antibiotics and comments appended to results can further inform clinical decision-making.

Nurses

Nursing is the largest health care profession in the United States,[13] and there is growing recognition of the importance of engaging nurses in ASP activities. Nurses affect antimicrobial use through diagnostic stewardship, by knowing both the appropriate indications and proper techniques for specimen collection. Nurses can also improve the evaluation of penicillin allergies, assist with intravenous to oral transitions, and prompt antibiotic reviews with the care team. In addition, nurses can play a key role for patient education efforts.[1]

Informaticists

Informaticists play roles in both internal and external stewardship activities. Internally, informaticists support stewardship by updating the hospital electronic health record with institution-specific treatment guidelines and protocols. They develop reports and prompts in the system, which function as triggers for stewardship program review of antibiotic use. Externally, informatics helps to facilitate the reporting of antimicrobial usage data to the National Healthcare Safety Network (NHSN) Antimicrobial Use and Resistance (AUR) program.[1]

Epidemiologists

The Association for Professionals in Infection Control and Epidemiology alongside SHEA has outlined the reciprocal relationship between ASP and infection preventionists and hospital epidemiologists. ASP programs can assist infection prevention and epidemiology to identify trends and outbreaks of significant organisms. Infection prevention/epidemiology can provide support and guidance regarding surveillance of

---

Box 1
Key support offered by microbiologists in stewardship efforts

- Guide proper test utilization (diagnostic stewardship).

- Help optimize antibiotic prescribing by providing institutional antibiogram.

- Guide in implementation of rapid diagnostics and changes to susceptibility breakpoints.

- Help create guidance when testing changes take place that affect clinical decisions.

- When microbiology is an externally contracted service, ensure information is available to the institution's ASP.

Data from CDC. Core elements of hospital antibiotic stewardship programs. Available at: https://www.cdc.gov/antibiotic-use/core-elements/hospital.html. Published 2019. Accessed February 4, 2020.

syndromes of interest, drive compliance with hand hygiene, and analyze/report data on infection rates to administrators. In addition, these groups can assist with education of staff.[1,14]

TECHNOLOGY AND DATA
Role of Diagnostics

One of the most important phases of testing for obtaining the correct diagnosis occurs in the preanalytical phase, before a specimen reaches the laboratory. This phase of testing is a shared responsibility between clinicians, staff, and the laboratory. It also requires ongoing education, clear instructions that reach nursing and house staff, and frequent communication, as it has a first and direct impact on the quality of results and thus on patient care decisions, outcome, and stewardship efforts.[15] A joint guide was issued in 2018, by the IDSA and American Society for Microbiology (ASM) to assist in the proper utilization of the microbiology laboratory. Ten key points for specimen management were specified and serve to improve patient outcome and strengthen stewardship efforts (summarized in **Box 2**).[15]

Traditionally, long turnaround times (TAT) in culture and susceptibility testing made further optimization of the standard analytical and postanalytical phases difficult to achieve. Attempts to circumnavigate these limitations have a long history in the field, with automation in blood culture instruments, biochemical identification, and susceptibility testing. With the introduction of rapid molecular methods and mass spectrometry platforms, however, came a substantially expanded array of options for what improvements are possible in the realm of rapid diagnostic testing (RDT).

Given the significant morbidity associated with bloodstream infections (BSI), early attempts at RDT occurred in direct-from-blood preliminary susceptibility testing.[16–18] Although multiplex molecular diagnostic assays, now widely in use, have shortened the window for both organism identification and detection of resistance gene targets, their utility for timely decisions in escalation/deescalation of antibiotics for gram-

---

Box 2
Ten key points in specimen management recommended by the Infectious Diseases Society of America and American Society for Microbiology

- Do not send swabs; tissue, aspirates, and fluids are specimens of choice.
- Specimens should be collected before administration of antibiotic.
- Avoid contamination by ensuring appropriate collection.
- Specimens must be accurately labeled with site, and clinical information should be specified.
- Do not request or report "everything that grows."
- Poor-quality specimens must be rejected.
- The laboratory is responsible for establishing technical policy.
- The laboratory must follow its procedure manual; requests for deviation from protocol is risky.
- Susceptibility testing should only be done on clinically significant isolates.
- Reported results should be accurate, significant, and clinically relevant.

Data from Miller JM, Binnicker MJ, Campbell S, et al. A guide to utilization of the microbiology laboratory for diagnosis of infectious diseases: 2018 update by the Infectious Diseases Society of America and the American Society for Microbiology. Clin Infect Dis. 2018;67(6):e1-e94.

negative infections has been less affected due to the limitations of molecular prediction of phenotypic susceptibility.[19] This led a Clinical and Laboratory Standards Institute (CLSI) working group to consider the feasibility of a standardized disk diffusion susceptibility method direct-from-blood culture for gram-negative organisms, over 4 decades after initially being described in the literature. This methodology has the potential for a less costly approach with a wider array of gram-negative organism testing possible.

For BSI, more robust evidence exists showing improvements in appropriate antibiotic therapy, mortality, and length of stay with the use of molecular RDT.[20] A meta-analysis showed an association between molecular RDT and significant decreases in mortality only in the presence of an ASP.[21] The 2016 IDSA/SHEA guidelines recommend combining RDT with ASP interventions for BSI.[4]

A newer automated system (Accelerate PhenoTest BC Kit) combines rapid identification and phenotypic susceptibility for positive blood cultures and has been shown to improve TAT in blood culture results.[22–24] Early studies thus far have also shown potential for improvement in time to appropriate antibiotic therapy and length of stay.[25,26]

Another area where RDT coupled with ASP may serve to reduce inappropriate antibiotic usage is rapid testing for respiratory pathogens, although the data thus far have been conflicting. A recent meta-analysis reviewed clinical outcomes of multiple rapid molecular assays.[27] Although all analyzed studies showed improved TAT, and most of the studies found reduced hospital length of stay, increased appropriate use of oseltamivir, and reduced costs, no impact was seen on antibiotic use or duration. One retrospective study found an association between switching to a more rapid molecular assay (<3 hours to result) from one with a longer TAT (27.9 hours on average) and a reduction in antibiotic initiation in adult patients without focal findings on chest radiography.[28] Combination of respiratory RDT with the biomarker, procalcitonin, has shown inconsistent results, and what the impact might be in combination with ASP is still not firmly established.

ANTIBIOGRAM

The laboratory is frontline not only in detecting emerging antimicrobial resistance but also in generating timely cumulative susceptibility data. Such data serve to assist in proper choice of empirical antibiotic therapy for a given organism identification in an individual patient, inform institutional guidelines for empirical disease-specific management, and assist in infection control interventions. Reporting of the antibiogram relies on the careful prerelease analysis of the validity of the data. The CLSI guideline, M39, assists in generating accurate and standardized antibiograms.[29]

It has been previously suggested that antibiograms have value not only in clarifying susceptibility patterns within an institution but may offer interinstitutional insight.[30] One study demonstrated the feasibility of collecting and synthesizing antibiograms of 45 institutions into a regional cumulative antibiogram within one state.[31] Although promising, such compilation of antibiograms requires strict adherence to CLSI-M39 standards as well as consistent utilization of updated breakpoints, which have proved challenging for laboratories, as illustrated in past surveys.[30,32,33] Others have demonstrated utility of composite regional antibiograms after pooled testing of specific organisms in a single laboratory, which although is a potential solution for problems of inconsistency, is likely feasible only in a targeted manner.[33,34] Aggregation of data may also be more feasible in multihospital institutions with shared information technology and other resources.[12]

Combining data from external sites is also caveated in that similar institutions within a geographic area should be compared and is only appropriate if the percentage susceptibility is similar at those sites. Another issue in using antibiograms for regional public health applications is the risk of missing emergence of new resistance trends. In using the first isolate per patient per reporting period to assist in empirical approach to antibiotic therapy, subsequent changes in susceptibility for later isolates would not be evident in the data. Resistance trends analyses require a more complete dataset not delimited to the first patient isolate. In addition, recommendations are to consider adding further statistical analyses in order to more broadly generalize from the data.[29]

Decision Support Tools

The IDSA 2016 guidelines recommend incorporation of computerized clinical decision support systems (CDSS) at the time of antimicrobial prescribing. Systems should be designed to provide treatment recommendations to clinicians, based on national or local guidelines. Decision support programs targeted at prescribers have demonstrated decreases in antibiotic use, cost, length of stay, and mortality. In addition to the costs and time requirements to implement such tools, a disadvantage is the concern for "alert fatigue" on prescribers when programs generate many nonactionable alerts. Alert fatigue is defined as inadvertent disregard of alerts leading to missed opportunities for intervention.[4,35]

CDSS for ASPs have been created both by major electronic health record companies as well as by third party vendors. CDSS software analyze hospital antimicrobial information via algorithms, which result in actionable data for ASPs. These programs can alert clinicians to drug-drug interactions, dose checking, bug-drug mismatches, or opportunities for deescalation. CDSS can be customized to aid in compliance with hospital guidelines for disease states by incorporating evidence-based treatment guidelines and best practice pathways. Such customization requires close collaboration between ASPs and IT personnel.[35,36] CDSS have been shown to increase the number of charts ASPs are able to review and increase the number of antimicrobial recommendations that program personnel make leading to decreased antimicrobial use.[35] Data on the direct impact of CDSS on patient outcomes (rather than process measures) are still lacking.

TEAM ACTION

The IDSA guideline for implementation of ASPs recommend 2 main strategies as the core interventions for stewardship programs: preauthorization and prospective audit and feedback.[4]

Prospective Audit

Prospective audit with feedback, sometimes called postprescription review, entails review of antibiotic therapy by an expert in antibiotic use followed by suggestions to optimize use; this activity may occur at any point after the antimicrobial agent has been prescribed. The primary focus of prospective audit is antimicrobial deescalation—defined as a strategy to reduce spectrum of antimicrobials. Guidelines recommend daily assessment for the opportunity to deescalate antimicrobials to narrower spectrum therapy based on microbiologic and radiologic data and clinical response. The goal of deescalation is to reduce the development of bacterial resistance.[37]

Prior Authorization

Prior authorization, also called preauthorization, requires prescribers to gain approval to use certain antimicrobials before initiating therapy. Prior authorization may be implemented in several ways (ie, telephone approval, electronic antibiotic order forms, etc.), however without leading to delays in therapy for serious infections. Personnel must be available in real time; often programs allow overnight administration of restricted antibiotics pending approval the following day.[4]

Prospective audit allows for a collaborative relationship between front line providers and the ASP team. Interventions can have a greater focus on de-escalation and duration of therapy. However, compliance with prospective audit recommendations is voluntary and it takes longer to achieve reductions in antibiotic use. IT support may be needed to set up tools for the ASP team to identify patients requiring review. Prior authorization ensures the appropriateness of empiric therapy and provides more direct control over antibiotic use, decreasing use of high cost agents. However, it has less impact on de-escalation and often results in a shift of antibiotic prescribing patterns to unrestricted drugs which may not be appropriate. Front line providers report a loss of autonomy under prior authorization programs.

Few studies have compared prospective audit and prior authorization directly. In a quasi-experimental crossover trial, there were greater decreases in antibiotic use (as measured by days of therapy) with postprescription review with feedback compared with preprescription authorization.[38]

Handshake Stewardship

Handshake stewardship entails active engagement of frontline providers by providing face-to-face feedback.[1] It differs from prospective audit and prior authorization in 3 ways:

o Lack of restriction and preauthorization.
o Review of all prescribed antimicrobials.
o Rounding-based in-person approach with feedback provided by a pharmacist-physician team.

Although this method is more resource intensive, it allows a more collaborative relationship between ASP and front-line providers.[39]

Disease State Surveillance

Disease state surveillance is also called infection-based interventions. The 3 most frequently targeted infections are lower respiratory tract infection, urinary tract infection, and skin and soft tissue infection. Interventions may focus on diagnosis, deescalation of antibiotic therapy based on culture results, and/or optimization of treatment duration.[1] Specific examples include development of antibiotic guidelines for sepsis based on local microbiology data, recommendations to stop unnecessary antibiotics in patients with *Clostridium difficile* infections, and requirement for ID consultation for patients with *Staphylococcus aureus* BSI.[1]

Education

The ASP should educate prescribers, pharmacists, and nurses about adverse reactions from antibiotics, antibiotic resistance, and optimal prescribing.[1] Teams may elect to use a broad range of educational modalities, including didactic lectures, flyers and newsletters, program Websites, and case-based education. Preauthorization, prospective audit, and handshake stewardship all provide opportunities for clinician education. Physicians, nurses, and pharmacists can also perform patient education. Patients should know what antibiotics were prescribed, why they were prescribed, and what potential adverse effects may occur. Community education regarding the importance of appropriate antimicrobial use and the global impact of antimicrobial resistance is also important.

PERFORMANCE METRICS AND SELF-EVALUATION

ASP metrics include both process and outcome measures. Frequently used process measures include compliance with hospital treatment guidelines and assessment of the types of interventions performed by ASP personnel. Outcome measures include both patient clinical outcomes, antibiotic resistance, and antibiotic use.[1]

The IDSA 2016 guidelines recommend days of therapy (DOT) as the preferred metric for measuring antibiotic use. DOT is a metric based on patient level data for both adult and pediatric populations. Institutions should use DOT as both an internal monitor and for interfacility comparisons.[4] The CDC recommends hospitals submit data electronically to the NHSN AU option. These data are used to monitor antibiotic use nationally and to allow hospitals to benchmark their inpatient antibiotic use against comparable institutions.[1]

Measuring financial outcomes (such as antibiotic costs) can help demonstrate the value of ASP and secure resources. Antibiotic costs should be expected to decrease initially after the implementation of an ASP and stabilize after several years but can increase again if ASPs are discontinued.[1]

IMPACT OF ANTIMICROBIAL STEWARDSHIP PROGRAMS

Measuring the impact of ASP interventions on antibiotic resistance is challenging and has generated mixed results.[40] In general, interventions have been shown to decrease overall antimicrobial use, increase appropriate antimicrobial use, reduce health care costs, and reduce antimicrobial resistance, all while improving patient outcomes and safety.[40] Importantly, interventions have not been associated with negative impacts on mortality, length of stay, or readmission rates. Effective ASPs have been associated with improved rates of C difficile infection and decreased rates of health care–associated infections with resistant gram-negative pathogens.[37,41–44]

FUTURE DIRECTION

The need for a greater ASP footprint in improving antibiotic prescribing in all health care settings is critical. Patients in nursing homes, skilled postacute care facilities, and long-term acute care hospitals are frequently prescribed antibiotics. Up to 70% of residents in a nursing home receive one or more courses of antibiotics over a given year, and 40% to 75% of these antibiotics are either unnecessary or inappropriate.[45] An expanded presence of ASP is also required in primary care clinics, specialty care clinics, urgent care clinics, and emergency departments, as approximately 60% of US antibiotic expenditures for humans are related to outpatient care.[46] Each of these settings provides unique challenges for ASPs. Looking ahead, there exists potential in the utilization of telemedicine, including teleconsultation and remote stewardship monitoring.[47]

SUMMARY

A commonly heard and succinct expression is that ASPs promote the use of the right antibiotic, for the right patient, at the right time, with the right dose, and the right route, causing the least harm to the patient and future patients. ASPs use a multidisciplinary collaborative approach, and each ASP member must understand the valuable role they play. The success of the initiative at each institution requires a clear understanding of the available technology, sources of data, and possible actions an ASP may take in aligning with regulatory and clinical standards. A critical need remains in expanding ASP initiatives to other care settings and opportunities exist in the emerging field of telemedicine.

DISCLOSURE

The authors have nothing to disclose.

REFERENCES

1. CDC. Core elements of hospital antibiotic stewardship programs. Atlanta (GA): US Department of Health and Human Services, CDC; 2019. Available at: https://www.cdc.gov/antibiotic-use/core-elements/hospital.html. Accessed February 4, 2020.
2. Fridkin S, Baggs J, Fagan R, et al. Vital signs: improving antibiotic use among hospitalized patients. MMWR Morb Mortal Wkly Rep 2014;63(9):194–200.
3. CDC. Antibiotic resistance threats in the United States, 2019. Atlanta (GA): U.S. Department of Health and Human Services, CDC; 2019. Available at: https://www.cdc.gov/DrugResistance/Biggest-Threats.html. Accessed February 10, 2020.
4. Barlam TF, Cosgrove SE, Abbo LM, et al. Implementing an antibiotic stewardship program: guidelines by the Infectious Diseases Society of America and the society for healthcare epidemiology of America. Clin Infect Dis 2016;62(10):e51–77.
5. Centers for Medicare & Medicade Services. Medicare and Medicaid programs; regulatory provisions to promote program efficiency, transparency, and burden reduction; fire safety requirements for certain dialysis facilities; hospital and critical access hospital (CAH) changes to promote innovation, flexibility, and improvement in patient care. Fed Regist 2019;84:189. Available at: https://federalregister.gov/d/2019-20736. Accessed February 4, 2020.
6. Heil EL, Kuti JL, Bearden DT, et al. The essential role of pharmacists in antimicrobial stewardship. Infect Control Hosp Epidemiol 2016;37(7):753–4.
7. Buckel WR, Cosgrove SE. Structure of an antibiotic stewardship team and core competencies. In: Barlam TF, Neuhauser MM, Tamma PD, et al, editors. Practical implementation of an antibiotic stewardship program. Cambridge, UK: Cambridge University Press; 2018. p. 24–5.
8. Ostrowsky B, Banerjee R, Bonomo RA, et al. Infectious diseases physicians: leading the way in antimicrobial stewardship. Clin Infect Dis 2018;66(7):995–1003.
9. Septimus EJ, Owens RC. Need and potential of antimicrobial stewardship in community hospitals. Clin Infect Dis 2011;53(Suppl 1):S8–14.
10. Garau J, Bassetti M. Role of pharmacists in antimicrobial stewardship programmes. Int J Clin Pharm 2018;40(5):948–52.
11. Thomson RB, Doern GV. What will the role of the clinical microbiology laboratory director be in 2015? J Clin Microbiol 2011;49(9 Supplement):S68–71.
12. Morency-Potvin P, Schwartz DN, Weinstein RA. Antimicrobial stewardship: how the microbiology laboratory can right the ship. Clin Microbiol Rev 2017;30(1):381–407.

13. American Association of Colleges of Nursing (AACN) > News & information > Fact sheets > Nursing fact sheet. Available at: https://www.aacnnursing.org/News-Information/Fact-Sheets/Nursing-Fact-Sheet. Accessed February 18, 2020.

14. Moody J, Cosgrove SE, Olmsted R, et al. Antimicrobial stewardship: a collaborative partnership between infection preventionists and healthcare epidemiologists. Infect Control Hosp Epidemiol 2012;33(4):328–30.

15. Miller JM, Binnicker MJ, Campbell S, et al. A guide to utilization of the microbiology laboratory for diagnosis of infectious diseases: 2018 update by the Infectious Diseases Society of America and the American Society for Microbiology. Clin Infect Dis 2018;67(6):e1–94.

16. Mirrett S, Reller LB. Comparison of direct and standard antimicrobial disk susceptibility testing for bacteria isolated from blood. J Clin Microbiol 1979;10(4):482–7.

17. Fay D, Oldfather JE. Standardization of direct susceptibility test for blood cultures. J Clin Microbiol 1979;9(3):347–50.

18. Coyle MB, McGonagle LA, Plorde JJ, et al. Rapid antimicrobial susceptibility testing of isolates from blood cultures by direct inoculation and early reading of disk diffusion tests. J Clin Microbiol 1984;20(3):473–7.

19. Chandrasekaran S, Abbott A, Campeau S, et al. Direct-from-Blood-Culture disk diffusion to determine antimicrobial susceptibility of gram-negative bacteria: preliminary report from the clinical and laboratory standards Institute methods development and standardization working group. J Clin Microbiol 2018;56(3). https://doi.org/10.1128/JCM.01678-17.

20. Zeitler K, Narayanan N. The present and future state of antimicrobial stewardship and rapid diagnostic testing: can one ideally succeed without the other? Curr Treat Options Infect Dis 2019;11(2):177–87.

21. Timbrook TT, Morton JB, McConeghy KW, et al. The effect of molecular rapid diagnostic testing on clinical outcomes in bloodstream infections: a systematic review and meta-analysis. Clin Infect Dis 2017;64(1):15–23.

22. Marschal M, Bachmaier J, Autenrieth I, et al. Evaluation of the accelerate pheno system for fast identification and antimicrobial susceptibility testing from positive blood cultures in bloodstream infections caused by gram-negative pathogens. J Clin Microbiol 2017;55(7):2116–26.

23. Charnot-Katsikas A, Tesic V, Love N, et al. Use of the accelerate pheno system for identification and antimicrobial susceptibility testing of pathogens in positive blood cultures and impact on time to results and workflow. J Clin Microbiol 2018;56(1). https://doi.org/10.1128/JCM.01166-17.

24. Pancholi P, Carroll KC, Buchan BW, et al. Multicenter evaluation of the accelerate phenotest BC kit for rapid identification and phenotypic antimicrobial susceptibility testing using morphokinetic cellular analysis. J Clin Microbiol 2018;56(4). https://doi.org/10.1128/JCM.01329-17.

25. Elliott G, Malczynski M, Barr VO, et al. Evaluation of the impact of the Accelerate Pheno™ system on time to result for differing antimicrobial stewardship intervention models in patients with gram-negative bloodstream infections. BMC Infect Dis 2019;19(1):942.

26. Henig O, Cooper CC, Kaye KS, et al. The hypothetical impact of Accelerate Pheno™ system on time to effective therapy and time to definitive therapy in an institution with an established antimicrobial stewardship programme currently utilizing rapid genotypic organism/resistance marker identification. J Antimicrob Chemother 2019;74(Supplement_1):i32–9.

27. Vos LM, Bruning AHL, Reitsma JB, et al. Rapid molecular tests for influenza, respiratory syncytial virus, and other respiratory viruses: a systematic review of diagnostic accuracy and clinical impact studies. Clin Infect Dis 2019;69(7):1243–53.
28. Weiss ZF, Cunha CB, Chambers AB, et al. Opportunities revealed for antimicrobial stewardship and clinical practice with implementation of a rapid respiratory multiplex assay. J Clin Microbiol 2019;57(10). https://doi.org/10.1128/JCM.00861-19.
29. CLSI. Analysis and presentation of cumulative antimicrobial susceptibility test data; approved guideline - fourth edition. CLSI document M39-A4. Wayne (PA): Clinical and Laboratory Standards Institute.; 2014.
30. Avdic E, Carroll KC. The role of the microbiology laboratory in antimicrobial stewardship programs. Infect Dis Clin North Am 2014;28(2):215–35.
31. Guarascio AJ, Brickett LM, Porter TJ, et al. Development of a statewide antibiogram to assess regional trends in antibiotic-resistant ESKAPE organisms. J Pharm Pract 2019;32(1):19–27.
32. Humphries RM, Hindler JA, Epson E, et al. Carbapenem-resistant enterobacteriaceae detection practices in California: what are we missing? Clin Infect Dis 2018;66(7):1061–7.
33. Durante AJ, Maloney M, Leung VH, et al. Expanded susceptibility and resistance mechanism testing among carbapenem-resistant Enterobacteriaceae through a statewide antibiogram, a clinical and public health partnership. Infect Control Hosp Epidemiol 2019;40(9):1071–3.
34. Humphries R, Mendez J, Miller LG, et al. The regional antibiogram is an important public health tool to improve empiric antibiotic selection, stenotrophomonas maltophilia as A case example. Open Forum Infect Dis 2017;4(suppl_1):S258.
35. Forrest GN, Van Schooneveld TC, Kullar R, et al. Use of electronic health records and clinical decision support systems for antimicrobial stewardship. Clin Infect Dis 2014;59(Suppl 3):S122–33.
36. Kullar R, Goff DA, Schulz LT, et al. The "epic" challenge of optimizing antimicrobial stewardship: the role of electronic medical records and technology. Clin Infect Dis 2013;57(7):1005–13.
37. Tabah A, Cotta MO, Garnacho-Montero J, et al. A systematic review of the definitions, determinants, and clinical outcomes of antimicrobial de-escalation in the intensive care unit. Clin Infect Dis 2016;62(8):1009–17.
38. Tamma PD, Avdic E, Keenan JF, et al. What is the more effective antibiotic stewardship intervention: preprescription authorization or postprescription review with feedback? Clin Infect Dis 2017;64(5):537–43.
39. Baker DW, Hyun D, Neuhauser MM, et al. Leading practices in antimicrobial stewardship: conference summary. Jt Comm J Qual Patient Saf 2019;45(7):517–23.
40. Spivak ES, Hicks LA, Srinivasan A. The need for antibiotic stewardship programs. In: Barlam TF, Neuhauser MM, Tamma PD, et al, editors. Practical implementation of an antibiotic stewardship program. Cambridge, UK: Cambridge University Press; 2018. p. 5–6.
41. Carling P, Fung T, Killion A, et al. Favorable impact of a multidisciplinary antibiotic management program conducted during 7 years. Infect Control Hosp Epidemiol 2003;24(9):699–706.
42. Valiquette L, Cossette B, Garant M-P, et al. Impact of a reduction in the use of high-risk antibiotics on the course of an epidemic of Clostridium difficile-associated disease caused by the hypervirulent NAP1/027 strain. Clin Infect Dis 2007;45(Suppl 2):S112–21.

43. Davey P, Marwick CA, Scott CL, et al. Interventions to improve antibiotic prescribing practices for hospital inpatients. Cochrane Database Syst Rev 2017;(2):CD003543.
44. Karanika S, Paudel S, Grigoras C, et al. Systematic review and meta-analysis of clinical and economic outcomes from the implementation of hospital-based antimicrobial stewardship programs. Antimicrob Agents Chemother 2016;60(8): 4840–52.
45. CDC. The core elements of antibiotic stewardship for nursing homes. Atlanta (GA): US Department of Health and Human Services, CDC; 2015. Available at: http://www.cdc.gov/longtermcare/index/html. Accessed February 18, 2020.
46. Suda KJ, Hicks LA, Roberts RM, et al. Antibiotic expenditures by medication, class, and healthcare setting in the United States, 2010-2015. Clin Infect Dis 2018;66(2):185–90.
47. Sanchez GV, Fleming-Dutra KE, Roberts RM, et al. Core elements of outpatient antibiotic stewardship. MMWR Recomm Rep 2016;65(6):1–12.

Fellowship Training for the Future Clinical Microbiology Laboratory Director

Bobbi S. Pritt, MD, MSc[a,b,]*, Carrie A. Bowler, MS[b], Elitza S. Theel, PhD[a]

KEYWORDS

- Graduate Medical Education • Clinical Microbiology • Fellowship • Public Health
- Training

KEY POINTS

- Clinical microbiology laboratory directors play an essential role in ensuring high-quality, relevant, cost-effective, and safe diagnostic testing, compliant across regulatory bodies.
- Medical and public health microbiology (MPHM) fellowship training plays a highly valuable role in preparing future clinical microbiology laboratory directors for their leadership and management responsibilities.
- Given the continually evolving MPHM field, fellowships must remain adaptable to such changes and advances, providing trainees with the opportunity to engage with newly emerging diagnostic modalities, while continuing to emphasize the "bread and butter" techniques of clinical microbiology.

INTRODUCTION

The clinical microbiology laboratory occupies an essential role in the health care system, contributing to the diagnosis, treatment, prevention, and control of infectious diseases.[1] Full-service laboratories provide a broad spectrum of low, moderate, and high complexity tests for the detection and characterization of bacterial, viral, fungal, and parasitic pathogens using conventional and advanced diagnostic techniques. Testing services directly support patient care, guide institutional antimicrobial stewardship efforts,[2] sustain systems for infectious disease surveillance,[3] aid in the detection of

Funding: The authors receive internal funding from Mayo Clinic.
[a] Department of Laboratory Medicine and Pathology, Division of Clinical Microbiology, Mayo Clinic, 200 1st Street Southwest, Rochester, MN 55905, USA; [b] Department of Laboratory Medicine and Pathology, Graduate Medical Education, Mayo Clinic, 200 1st Street Southwest, Rochester, MN 55905, USA
* Corresponding author. Department of Laboratory Medicine and Pathology, Division of Clinical Microbiology, Mayo Clinic, 200 1st Street Southwest, Rochester, MN 55905.
E-mail address: Pritt.bobbi@mayo.edu
Twitter: @ParasiteGal (B.S.P.); @cabowler1 (C.A.B.); @ElliTheelPhD (E.S.T.)

outbreaks, and support public health disease reporting. Collectively, these services directly support patient care, while also shaping policy and practice decisions across the institutions and communities that it serves.

Given the complexity and scope of services provided, it is essential that the clinical microbiology laboratory director have the skills, knowledge, and experience needed to carry out their responsibilities in support of the institution's mission. These responsibilities are numerous[4] and are outlined at the most basic level by Standard 493 Subpart M of the Clinical Laboratory Improvement Amendments (CLIA) of 1988 in its description of *Technical Supervisor* responsibilities for non-waived testing.[5] First and foremost, the clinical microbiology laboratory director (ie, CLIA technical supervisor) serves as an essential member of the clinical care team, ensuring that the laboratory provides high-quality, timely, relevant, cost-effective, and safe testing in compliance with local and federal regulatory bodies. In this role, the laboratory director defines the scope and contents of the laboratory test menu, establishes or verifies test performance characteristics before clinical implementation, designs and implements a quality management system to ensure ongoing accurate and timely test results, and provides consultative services to aid in test selection, specimen collection, and result interpretation. The laboratory director also works with other members of the patient care team to create testing algorithms, design and implement microbial screening protocols, and coordinate public health reporting. Finally, the laboratory director takes on a myriad of other less-defined but essential roles and responsibilities, such as representing the laboratory on institutional committees (eg, antimicrobial stewardship committee, hospital infection prevention, and control committee), conducting clinically relevant research, and providing clinical microbiology education to trainees, laboratory staff, and other members of the health care team.

To qualify as a clinical microbiology laboratory director in the United States, individuals must fulfill specific educational requirements and have appropriate training and/or experience.[5] Although completion of a clinical microbiology fellowship is not an absolute requirement for the role, the authors believe that the specialized training provided by a fellowship is exceedingly beneficial for preparing future laboratory directors for their responsibilities and is highly valued by potential employers. In this article, the authors discuss the essential components of a clinical microbiology fellowship and share best practices gleaned from their combined 68 years of operating 2 doctoral-level clinical microbiology fellowships at Mayo Clinic, Minnesota. Although the focus is on the training provided in the United States, the general principles discussed herein are applicable to clinical microbiology laboratory director training programs worldwide.

OVERVIEW OF FELLOWSHIP PROGRAMS

There are 2 types of formal, medical and public health microbiology (MPHM) fellowship programs in the United States. Although each has slightly different requirements, the training provided and postgraduation qualifications have many similarities. Both aim to train postdoctoral level graduates to become successful clinical microbiologists, able to run a clinical or public health microbiology laboratory. Alternatively, graduates may find employment in industry, as scientific or research leaders for the development of diagnostic assays or equipment, or they may pursue roles in government agencies associated with public health (eg, Centers for Disease Control and Prevention [CDC]) or with oversight of diagnostic products or regulation of clinical laboratories (eg, Food and Drug Administration [FDA], Centers for Medicare and

Medicaid Services). The following sections discuss important details of each fellowship pathway.

Accreditation Council of Graduate Medical Education for Committee Pathology

The Accreditation Council of Graduate Medical Education (ACGME) provides accreditation for fellowship programs in medical microbiology, as well as 9 other subspecialties under the medical specialty of pathology.[6] Fellowships must be 12 months in length and are typically located at large hospitals or academic medical centers. There are currently 15 ACGME-accredited medical microbiology fellowship programs in the United States, the details for which can be found on the ACGME Website.[6] Application to these fellowships is limited to physicians who have successfully completed training in specific pathology or infectious diseases training programs accredited by the ACGME, ACGME-International, American Osteopathic Association, Royal College of Physicians and Surgeons, or College of Family Physicians of Canada.[6] Special exceptions to these eligibility requirements may be considered for exceptionally qualified applicants. Following completion of an ACGME-accredited medical microbiology fellowship, graduates are eligible to take the subspecialty board examination through the American Board of Pathology, a member board of the American Board of Medical Specialties.[7] Graduates are also eligible to take the American Board of Medical Microbiology (ABMM) examination, which "certifies doctoral-level microbiologists to direct medical and public health microbiology laboratories."[8]

Medical and Public Health Microbiology Fellowship Programs Endorsed by the Committee on Postgraduate Educational Programs

The Committee on Postgraduate Educational Programs (CPEP) is authorized by the American Society for Microbiology (ASM) to oversee 2 different postgraduate education programs, one concentrated on Medical Immunology, and the other on MPHM. Focusing on MPHM programs, these are 2 years in duration and are typically located at large hospitals or academic medical centers. There are currently 18 MPHM programs accredited by the CPEP across the United States, details of which can be found on the ASM Website.[9]

Application to CPEP-accredited MPHM fellowships is open to most postdoctoral level graduates, including those with a PhD, MD, ScD, DO, or a DrPH; individuals with a Doctorate of Clinical Laboratory Sciences or those with a Doctorate of Pharmacology do not currently meet CPEP eligibility criteria. In addition, each fellowship may have program-specific requirements (eg, external funding) or eligibility criteria (eg, visa requirements), which applicants should be cognizant of, alongside the varied program cycles and application deadlines among fellowships, with some programs interviewing for positions over 1 year in advance of the start date. Although each MPHM program has their own unique applicant evaluation criteria, common areas of overlap include a focus on microbiology or a related discipline (not necessarily clinical), budding academic achievement, including presentation at regional or national scientific conferences, and exhibiting efforts to interact with the clinical microbiology field (eg, meeting with a local clinical microbiologist, attending rounds, or completing a rotation in a clinical microbiology laboratory, etc.). Although differences across the 18 MPHM fellowship programs exist with respect to a variety of training aspects, including the methods and types of diagnostic assays maintained by the laboratory, on-call responsibilities, and the level of emphasis on research/assay development projects, they all meet *at least* the "minimum standards of quality in education programs" required for CPEP accreditation.[10] These CPEP criteria, referred to as the *Essentials*, are mandatory for accredited programs to adhere to and cover all required aspects of a clinical microbiology training program, including setting the curriculum, establishing the methodologies trainees should be exposed to, outlining important laboratory management concepts, defining fellowship director responsibilities, and delineating reaccreditation requirements, among others. As a result of the CPEP *Essentials*, trainees can be assured that irrespective of which CPEP-accredited program they enter, the educational curriculum and expectations are standardized across the MPHM fellowships. Finally, to ensure that accredited programs maintain adherence to these *Essentials*, reaccreditation of each MPHM fellowship occurs every 7 years and includes an on-site inspection by a member of the CPEP committee.

Following completion of a CPEP MPHM fellowship, graduates are eligible to take the ABMM examination to gain qualifications for directing a medical or public health microbiology laboratory.

IMPORTANCE OF DEFINING THE PROGRAM MISSION AND AIMS

To enhance transparency of the fellowship program both within the institution and externally, development of a program mission statement and supporting aims are essential, as they define the program's purpose, scope of training, and the prospective applicants.

Mission Statement

Simply defined, a mission statement is a "formal summary of the aims and values" of a particular group.[11] They are used by companies and organizations to convey their overall purpose, identifying the scope, services, intended users, and internal guiding principles to the interested public. For accredited fellowships, a well-defined mission statement can be used to succinctly frame the program's objectives. As an example, the following mission statement is currently used for both the CPEP- and ACGME-accredited MPHM fellowship programs at Mayo Clinic:

> *Develop post-graduate trainees into self-sufficient, academically productive, lifelong learning, board-certified clinical microbiologists, who are fully prepared to provide the full spectrum of diagnostic testing and interpretive guidance to clinicians to meet the needs of their patients.*

Program Aims

Stemming from the mission statement, program aims serve the purpose of conveying how the program will carry out the organization's mission. They provide a well-defined framework of the program's and institution's expectations and define the intended learning outcomes, with measurable actions. Examples of currently used aims for both the CPEP- and ACGME-accredited MPHM programs at Mayo Clinic include:

1. Foster an environment of learning and mentorship that prepares trainees to contribute to and advance the field of medical and public health microbiology.
   a. Activities/Criteria to Advance the Aim:
      1. All trainees will publish or submit for publication at least one peer-reviewed article, review article, or book chapter during their fellowship or within 1 year of graduation from the program.
      2. All trainees will participate in diagnostic assay development or an alternative MPHM-related research project during their fellowship.
2. Provide a clinical and didactic learning environment that supports the educational needs of all trainees.
   a. Activities/Criteria to Advance the Aim:

1. The fellowship program will provide at least 200 hours of didactic content related to MPHM to all trainees.
2. The fellowship program will provide experiences in all specialty areas of clinical microbiology (eg, bacteriology, mycobacteriology, virology, mycology, parasitology, infectious diseases serology, public health microbiology, epidemiology, etc.) and in select areas of the Infectious Diseases clinical practice (eg, antimicrobial stewardship, infection prevention and control, rotation with infectious diseases services, etc.).
3. Produce future leaders in medical and public health microbiology.
   a. Activities/Criteria to Advance the Aim:
      1. All trainees will present a poster or oral presentation at least once before graduation at a regional, national, or international conference.
      2. At least half of all program graduates will assume a leadership role (eg, laboratory or associate laboratory director, senior scientist in industry, etc.) within 5 years of graduation from the fellowship

SCOPE OF TRAINING
Clinical and Analytical Microbiology

At their core, accredited programs are designed to provide in-depth training focused on pathogen identification strategies and interpretive guidance for acquired results in all areas of clinical microbiology. These programs also provide trainees the opportunity to practice these learned skills in a supportive and safe environment, through interactions with laboratory directors, laboratory technologists, patient-facing clinicians, and other trainees. Generally, the training areas include the following:

- Bacteriology
- Mycobacteriology
- Mycology
- Virology
- Parasitology
- Infectious diseases serology
- Public health microbiology
- Fundamentals of pathogenesis
- Infection prevention and control
- Laboratory leadership and management (see later discussion)
- Laboratory biosafety and biosecurity
- Laboratory regularly oversight
- Antimicrobial stewardship

The field of MPHM is continually evolving, with optimization of classic techniques and introduction of novel methods occurring constantly. Given these advancements, it is essential that accredited programs provide trainees with the opportunity to engage with as many of the newly emerging diagnostic modalities as possibly, while continuing to emphasize the "bread and butter" techniques of clinical microbiology. Education related to the following diagnostic modalities should be included in any accredited MPHM program:

- Specimen collection, collection devices, and transport/storage conditions
- Direct-from-specimen or culture stains
- Bacterial, mycobacterial, fungal liquid, and solid media culture methods
- Common biochemical reactions for microbial identification
- Antimicrobial susceptibility testing

- Matrix-assisted laser desorption-ionization time-of-flight mass spectrometry
- Molecular diagnostics
  - Automated extraction platforms
  - Nonamplifying methods
  - Nucleic acid amplification methods
  - Traditional (Sanger) sequencing
  - Next-generation sequencing techniques and associated bioinformatics pipelines
- Common and esoteric serologic tests for antibody and antigen detection
- Familiarity with common molecular and serologic automated instruments
- Laboratory automation and information systems
- Infectious disease rapid diagnostic assays available at the point of care
- Infectious diseases histopathology (see Infectious Disease Histopathology)

The educational techniques used to relay these concepts should range beyond classic didactic lectures and bench work, to include increasingly hands-on, problem solving opportunities as the fellow advances in his/her training. Similarly, fellows should be given graduated responsibility as they demonstrate competence in key training milestones (see Assessment and Feedback). Commonly used educational methods of successful programs, in addition to didactic lessons, include the following:

- Guided self-learning using laboratory director–recommended reading
- Group discussion (fellow or director-lead) of reading materials
- On-call responsibilities, including clinical consultation
- Presentation at laboratory rounds (ie, "plate" rounds)
- Case-based oral presentations by fellows
- Journal club discussions led by fellows
- Rotation-specific case review sets
- Laboratory directorship rotation (see Leadership and Management Training)

Finally, equally important to mastering content related to pathogen detection, identification, and interpretation of clinical significance, is comprehension of all aspects related to diagnostic assay development, evaluation, validation, and verification. An understanding of the different regulatory classifications of diagnostic assays (eg, Food and Drug Administration [FDA]-waived, FDA-cleared, FDA-approved, laboratory-developed tests, etc.), the different requirements for validation and/or verification studies (eg, accuracy, precision, reference range, reportable range, analytical sensitivity, analytical specificity, etc.), and how to select, evaluate, and implement an assay into the clinical laboratory workflow is essential. Ideally, MPHM programs will offer trainees opportunities to participate in assay development or implementation activities as they become available.

Leadership and Management Training

Training fellows to become future leaders is an essential role of all MPHM fellow programs and should therefore be approached in a thoughtful and deliberate manner, similar to other aspects of their training. To specifically focus on this area, one approach the MPHM programs at Mayo Clinic have taken is to require trainee attendance of a monthly, full-day course on relevant leadership and management topics covering accreditation, reimbursement, human resources, diversity and inclusion, finance, laboratory informatics, and the quality system essentials. During this course, trainees also complete a quality improvement project, which they entirely envision, complete, and present on, to both the affected laboratory and class faculty. Aside from this dedicated course, fellows participate in monthly small group discussions on microbiology-specific quality management topics, participate in the critical analysis of laboratory errors/events, and complete a 1 month or longer laboratory directorship rotation.

Infectious Diseases Histopathology

Although not a standard part of all training programs, basic knowledge of how bacteria, fungi, viruses, and parasites appear in histopathology preparations is a useful skill for clinical microbiology laboratory directors. Feedback from Mayo Clinic's MPHM program graduates indicate that many are commonly asked to look at histopathology preparations, despite the lack of dedicated pathology training. To address this need, the Mayo Clinic programs have incorporated a monthly slide-based conference for all MPHM fellows covering a spectrum of common infectious entities, as well as important esoteric microorganisms in histopathology preparations. Fellows are also regularly shown routine clinical cases from the Mayo Clinic Infectious Diseases pathology consult service. For programs in which this type of training is not available, graduates should be made aware of the valuable online resources such as formal consultative services offered through the CDC's Infectious Diseases Pathology Branch (https://www.cdc.gov/ncezid/dhcpp/idpb/specimen-submission/index.html) and the Division of Parasitic Diseases and Malaria (https://www.cdc.gov/dpdx/dxassistance.html). Informal opinions on current cases can also be rapidly obtained from members of ASM's listserv, ClinMicroNet (see later discussion).

External Resources for Training

Although CPEP- and ACMGE-accredited programs will have a well-curated repository of didactic (eg, library of relevant MPHM manuals, textbooks, etc.) and hands-on training materials (eg, fixed and stained slides, specimens, etc.), external resources are also frequently accessed and used for educational purposes. Although not an exhaustive list, the resources in **Table 1** offer additional case-based educational or training opportunities.

Finally, social media and blog Websites are providing increased access to MPHM educational content. However, it is important for programs to critically vet any site for content accuracy. **Table 2** is a select listing of several social media, listservs and blog sites that are frequented by the MPHM community.

LEARNER ASSESSMENT

Assessment is critical to the development of a learner and provides a substantial source of data for program evaluation purposes.[12] The terms "assessment" and "evaluation" are frequently used interchangeably, yet are distinct entities. Assessment is focused on the *learner*, helping inform them on how well they are doing, whereas evaluation is focused on *program-related activities* to inform training outcomes.[13,14] Both learner assessment and program evaluation make use of formative and summative practices.

Formative practices are focused on the real-time provision of feedback for immediate improvement, whereas summative practices are meant to provide a final determination, without the ability to demonstrate improvement.[13] The process of formative assessment provides faculty members the opportunity to understand a learner's knowledge acquisition and comprehension, provide feedback, and subsequently tailor an optimized plan to achieve the intended learning outcomes.[12] Formative assessments are measures *for* learning and therefore occur before and during the

Table 1 Education and training resources		
Organization	**Selected Topics**	**Website/Resource**
American Society for Microbiology (ASM)	• Variety of MPHM webinars and journal clubs available for purchase or free to ASM members	https://www.asm.org/
Association of Public Health Laboratories (APHL)	• Essentials for Mycobacteriology • Introduction to Laboratory Informatics • Specimen Packaging and Shipping • Biothreat Preparedness for *Bacillus anthracis, Brucella* spp., *Burkholderia* spp., *Yersinia pestis, Francisella tularensis,* etc.	https://www.aphl.org/training/Pages/online.aspx
College of American Pathologists (CAP)	• Information related to CAP Laboratory Accreditation • Information related to Proficiency Testing	https://www.cap.org/laboratory-improvement/accreditation https://www.cap.org/laboratory-improvement/proficiency-testing
Centers for Disease Control and Prevention (CDC)	• Packing and Shipping Materials: What the Laboratory Professional Should Know	https://www.cdc.gov/labtraining/training-courses/packing-shipping-division-6.2-materials.html
	• Basic to intermediate courses on a variety of clinical microbiology topics ranging from culture and identification techniques, to molecular assays, biothreat preparedness, and working in biological safety cabinets, among others	https://www.cdc.gov/labtraining/index.html
	• General list of MPHM training/educational material offered through the CDC or CDC partner organizations	https://www.cdc.gov/learning/training-resources/index.html
	• Laboratory Identification of Parasites of Public Health Concern (DPDx)	https://www.cdc.gov/dpdx/index.html
	• Information related to the Clinical Laboratory Improvement Amendments (CLIA)	https://www.cdc.gov/clia/about.html

(continued on next page)

Table 1
(continued)

Organization	Selected Topics	Website/Resource
Centers for Medicare and Medicaid Services (CMS)	• Information related to CLIA	https://www.cms.gov/Regulations-and-Guidance/Legislation/CLIA/index?redirect=/clia/
Clinical Laboratory Standards Institute (CLSI)	• Access to antimicrobial susceptibility testing and other diagnostic microbiology standards and related education webinars	https://clsi.org/
Emory Pathology e-Learning Portal	• Case-based quiz modules for bacteria, mycobacteria, fungi, parasites, and viruses	http://www.path.emory.edu/EPeP/microbiology.cfm
Pan American Society for Clinical Virology	• Case-based virology educational content and webinars	https://www.pascv.org/
Society for Healthcare Epidemiology of America (SHEA)	• Online courses on Antimicrobial Stewardship, Epidemiology, and Infection Prevention and Control topics	https://learningce.shea-online.org/course-catalog-list
University of Adelaide Mycology Online	• Provides extensive educational content related to fungi, including descriptions, antifungal susceptibility information, and virtual self-assessments	https://mycology.adelaide.edu.au/

learning cycle (eg, rotation). Examples of formative assessment practices include verbal feedback (the hallmark of such assessment), discussions, case studies, and low-stakes quizzes, among others.

Summative assessments are measures *of* learning and therefore occur at the end of the learning cycle.[12] Examples of summative assessments include final examinations, papers, and direct observations, among others, and are often characterized by documentation and written feedback provided to the trainee from the rotation director and/or program director. Ideally, programs will have a mechanism to provide learners with feedback using both formative and summative assessments. One such mechanism is through the use of rubrics, which are assessment tools that can help provide an objective appraisal using both types of practices. A rubric identifies performance levels or criteria and the specific performance descriptions and tasks that must be accomplished to achieve each level.[15] As a result, the assessment process is more objective and standardized and provides transparency to trainees regarding the assessment practice.[15] The ACGME requires the formation of Clinical Competency Committees, to biannually evaluate a trainee's progress through an evaluation of competency-based milestones.[16] The ACGME milestones are a narrative trajectory of performance

Table 2 Select listing of medical and public health microbiology community social media, listservs, and blog sites		
Organization (Type)	**Topics Covered**	**Additional Information**
ClinMicroNet (Listserv)	• Available for MPHM laboratory directors and trainees • General listserv used to pose and receive feedback of MPHM-related diagnostic questions, including informal opinions on histopathology cases	• Requires American Society for Microbiology (ASM) membership
DivC (Listserv)	• Available for MPHM laboratory directors, trainees and laboratory supervisors, technologists, etc. • General listserv used to pose and receive feedback of MPHM related questions	• Requires American Society for Microbiology (ASM) membership
Creepy Dreadful Wonderful Parasites	• Weekly cases and answers posted related to parasitic infections in humans	https://parasitewonders.blogspot.com/
Twitter (Social Media)	• Variety of MPHM-related content posted by laboratory directors, trainees, infectious disease clinicians, etc.	• Identify and follow individual MPHM directors or fellows, ID clinicians • Suggested hashtags to follow (not an exhaustive list): 　○ #ASMClinMicro 　○ #MicroRounds 　○ #IDTwitter

levels a trainee is expected to demonstrate competence throughout their training program. A rubric-based assessment process aligns with the evaluation of these performance levels. The Mayo Clinic MPHM programs apply these milestones to both their ACGME- and CPEP-accredited fellowships, providing feedback to both the program director and trainee.

PROGRAM EVALUATION AND CONTINUOUS IMPROVEMENT

Program evaluation is a necessary activity to provide evidence that a training program achieves successful outcomes. The intent of program evaluations is to monitor and improve the quality and effectiveness of training through the use of a systematic measurement plan.[14] There are numerous program evaluation models that can be used to provide program stakeholders with the data needed to make informed decisions related to curricular change, such as Kirkpatrick's 4-level evaluation model, Logic Model, and the Context, Input, Process, Product model.[14] The measurements selected for program evaluation can be collected from many sources, including data linked to trainee assessments (eg, first-time pass rate for board examinations, milestone progression, etc.), assessment of the program curriculum by faculty and learners, feedback from employer and graduate surveys, and patient safety events.[6,13,14] The ACGME mandates appointment of a Program Evaluation Committee (PEC) responsible for program oversight via review of the program's self-determined goals and progress toward achievement, ongoing program improvement, including the development of new goals, and review of the operating environment to identify strengths, challenges, opportunities, and threats as they relate to the program's mission and aims.[6] This Annual Program Evaluation (APE) provides the opportunity for program leadership to determine the need for actions or changes, which are the basis for ongoing program improvement. As with the ACGME milestones, a PEC and APE can be adopted by both ACMGE- and CPEP-accredited programs.

ROLE OF THE PROGRAM DIRECTOR

The MPHM fellowship program director serves many roles, ensuring program accreditation, delivery of high-quality education, and successful recruitment and graduation of fellows. Although many of these roles are specifically defined by the fellowship accrediting bodies, others are "unwritten" but equally important—and sometimes harder than written requirements! For example, the program director must maintain morale of the fellows; support open lines of communication among fellows and faculty; set clear performance expectations; hold fellows and faculty accountable for their actions; advocate for the fellowship program and trainees; and serve as a clinician, teacher, researcher, and professional role models.

ADVICE FOR CURRENT AND FUTURE FELLOWS

Entering into an MPHM fellowship is an exciting time, full of opportunities to learn from experts in the field and to contribute to the constantly evolving diagnostic arena. However, this can also be a challenging time for trainees, especially for those without prior exposure to the clinical laboratory or medical field. It is therefore important for fellows to strive to maintain their physical health and mental well-being for the duration of the program. Toward that end, programs and program directors should ensure that trainees have access to educational material, local resources, and support networks, as necessary.

Beyond bench rotations, reading textbooks and manuals, reviewing case studies, participating in rounds, and attending relevant institutional meetings, successful fellowships also set trainees up for independent advancement following graduation. There are multiple avenues that can be pursued to achieve this, many of them revolving around increasing trainee visibility and recognition in the MPHM community. Trainee engagement in these areas is strongly encouraged and will be of significant benefit as they begin to consider postgraduation employment options. Opportunities to consider participating in during fellowship include, but are not limited to, the following:

- Trainee membership in MPHM-related societies and organizations including, but not limited to
  - American Society for Microbiology (ASM)
  - Pan American Society for Clinical Virology (PASCV)
  - College of American Pathologists (CAP)

- o American Society for Clinical Pathology (ASCP)
- o Infectious Diseases Society of America (IDSA)
- Trainee networking at regional/national/international MPHM-related conferences:
  - o Attending networking opportunities that are organized by many of the annual MPHM-related conferences (eg, ASM, Clinical Virology Symposium, etc.)
  - o Attending conference poster sessions and interacting with scientists and vendors
  - o Submitting conference abstracts and applying for travel awards
- As appropriate, meeting formally or informally, with external invited speakers and/or industry representatives
- Joining MPHM-related listservs (eg, ClinMicroNet, DivC, etc.) and social media (eg, Twitter, MPHM-related blogs) to follow relevant content
- Participating in miscellaneous manuscript-writing opportunities in addition to publication of scientific research (eg, book/manual chapters, review articles, case reports, etc.)

FUTURE DIRECTIONS

As the field of MPHM continues to evolve, expanding into increasingly advanced diagnostic methodologies and responding to needs of clinicians and patients, accredited programs will likewise have to adapt to the changing educational content needed by trainees, which will ensure that trainees remain competitive in the job market and more importantly, that they are successfully postgraduated. Several areas that the authors foresee MPHM training programs having to enhance their educational content for, both in didactic and practice formats, include the following:

- Point-of-care diagnostic assay oversight
- Digital consultation
- Outreach
- Laboratory consolidation and centralization
- Bioinformatics and big data analytics
- Direct-to-consumer testing

In conclusion, with diligence, careful planning, strong leadership, and dedicated faculty, accredited MPHM fellowships can continue to provide trainees with the necessary education and skillsets to become successful leaders of their own accord.

ACKNOWLEDGMENTS

The authors would like to acknowledge the contributions of the Mayo Clinic education program coordinator, Ms. Tasha Gilbertson, and the Associate Program Directors of the Mayo Clinic Clinical Microbiology fellowship programs, Drs. Matthew Binnicker and Audrey Schuetz.

DISCLOSURE

Dr B.S. Pritt receives an editor's stipend from the Journal of Clinical Microbiology, Clinical Microbiology Reviews, and The Manual of Clinical Microbiology, and also receives royalties from the College of American Pathologists Press. Dr E.S. Theel receives a stipend from the Clinical Microbiology Newsletter. C.A. Bowler has nothing to disclose.

REFERENCES

1. Miller JM, Binnicker MJ, Campbell S, et al. A guide to utilization of the microbiology laboratory for diagnosis of infectious diseases: 2018 update by the infectious diseases society of America and the American Society for Microbiology. Clin Infect Dis 2018;67(6):813–6.
2. Avdic E, Carroll KC. The role of the microbiology laboratory in antimicrobial stewardship programs. Infect Dis Clin North Am 2014;28(2):215–35.
3. Canton R. Role of the microbiology laboratory in infectious disease surveillance, alert and response. Clin Microbiol Infect 2005;11(Suppl 1):3–8.
4. Thomson RB Jr, Wilson ML, Weinstein MP. The clinical microbiology laboratory director in the United States hospital setting. J Clin Microbiol 2010;48(10):3465–9.
5. Department of Health and Human Services, Centers for Medicare and Medicaid Services. Clinical laboratory improvement amendments of 1988; final rule. Fed Regist. 2003. Subpart M - Personnel for Nonwaived Testing. Available at: https://www.ecfr.gov/cgi-bin/text-idx?SID=1248e3189da5e5f936e55315402bc38b&node=pt42.5.493&rgn=div5#sp42.5.493.m.
6. Accreditation Council for Graduate Medical Education (ACGME). Pathology. 2020. Available at: https://www.acgme.org/Specialties/Program-Requirements-and-FAQs-and-Applications/pfcatid/18/Pathology. Accessed February 16, 2020.
7. The American Board of Pathology. Medical microbiology. 2015. Available at: https://www.abpath.org/index.php/to-become-certified/requirements-for-certification?id=45. Accessed February 16, 2020.
8. American Society for Microbiology. American Board of Medical Microbiology Certification. 2020. Available at: https://www.asm.org/Certifications/American-Board-of-Medical-Microbiology. Accessed February 16, 2020.
9. American Society for Microbiology. Fellowships. 2020. Available at: https://www.asm.org/Fellowships/CPEP. Accessed February 16, 2020.
10. American Society for Microbiology. CPEP essentials: essentials and guidelines of an accredited postgraduate fellowship program in medical and public health laboratory microbiology. Est. by the Committee on Postgraduate Educational Programs. 2018. Available at: https://www.asm.org/getattachment/2a162a8b-5b09-4c02-9088-37020e30b9c9/Essentials-and-Guidelines_Microbiology-2018.pdf?lang=en-US. Accessed February 16, 2020.
11. Lexico: powered by Oxford. Mission statement. 2020. Available at: https://www.lexico.com/definition/mission_statement, 2/16/2020. Accessed February 16, 2020.
12. Shumway JM, Harden RM, Association for Medical Education in E. AMEE Guide No. 25: the assessment of learning outcomes for the competent and reflective physician. Med Teach 2003;25(6):569–84.
13. Cook DA. Twelve tips for evaluating educational programs. Med Teach 2010;32(4):296–301.
14. Frye AW, Hemmer PA. Program evaluation models and related theories: AMEE guide no. 67. Med Teach 2012;34(5):e288–99.
15. Boateng BA, Bass LD, Blaszak RT, et al. The development of a competency-based assessment rubric to measure resident milestones. J Grad Med Educ 2009;1(1):45–8.
16. Accreditation Council for Graduate Medical Education (ACGME). Milestones. 2020. Available at: https://www.acgme.org/Specialties/Milestones/pfcatid/36Nikhil/Program%20Requirements%20and%20FAQs%20and%20Applications. Accessed February 16, 2020.

Novel Assays/Applications for Patients Suspected of Mycobacterial Diseases

Niaz Banaei, MD[a], Kimberlee A. Musser, PhD[b],
Max Salfinger, MD[c],*, Akos Somoskovi, MD, PhD, DSc[d],
Adrian M. Zelazny, PhD[e]

KEYWORDS

- *Mycobacterium tuberculosis* • Nontuberculous mycobacteria
- Minimal inhibitory concentration • Molecular drug resistance
- MALDI-TOF mass spectrometry • Nucleic acid amplification testing
- Whole genome sequencing • Tuberculosis

KEY POINTS

- The use of nucleic acid amplification testing should be an integral part of the workup of a patient with a tuberculosis suspicion.
- Non–sputum-based tests that detect all forms of tuberculosis have been declared by the World Health Organization as a top priority for tuberculosis diagnostics.
- Many newer polymerase chain reaction-based and sequencing-based molecular tests are available and can provide comprehensive characterization for culture-positive *Mycobacterium tuberculosis*.
- An adequate combination of quantitative antimicrobial susceptibility testing and molecular testing are indispensable to determining drug resistance, cross-resistance, and predicting achievable drug concentrations.
- Matrix-assisted laser desorption ionization time-of-flight mass spectrometry is becoming a reliable tool for nontuberculous mycobacterial identification.

INTRODUCTION

Mycobacteria are the causative organisms for diseases such as tuberculosis (TB), leprosy, Buruli ulcer, and pulmonary nontuberculous mycobacterial (NTM) disease. In 2018, globally,[1] almost 10 million people developed TB, and almost one-half of a

[a] Stanford University School of Medicine, Room 1602, 3375 Hillview Avenue, Palo Alto, CA 94304, USA; [b] Wadsworth Center, New York State Department of Health, 120 New Scotland Avenue, Albany, NY 12208, USA; [c] University of South Florida College of Public Health and Morsani College of Medicine, 13201 Bruce B. Downs Boulevard, MDS 56, Tampa, FL 33612, USA; [d] Roche Molecular Systems Inc., Pleasanton, CA 94588, USA; [e] National Institutes of Health, Building 10, Room 2C-385, 10 Center Drive MSC 1508, Bethesda, MD 20892-1508, USA
* Corresponding author.
E-mail address: max@usf.edu

Clin Lab Med 40 (2020) 535–552
https://doi.org/10.1016/j.cll.2020.08.010
0272-2712/20/© 2020 Elsevier Inc. All rights reserved.

labmed.theclinics.com

million patients suffered from its multidrug-resistant form. In 2019, a total of 8920 new TB cases were reported in the United States.[2] TB is defined not only by latent TB infection and active disease, but is also a spectrum of infection where latent TB infection and active TB disease are 2 snapshots in the continuum of the pathophysiologic status of the patient. Drain and colleagues[3] propose a new framework with 5 discrete categories: eliminated TB infection, latent TB infection, incipient TB infection, subclinical TB disease, and active TB disease. This 5-state framework incorporates a recent understanding of clinical TB pathogenesis as well as advances in the diagnostic approaches to detecting viable TB and predicting the progression of disease activity.

Pulmonary NTM disease is an emerging public health challenge. The US National Institutes of Health reported an increase during 1997 to 2007 from 20 to 47 cases per 100,000 persons[4] (or an 8.2% increase per year) of pulmonary NTM disease among adults aged 65 years or older throughout the United States, with 181,037 national annual cases estimated in 2014. Although *Mycobacterium avium* complex is most frequently isolated in pulmonary NTM patients in North America,[5] the second-most common species depend on the geographic region, for example, *Mycobacterium kansasii* in the Midwest,[6] *Mycobacterium abscessus* in all other regions, and *Mycobacterium xenopi* in Canada.[7] In this article, we focus on novel assays, applications, and procedures for diagnosing TB, including drug-resistant TB, incipient TB, and pulmonary NTM disease and its molecular drug resistance markers.

TAXONOMY

The only genus *Mycobacterium* in the family *Mycobacteriaceae*[8] is a diverse group of bacteria with varying traits, including their potential to be pathogens in humans and animals, their reservoirs, and their ability to grow (or not grow) in culture. Mycobacteria can be divided into 4 major groups: those that belong to the *Mycobacterium tuberculosis* complex (MTBC), *Mycobacterium leprae*, and *Mycobacterium ulcerans*, and those referred to as NTM. They differ in their epidemiology, their ability to cause disease, type of disease they cause, and their ability to grow within the laboratory.

A common characteristic among the *Mycobacterium* spp. are the presence of mycolic acids in their cell wall. They share this characteristic with bacteria of other genera, including *Gordonia, Nocardia, Rhodococcus*, and *Tsukamurella*. Mycolic acids enable differentiation of these bacteria from other bacteria using staining techniques. The high mycolic acid content in the bacterial cell wall creates resistance to decolorization with acid alcohol (ie, "acid fast") during acid-fast bacilli (AFB) staining.

According to the List of Prokaryotic names with Standing in Nomenclature (https://lpsn.dsmz.de/genus/mycobacterium [accessed July 19, 2020]), there are 192 distinct species recognized in the genus *Mycobacterium*. The species within the MTBC with validly published names are *M tuberculosis, Mycobacterium bovis, Mycobacterium africanum, Mycobacterium caprae, Mycobacterium microti,* and *Mycobacterium pinnipedii* (note that *Mycobacterium canettii* is not a validly published species). Using next-generation sequencing, digital DNA–DNA hybridization, and average nucleotide identity determination, Riojas and colleagues[9] investigated the various type strains of the MTBC and proposed that currently recognized species of the MTBC be united as *M tuberculosis*. For example, *M tuberculosis* complex would be *M tuberculosis*, *M tuberculosis* would be *M tuberculosis* var. tuberculosis, *M bovis* would be *M tuberculosis* var. bovis, and *M bovis* BCG would be *M tuberculosis* var. BCG. We use the more familiar names in this article.

According to the web site, *M avium* includes the following subspecies: subsp. *avium*, subsp. *paratuberculosis*, and subsp. *silvaticum*. *Mycobacterium intracellulare* has the subsp. *chimaera* (formerly a species) and subsp. *intracellulare*. *M abscessus* has 3 subspecies: subsp. *abscessus*, subsp. *massiliense*, and subsp. *bolletii*. In 2019, Christine Turenne[10] wrote a comprehensive review article entitled "Nontuberculous mycobacteria: Insights on taxonomy and evolution" for those interested in more detailed information about rules and processes in taxonomy.

NUCLEIC ACID AMPLIFICATION TESTING AND ITS ROLE OF RELEASING TUBERCULOSIS SUSPECTS FROM AIRBORNE INFECTION ISOLATION

There are several review articles[8,11,12] analyzing the technical performance of the various nucleic acid amplification tests (NAAT). Data on the use of NAAT in the United States, however, are sparse because not all states are tracking it. In Florida,[13] a NAAT result was available in 2770 out of 3409 (81.2%) TB cases with positive sputum culture reported between 2009 and 2017. The percentage of NAAT results that were available increased from 74.6% (2009–2011) to 84% (2012–2014) to 87% (2015–2017). Among cases with a positive AFB smear result, NAAT was performed on 1942 of 2156 (90%). In the same 3-year intervals, the percentage of NAAT results increased from 83.4% to 93.1% to 94.6%, respectively. In California,[14,15] NAAT results were available in 74% of all TB cases reported in 2018, including cases for which there is a clinical diagnosis only. In 2019, for AFB smear-positive cases, 77% had a NAAT result whereas in AFB smear-negative cases, only 49% had NAAT results.

It is most important to confirm that the AFB seen in the smear is indeed TB and not NTM because nationwide pulmonary NTM disease is about ten times more prevalent than TB.[16] This goal can be accomplished using NAAT. In the 2005 American Thoracic Society, the Centers for Disease Control and Prevention, and the Infectious Disease Society of America statement,[17] "*Controlling TB in the United States*," suspicion of TB is higher than actual cases. An estimated 10 (in Grady Memorial Hospital, Atlanta, Georgia) to 100 (in the province of Alberta, Canada) persons were suspected of having TB for every case of actual diagnosed pulmonary TB. Based on clinical criteria, patients are placed in airborne infection isolation and must be evaluated. When TB is ruled out using molecular assays, the patients can be more quickly released from airborne infection isolation.

Campos and colleagues[18] determined the accuracy of the first sputum NAAT result and the use of serial smears for identifying patients with potentially infectious TB who truly require airborne infection isolation. Forty-six of 493 patients (9.3%) had TB confirmed by culture. A first sputum NAA test detected all patients with TB who had a positive AFB smear (n = 35), even when the first of the 3 specimens was AFB smear negative. In another study, Lippincott and colleagues[19] compared the use of the 3-AFB smear strategy with a 1-, 2-, and 3-specimen GeneXpert MTB/RIF (Xpert; Cepheid, Sunnyvale, CA) test at the University of North Carolina Hospitals. The 830-bed tertiary medical center provides care to 200 to 300 patients with presumptive TB annually. An average of 8 of these 200 to 300 patients are diagnosed with pulmonary TB. Among 207 subjects in the study, the median duration of airborne infection isolation was 68.0 hours for patients with only AFB smear microscopy compared with 20.8 hours for the 1-specimen Xpert, 41.2 hours for the 2-specimen Xpert, and 54.0 hours for the 3-specimen Xpert strategies ($P \leq .004$). The median laboratory processing time for AFB smear microscopy was 2.5 times as long as Xpert ($P < .001$). The use of the 2- and 3-specimen Xpert and AFB smear microscopy strategies captured all 6 TBs cases (3% of the suspects). The 1-specimen Xpert strategy missed 1 TB case. Use of the 2-specimen Xpert strategy was the most efficient to minimize airborne infection isolation time and identified all TB cases among those presumptive TB-positive individuals in this low-burden setting.

Chaisson and colleagues[20] describe the implementation of a molecular testing algorithm using Xpert on sputum to provide information to discontinue airborne infection isolation for patients with suspected TB. In a prospective cohort study, the authors analyzed 621 consecutive hospitalized patients with suspected TB undergoing sputum examination from January 2014 to January 2016 at the Zuckerberg San Francisco General Hospital and Trauma Center. In this study, NAAT assays significantly decreased the median time to discontinuation of airborne infection isolation from 2.9 to 2.5 days and hospital discharge time from 6.0 to 4.9 days. The savings from these seemingly minor stay differences were meaningful. Implementing the algorithm, the mean hospital costs per molecular TB test-negative patient decreased from $46,921 to $33,574, providing an average savings of $13,347 per patient. The estimated use and evaluation costs for approximately 250 patients with active TB each year were an annual savings to the hospital of $3.3 million.

The evidence from the study showed that stakeholders, including clinicians, infection preventionists, and hospital administrators, should work together to identify barriers at their institution to the implementation of NAAT. These barriers include outdated electronic ordering algorithms and looking only at the laboratory expense, not the system-wide savings with implementation of tests such as NAAT. Using this new algorithm described in the Chaisson study[20], institutions can reap the potential substantial savings that result from using a NAAT for suspect patients with TB in airborne infection isolation.

MICROSCOPY

Molecular diagnostic assays have enabled faster diagnosis of TB, and although this type of detection is more sensitive than microscopy, microscopy is still widely used to diagnose TB in many parts of the world. AFB smear microscopy has been in use for more than 140 years, and there are still opportunities for improvement. Here we highlight a few recent developments. In 2011, the World Health Organization (WHO)[21] issued a report about conventional versus light-emitting diode (LED) microscopes. Compared with conventional mercury vapor fluorescence microscopes, LED microscopes are less expensive and have lower maintenance requirements that conventional fluorescent microscopy (FM). Furthermore, LED microscopy, unlike FM, does not require a darkroom. A WHO expert group found that LED microscopy was 5% (95% confidence interval [CI], 0%–11%) more sensitive and 1% (95% CI, −0.7% to 3.0%) more specific than conventional fluorescence microscopy. Based on findings by the expert group's assessment and the endorsement of the WHO Strategic and Technical Advisory Group for Tuberculosis, the WHO has recommended that conventional FM be replaced by LED-FM in all settings where FM is currently used, and that LED FM be phased in as an alternative to conventional Ziehl-Neelsen microscopy in all settings.

Besides the LED light source, 4 more interesting findings are mentioned here about the fluorescent stain. First, researchers at the Hartford Hospital in Hartford, Connecticut, compared the rhodamine-auramine staining performed at room temperature versus 37°C and found that the yield of positive smears and the number of bacilli per slides increased for M tuberculosis and for M avium complex when 782 clinical specimens stained at 37°C were compared with the conventional method at room temperature.[22] Currently at the University of Florida Health in Jacksonville, Florida, the auramine-rhodamine bottle is prewarmed in an ambient air 35°C incubator for 30 minutes before use (McCarter YS, Personal Communication,

May 29, 2020). Second, researchers at Johns Hopkins Medical Institutions in Baltimore, Maryland, compared a rapid auramine O fluorescent stain, which required 6 steps and 2 minutes to complete, with the conventional protocol, which requires 8 steps and 22 minutes to complete. Organisms included in the study were *M tuberculosis, M avium*, and *Mycobacterium fortuitum*. The 2-minute method[23] outperformed the standard method. Bacilli seemed to be brighter with the shorter method, whereas background debris fluorescence was markedly reduced. Also, the decrease in background fluorescence made the detection of AFB easier. Third, laboratory scientists at the Public Health Ontario Laboratory, one of the busiest mycobacteriology laboratories in North America with more than 200 AFB smears read per day, provided another example of how to improve fluorescent staining. They compared an in-house developed bulk container staining method incorporating an acetone rinse step with the standard auramine O/rhodamine B staining method using individual slide racks. Slides stained with acetone were consistently rated of better quality with less background debris and more intensely fluorescing bacilli. *M avium* yield increased from 53 AFB smear-positive slides with individual rack staining to 60 of 66 (10.6% increase) with acetone rinse staining. The results for *M tuberculosis* positive slides were about the same, with 47 and 48 AFB smear-positive slides out of 50, respectively. This finding is significant given that *M avium* complex organisms are typically smaller and more prone to masking from background fluorescence than *M tuberculosis*. This factor is especially true in North America, where many mycobacteriology laboratories experience more culture-positive respiratory samples owing to NTM than *M tuberculosis*.

Fourth, it is important to remember that NTM, especially rapidly growing mycobacteria, are less frequently detected when using a fluorescent stain versus Ziehl-Neelsen. The American Society for Microbiology Manual of Clinical Microbiology states[24]: "If the presence of a rapid grower is suspected and the results of acid-fast stains, in particular fluorochrome stains, are negative, it may be worthwhile to stain the smear with carbol fuchsin and to use a weaker decolorizing process."

As informatics progresses and allows for the analysis of very large datasets, artificial intelligence or machine learning is more and more used for diagnosis purposes, for example, reading chest radiographs for active pulmonary TB[25] or the interpretation of blood culture Gram stains.[26] Xiong and colleagues[27] built a convolutional neural network model specifically to recognize *M tuberculosis* complex organisms in formalin-fixed paraffin-embedded tissue blocks. The training set contained 45 samples (30 positive cases and 15 negative cases according to 2 pathologists' readings). Upon training the neural network model, 201 samples (108 positive cases and 93 negative cases) were collected as a test set to challenge the model. The artificial intelligence-assisted detection method achieved 97.9% sensitivity and 83.7% specificity. Convolutional neural networks have the potential to decrease pathologists' time of screening acid-fast stained slides and decrease chance of missed diagnoses.

New technologies can shorten turnaround times, improve quality, and ensure adherence to guidelines as can more experienced staff. Many times, TB or NTM disease may not be on the list of differential diagnoses for a patient. All that is sent to the microbiology laboratory is a sputum for Gram stain and culture to provide additional information for the clinician who is taking care of a patient with the clinical diagnosis of pneumonia. No AFB stain is ordered, only a Gram stain. It is in these situations where the experienced microscopist[28–30] recognizes Gram-labile, Gram-neutral, or Gram-ghost bacilli for which there is no culture correlation on the agar plate, and then performs an AFB stain, ultimately resulting in an AFB-positive organism—a Eureka moment!

NON–SPUTUM-BASED DIAGNOSIS OF TUBERCULOSIS

Despite recent advances in NAAT for direct detection of *M tuberculosis* in sputa, several million TB cases still go undiagnosed each year.[31] This is in part owing to the difficulty of diagnosing TB among children and individuals with human immunodeficiency virus (HIV)/AIDS and/or extrapulmonary TB. A diagnosis of TB in these groups often requires invasive sampling, such as gastric aspirate, bronchoalveolar lavage, and open biopsy, which are not available in many resource-limited settings and may result in medical complications. In response to this challenge, the WHO has developed target product profiles; first among these is a rapid, biomarker-based, non–sputum-based test to detect all forms of TB.[32]

Lipoarabinomannan (LAM) is an abundant branched lipoglycan in the outer wall of *M tuberculosis* that can be detected in the plasma and urine of patients with TB.[33] Over the past 2 decades, significant progress has been made to optimize the detection of LAM in urine using a simple lateral flow assay. The Alere Determine TB LAM Ag (AlereLAM, Waltham, MA) was the first lateral flow assay to receive WHO endorsement. In HIV-positive adults, AlereLAM showed pooled sensitivity 42% (95% CI, 31%–55%) and pooled specificity was 91% (95% CI, 85%–95%).[34] The pooled sensitivity was higher among inpatients compared with outpatient (62% vs 31%) and the sensitivity was higher in patients with a lower CD4 cell count.[34] Based on these findings, the WHO currently recommends the AlereLAM in inpatient settings for the diagnosis of active TB in HIV-positive adults, adolescents, and children with signs and symptoms of TB, or with advanced HIV disease, or who are seriously ill, or irrespective of signs and symptoms of TB and with a CD4 cell count of less than 200 cells/mm.[35] In the outpatient setting, the WHO recommends the AlereLAM in the same patient population with signs and symptoms of TB or seriously ill and/or with a CD4 cell count of less than 100 cells/mm. More recently, Fujifilm SILVAMP TB LAM (FujiLAM, Tokyo, Japan), a novel lateral flow assay based on Fujifilm technology, has been developed for detection of urine LAM. Compared with AlereLAM, FujiLAM was shown to be more sensitive in inpatients and outpatients with HIV.[36,37] The higher sensitivity of FujiLAM is likely to improve TB diagnosis in HIV-infected individuals. Preanalytical approaches that capture and concentrate urine LAM have shown high sensitivity in HIV-uninfected patients with TB and thus may render urine LAM a viable option for diagnosing TB in HIV-negative patients.[38]

Liu and colleagues[39] developed a novel assay (NanoDisk-MS) that can potentially rapidly diagnose active TB cases by direct detection of *M tuberculosis*-derived antigens in patients' blood samples. In this blood-based assay, nanoparticle-enriched peptides derived from the *M tuberculosis* virulence factors CFP-10 and ESAT-6 were analyzed by high-throughput mass spectrometry. The novel assay diagnosed 174 (88.3%) of the study's TB cases,[40] with 95.8% clinical specificity, and with 91.6% and 85.3% clinical sensitivity for culture-positive and culture-negative TB cases, respectively. The NanoDisk-MS also exhibited an 88% clinical sensitivity for pulmonary and a 90% for extrapulmonary TB, exceeding the diagnostic performance of mycobacterial culture for these cases. The detection and quantification of *M tuberculosis* antigens by such a method, requiring only a low-volume blood draw, may open up new possibilities for the diagnosis of TB.

Blood RNA signature represents another emerging nonsputum biomarker for diagnosis of active and incipient TB. The term "incipient TB" is used to classify patients who have no signs or symptoms of TB but are on their way to developing active TB.[3] Since the first study showing existence of a distinct blood RNA signature in patients with active TB versus a latent TB infection,[41,42] 27 unique blood RNA signatures have been reported. The immune transcripts mostly encode cytokines, transcription factors, and effectors downstream of regulators.[43] The best 4 signatures for active TB were shown to perform independent of age, sex, and HIV status and had sensitivities between 83.3% (95% CI, 71.3%–91.0%) and 90.7% (80.1%–96.0) at a specificity of 70% or higher (the minimum WHO target product profile specificity for a triage test).[42] No signature was sufficiently accurate to meet the WHO criteria of a triage test (95% sensitivity and 80% specificity) or a confirmatory test (65% sensitivity and 98% specificity).[42]

Blood RNA signatures have also been evaluated for diagnosis of incipient TB. The immune transcripts were shown to appear at least 18 months before a TB diagnosis in a dynamic manner.[44] The 8 best performing signatures have shown sensitivities of 24.7% to 39.9% at 24 months and of 47.1% to 81.0% at 3 months before a TB diagnosis was made, with corresponding specificities set at more than 90%.[42] At pretest probability of 2%, positive predictive values ranged from 6.8% to 9.4% at 24 months and 11.2% to 14.4% at 3 months.[42] At thresholds that maximize both sensitivity and specificity, no signature met the minimum WHO target product profile measures for incipient TB biomarkers (sensitivity ≥75% and specificity ≥75% over 2 years).[42] These findings raise important diagnostic questions for TB elimination plans regarding the implementation of blood RNA signature tests to diagnose and treat incipient TB. Given that they perform best proximally to a diagnosis of active TB, serial testing would be required. Thus, further research is needed to define the best population and frequency for testing and show the cost effectiveness of such testing strategy.

Cell-free DNA (cfDNA) in plasma and urine is another emerging biomarker for a sputum-free diagnosis of TB. Performance of published studies using various methods for collection, extraction, and testing for diagnosis of TB has been summarized previously.[45] The reported assays range in sensitivity from 29% to 79% and in specificity from 67% to 100%[45] for the diagnosis of TB. Although promising, current cfDNA assays suffer from significant variability, require significant assay time, and do not meet the minimum WHO target product profile. Several studies have recently investigated preanalytical and analytical variable effecting cfDNA testing to optimize and standardize cfDNA testing.[46,47] Further studies using optimized preanalytical extraction and analytical protocols are needed to assess the accuracy of TB cfDNA testing.

POSITIVE TUBERCULOSIS CULTURE: IDEAL NEXT STEPS?

Rapid detection and identification of the M tuberculosis complex is an important role of the microbiology laboratory. Laboratories use assays including commercial nucleic acid probes, laboratory-developed polymerase chain reaction–based DNA sequencing, or matrix-assisted laser desorption ionization time-of-flight mass spectrometry (MALDI-TOF MS). However, it is important to identify especially M tuberculosis, M bovis, and M bovis BCG within the M tuberculosis complex for epidemiologic, public health, and treatment reasons.

An important area of rapid improvements for laboratory tests are those for specimens determined to be culture positive for M tuberculosis and require antimicrobial susceptibility testing (AST) results. These tests include a range of polymerase chain reaction–based and sequencing-based molecular tests, which often provide improved turnaround times compared with culture-based test methods. Newer tests such as these are rapid and accurate, providing information to appropriately treat patients, weeks to even months before culture-based AST is available. This can greatly impact management of patients with multidrug-resistant TB or patients with extensively drug-resistant TB, especially when combined with epidemiology data to detect and track TB transmission.

Molecular testing methods for detection of mutations with resistance include some with market authorization from the US Food and Drug Administration, such as the Xpert as well as a new Cepheid Xpert MTB/RIF Ultra assay (Ultra), not currently available in the United States, which was developed with improved sensitivity and detection of resistance from mutations known to confer low-level resistance. Additional tests that can be validated in house for clinical testing are tests such as the GenoType MTBDR*plus* line probe assay (Hain Lifescience, Nehren, Germany) and other laboratory-developed tests using real-time polymerase chain reaction for detection and identification within the *M tuberculosis* complex,[48,49] or DNA sequencing methods,[50,51] or a combination of these methods. These assays can be performed and reported rapidly on culture-positive *M tuberculosis* complex isolates. Testing algorithms using these methods for patient management have been described elsewhere.[52]

Some documented challenges and issues have been reported for these tests. For the majority of documented gene mutations, there is a high correlation with growth-based AST. Some results from molecular assays, however, can be discordant with phenotypic results in some cases, or mutations can be associated with lower level resistance only detected with molecular or minimum inhibitory concentration testing, especially for rifampin and isoniazid.[53] Genotypic characterization of rifampin mutations and the association with phenotypic susceptibility testing have also been recently assessed for the MTBDR*plus* line probe assay, Deeplex-MycTB (Genoscreen, Lille, France), and Genoscholar™ NTM+MDRTB (Nipro, Osaka, Japan).[54–56]

For the Xpert, there are known issues with false-positive rifampin resistance detection owing to the identification of synonymous or silent mutations that should be considered in testing algorithms.[57,58] For this reason, and in general, it is recommended that DNA sequencing be performed to confirm mutations for this assay and for all other non–sequence-based molecular assays for analysis for mutations. If this testing cannot be performed at the laboratory performing the assay, samples may be sent to a reference testing program such as the Centers for Disease Control and Prevention. Reflex testing such as this will continue to inform the understanding of mutations associated with resistance and lead to improvements overall to improve molecular susceptibility testing.

Another important area of ongoing research is the development of whole genome sequencing (WGS)[59,60] and targeted next-generation sequencing (NGS) approaches[61,62] that provide comprehensive analysis of the *M tuberculosis* complex genome to more accurately assess genotypic AST. Sequencing all mutations simultaneously with a method such as WGS offers advantages over line probe assays and other commercial molecular assays. There is value in detecting all mutations, including those associated with first-line and second-line drug treatment regimens, because this can result in a higher sensitivity and provide more definitive data on which TB drugs to use. However, these methods typically require a grown culture and can take many days to test and report findings, compared with currently available polymerase chain reaction and pyrosequencing methods. WGS genotypic AST can be accomplished for additional and even novel drugs at no additional cost, contingent only on the knowledge base of characterized mutations. These testing data could be helpful when designing new treatment regimens. Reports of shorter turnaround times compared with growth-based AST with results available 7 to 8 days from a positive culture have also been described with the implementation of WGS.[63] Comprehensive WGS approaches and evaluation of data on low-level resistance mutations may continue to inform the best practices for treatment when strains harboring these mutations are present. Targeted NGS, although different, enables the detection of a significantly large enough portion of relevant mutations and could serve a similar role as WGS, but with the added benefit that testing may be applied directly to specimens, and provide results more quickly than WGS, and at a lower cost.

The WGS approach, when used to identify and predict susceptibility or resistance to TB drugs, can also provide a comprehensive genotyping approach with no additional testing.[64,65] Comparison studies have reported improvements of WGS over past genotyping methods. Studies comparing WGS and amplicon-based NGS methods as well as WGS analysis approaches, including WGS-derived spoligotyping, core genome multilocus sequence typing and single nucleotide polymorphism–based analysis, continue to be evaluated with positive outcomes. With NGS costs continuing to decrease over time and reduced turnaround times, a comprehensive WGS method will likely be used across the United States and globally in the years to come.

MINIMAL INHIBITORY CONCENTRATIONS TESTING FOR *M TUBERCULOSIS* COMPLEX

The potential diagnostic capacity of most phenotypic and molecular AST methods is significantly underused because they are used in a one size fits all approach that lumps patients into diagnostic boxes. Namely, in the absence of routine quantitative AST, TB strains are simply identified only as susceptible or resistant without trying to determine the level of drug resistance, the presence and level of cross-resistance, and the associated achievable drug concentration to enable a much-needed patient-centered and more effective regimen design.

At present, neither molecular nor phenotypic tests may stand alone to fulfill this unmet diagnostic need because different mutation types may be associated with different levels of phenotypic minimal inhibitory concentrations or clinically relevant levels of resistance. This factor may lead to unnecessary discontinuation of a key drug or incorrectly labeling a patient as a patient with multidrug-resistant TB or a patient with extensively drug-resistant TB (eg, in the case of low-level isoniazid or fluoroquinolone resistance).[66,67] Therefore, quantitative phenotypic AST is indispensable to validating the clinical significance of a specific mutation type in a particular patient or in newly identified mutations with an unknown phenotypic and clinical impact. Another reason to adequately combine the diagnostic capabilities of molecular and quantitative phenotypic AST for effective treatment monitoring is that most near-patient molecular methods do not provide information on the type of mutation or the viability of the strain. This information is required to predict the level of resistance or the efficacy of treatment. It is also important to keep in mind that the smart combination of quantitative molecular and phenotypic assays may enable the more accurate determination of any clinically significant proportion of drug-resistant strains associated with different levels of resistance in the sample that can better aid respective dose or treatment duration adjustments.[68]

However, molecular markers to predict drug resistance and adequately validated and widely implemented phenotypic tests are simply missing or incomplete for several drugs that are key in the recently WHO-prioritized therapeutic regimens (eg, linezolid, clofazimine, and bedaquiline).[67,69] Indeed, clinical evidence suggests that, with bedaquiline and clofazimine, where the genetic correlates of phenotypic resistance remain incomplete, there are cryptic or epistatic mutations leading to clinically meaningful resistance.[70] Moreover, resistance linked to known and novel genetic loci that have not yet been phenotypically characterized emerge despite standard or individualized therapy.[70] These emergent bedaquiline-resistant populations without a standardized molecular or phenotypic AST are concerning. We have little understanding of these populations as they relate to levels of phenotypic cross-resistance to clofazimine, or of potential differences in resistance levels for the same mutations in various geographic settings.[70,71] This complexity clearly underlines that neither molecular nor conventional phenotypic AST will stand alone. The commercially available, quality-controlled, and dry-form Sensititre Mycobacterium TB MIC Plate (Thermo Scientific, Waltham, MA), improved by the Automated Mycobacterial Growth Detection Algorithm (AMyGDA), which excludes manual observation and reading, may offer a cost-effective, high-throughput, and relatively fast interim solution in addition to the expensive automated BD BACTEC MGIT 960/EpiCenter TBeXiST quantitative AST system (Becton, Dickinson and Company, Franklin Lakes, NJ).[72,73] However, novel and potentially non–replication-dependent testing–based approaches with improvements in turnaround time, complexity, and sensitivity of nonconventional quantitative phenotypic AST are much needed to enable a truly patient-oriented viability and AST monitoring.

POSITIVE NONTUBERCULOUS MYCOBACTERIAL CULTURE: IDEAL NEXT STEPS?

MALDI-TOF MS has revolutionized microbial identification in clinical microbiology. Using MALDI-TOF MS, a spectral profile of the microorganism is created based on the abundance of proteins with specific mass-to-charge ratios. This microbial profile is then compared with a reference database and a match assessed to determine the organism's identity. Despite a late start in mycobacteriology, MALDI-TOF MS is becoming a reliable tool for NTM identification owing in part to improvements in mycobacterial extraction protocols and in commercial mycobacterial databases.[74] In reviewing studies evaluating MALDI-TOF MS for NTM, it is important to take into account the culture media used (solid vs liquid), extraction protocols, commercial system and type of library used (ie, version of a library), and the criteria for the acceptability of results (ie, match threshold, cutoff species vs group/complex-level reporting). Owing to their hardiness, extraction protocols for mycobacteria typically involve mechanical disruption via bead beating, sonication, and/or vortexing in ethanol, formic acid, and/or acetonitrile, which in some protocols are preceded by freeze–thaw cycles.[74–76] The extracted proteins are then spotted onto the target plate for MALDI-TOF MS analysis. There are currently 2 commercially available MALDI-TOF MS systems in the United States, the MALDI Biotyper (Bruker Daltonics, Billerica, MA) and the VITEK MS system (bioMérieux, Durham, NC). A review of recent MALDI Biotyper studies focused on (ie, included a large number of) NTM from colonies (solid media) revealed generally a greater than 90% agreement with the gold standard (range, 83.4%–98.4%), which included commercial hybridization methods (not available in United States) and/or gene sequencing.[75,77–79] Another large study with 291 NTM achieved approximately 88% agreement when using a combination of commercial and in-house databases.[80] In contrast, studies attempting direct identification from positive mycobacterial broth cultures showed variable outcomes (22.0%, 68.2%, 80.0%, and 97.4% correct identification from positive MGITs using a MALDI Biotyper).[75,81–83]

Studies with the VITEK MS system on NTM from solid media also showed a greater than 90% correct identification when using the IVD v3.0 database (range, 90%–95%) with sometimes lower percentages when using the Saramis v4.12 RUO database (range, 67%–90%).[77,84–87] Similar to the experience with Bruker, direct identification from mycobacterial broth cultures yielded variable outcomes with some studies showing similar performance to solid media, whereas others showed lower perfor-mance.[86-88] A recent multicenter study comparing the Bruker Biotyper system with RUO Mycobacteria Library v5.0.0 and VITEK MS IVD system with the v3.0 Knowledge Base shows similar performance with 92% and 95% of NTM strains (solid media), respectively, identified at least to complex/group level, and 62% and 57% identified to the highest taxonomic level.[77] It is clear that MALDI-TOF MS has a role in the myco-bacteriology laboratory and, in particular, in the identification of NTM, for which fewer commercial methods are available compared with *M tuberculosis*. However, there are current limitations of MALDI-TOF MS that should be addressed, including a lack of dif-ferentiation among some closely related species or subspecies and performance in liquid media. Studies of MALDI-TOF MS with NTM show limitations in differentiation among some related taxa, including subspecies of *M abscessus* (subsp. *abscessus, massiliense, bolletii*), members of the *M avium* complex (except *M avium*), *M fortuitum*, *Mycobacterium terrae*, and *Mycobacterium mucogenicum* groups/complexes, differ-entiation between *Mycobacterium chelonae/Mycobacterium salmoniphilum* (for Bruker), and between *Mycobacterium marinum/M ulcerans*. Identification within *M abscessus* and *M fortuitum* group has clinical relevance, because some taxa lack a functional *erm* gene conferring for inducible macrolide resistance (*M abscessus* subsp. *massiliense*; *Mycobacterium senegalense*, *Mycobacterium peregrinum*), whereas other members may harbor a functional gene (*M abscessus* subsp. *absces-sus* and subsp. *bolletii*; *M fortuitum*, *Mycobacterium porcinum*, *Mycobacterium septi-cum*). Identification of the species *M intracellulare* subsp. *chimaera* within *M avium* complex is critical owing to a recent outbreak of this species linked to heater-cooler units in cardiac surgery. Discrimination of *M intracellulare* subsp. *chimaera* from *M intracellulare* subsp. *intracellulare* by MALDI-TOF MS has been reported, but requires procedures not standard for a clinical microbiology laboratory.[89,90] In addition, rare or novel species not present or not well-represented in the database may not be identifiable (ie, *Mycobacterium frederickbergense*, *Mycobacterium hera-klionense*, *Mycobacterium madagascariense*),[75] and even some known species occa-sionally show low scores or match and require repeat testing or confirmation by an alternative method (*M xenopi*, *Mycobacterium gordonae*, *M kansasii*, and *Mycobacte-rium scrofulaceum*).[78] Identification of NTM directly from liquid media is challenging owing to several factors: low biomass of organisms at time of positivity, possible inter-ference from proteins from clinical specimen and/or media, and low efficiency of extraction protocols.[75,83] Improvements in extraction protocols, including concentra-tion of mycobacterial proteins and in sensitivity of MALDI-TOF MS systems, are warranted.

Although the focus of MALDI-TOF MS has been microbial identification, recent work with bacterial isolates (not AFB) highlight its potential use for detection antimicrobial resistance. The main approaches used to include measuring antibiotic modifications owing to the enzymatic activity of bacteria, analysis of changes in bacterial peak pat-terns, and semiquantification of bacterial growth upon exposure to a given antibiotic. Ceyssens and colleagues[91] applied mycobacterial identification combined with MBT-ASTRA methodology (Bruker) that measures the influence of antibiotics on *M tubercu-losis* and NTM as proof of concept of MALDI-TOF MS for AST in mycobacteria, noting that further validation and automation are required before routine implementation is possible. Commercial molecular assays for rapid AST of NTM are limited (when compared with *M tuberculosis*). One such assay, GenoType NTM-DR (Hain Life-science) allows detection of genes conferring macrolides (*erm*(41), *rrl*) or aminoglyco-sides (*rrs*) resistance to *M avium*, *M intracellulare* subsp. *intracellulare*, *M intracellulare* subsp. *chimaera*, *M abscessus* and its subspecies, and *M chelonae*. Evaluation of

GenoType NTM-DR showed promising results with 98% concordance with Sanger sequencing and 94.1% agreement with phenotypic susceptibility testing.[92]

SUMMARY

In this review, we focused on several assays to shorten turnaround times and increase diagnostic accuracy. More than 100 years ago, in 1908, Robert Koch, the discoverer of the TB bacterium visited Hermann Biggs, a physician, public health practitioner and the mastermind of the administrative control of TB in the United States in his New York City office. In his book about "The Life of Hermann M. Biggs, M.D., D. Sc., LLD. Physician and Statesman of the Public Health" by C.-E.A. Winslow,[93] the author describes the visit as follows:

> In the further course of his visit, Koch became enthusiastic about the many ways in which the health authorities in America gave practical assistance to the practicing physician. He was particularly impressed with the promptness and completeness of the service he saw rendered by the health department in New York City. That a physician could leave a throat culture at a drug store in his neighborhood at 5 PM and be sure of receiving a report by telephone before 10 AM the next morning was a remarkable achievement. 'You will agree, my dear Biggs, that most of these bacteriologic and serologic discoveries have come from Germany. For my part I must admit with shame that we in Germany are years and years behind you in their practical application. You have done marvelous work!'

If Robert Koch were to visit your laboratory or your office today, what would be his verdict?

ACKNOWLEDGMENTS

The authors are grateful to Shannon Mulhall for her thoughtful edits.

REFERENCES

1. World Health Organization. Global tuberculosis report 2019. Geneva (Switzerland): World Health Organization; 2019.
2. Schwartz NG, Price SF, Pratt RH, Langer AJ. Tuberculosis - United States, 2019. MMWR Morb Mortal Wkly Rep 2019;69(11):286–9.
3. Drain PK, Bajema KL, Dowdy D, et al. Incipient and subclinical tuberculosis: a clinical review of early stages and progression of infection. Clin Microbiol Rev 2018;31(4). e00021-18.
4. Strollo SE, Adjemian J, Adjemian MK, et al. The burden of pulmonary nontuberculous mycobacterial disease in the United States. Ann Am Thorac Soc 2015; 12(10):1458–64.
5. Spaulding AB, Lai YL, Zelazny AM, et al. Geographic distribution of nontuberculous mycobacterial species identified among clinical isolates in the United States, 2009-2013. Ann Am Thorac Soc 2017;14(11):1655–61.
6. Abate G, Stapleton JT, Rouphael N, et al. Variability in the management of adults with pulmonary nontuberculous mycobacterial disease. Clin Infect Dis 2020;ciaa252. https://doi.org/10.1093/cid/ciaa252. Online ahead of print.
7. Brode SK, Chung H, Campitelli MA, et al. The impact of different antibiotic treatment regimens on mortality in Mycobacterium avium complex pulmonary disease (MAC-PD): a population-based cohort study. Eur Respir J 2020;1901875. https://doi.org/10.1183/13993003.01875-2019. Online ahead of print.

8. Forbes BA, Hall GA, Miller MB, et al. Practice guidelines for clinical microbiology laboratories-Mycobacteria. Clin Microbiol Rev 2018;31(2):e00038-17.
9. Riojas MA, McGough KJ, Rider-Riojas CJ, et al. Phylogenomic analysis of the species of the *Mycobacterium tuberculosis* complex demonstrates that *Mycobacterium africanum, Mycobacterium bovis, Mycobacterium caprae, Mycobacterium microti* and *Mycobacterium pinnipedii* are later heterotypic synonyms of *Mycobacterium tuberculosis.* Int J Syst Evol Microbiol 2018;68(1):324–32.
10. Turenne CY. Nontuberculous mycobacteria: insights on taxonomy and evolution. Infect Genet Evol 2019;72:159–68.
11. Schumacher SG, Sohn H, Qin ZZ, et al. Impact of molecular diagnostics for tuberculosis on patient-important outcomes: a systematic review of study methodologies. PLoS One 2016;11(3):e0151073.
12. Shinnick TM, Starks AM, Alexander HL, et al. Evaluation of the Cepheid Xpert MTB/RIF assay. Expert Rev Mol Diagn 2015;15(1):9–22.
13. Bootseta R, Johnson L, Zabala J, et al. NAAT testing for TB and NTM in Florida. Atlanta (GA): National TB Controllers Association; 2019.
14. California Department of Public Health. California tuberculosis data tables. 2018. Available at: https://www.cdph.ca.gov/programs/cid/dcdc/pages/TB-disease-data.aspx. Accessed July 19, 2020.
15. California Department of Public Health. TB performance trends for National and California objectives 2018. Available at: https://www.cdph.ca.gov/Programs/CID/DCDC/CDPH%20Document%20Library/TBCB-Performance-Trends-for-US-CA-Objectives.pdf. Accessed June 16 2020.
16. Adjemian J, Daniel-Wayman S, Ricotta E, et al. Epidemiology of nontuberculous mycobacteriosis. Semin Respir Crit Care Med 2018;39(3):325–35.
17. Taylor Z, Nolan CM, Blumberg HM. Controlling tuberculosis in the United States. Recommendations from the American Thoracic Society, CDC, and the Infectious Diseases Society of America. MMWR Recomm Rep 2005;54(Rr-12):1–81.
18. Campos M, Quartin A, Mendes E, et al. Feasibility of shortening respiratory isolation with a single sputum nucleic acid amplification test. Am J Respir Crit Care Med 2008;178(3):300–5.
19. Lippincott CK, Miller MB, Popowitch EB, et al. Xpert MTB/RIF assay shortens airborne isolation for hospitalized patients with presumptive tuberculosis in the United States. Clin Infect Dis 2014;59(2):186–92.
20. Chaisson LH, Duong D, Cattamanchi A, et al. Association of rapid molecular testing with duration of respiratory isolation for patients with possible tuberculosis in a US hospital. JAMA Intern Med 2018;178(10):1380–8.
21. World Health Organization. Fluorescent light-emitting diode (LED) microscopy for diagnosis of tuberculosis policy. WHO/HTM/TB/2011.8. Geneva (Switzerland): World Health Organization; 2011.
22. McCarter YS, Robinson A. Detection of acid-fast bacilli in concentrated primary specimen smears stained with rhodamine-auramine at room temperature and at 37 degrees C. J Clin Microbiol 1994;32(10):2487–9.
23. Hendry C, Dionne K, Hedgepeth A, et al. Evaluation of a rapid fluorescent staining method for detection of mycobacteria in clinical specimens. J Clin Microbiol 2009;47(4):1206–8.
24. Martin I, Pfyffer GE, Parrish N. *Mycobacterium*: general characteristics, laboratory detection, and staining procedures. In: Carroll KC, Pfaller MA, Landry ML, et al, editors. Manual of clinical microbiology. 12th edition. Washington DC: American Society for Microbiology Press; 2019. p. 564.

25. Hwang EJ, Park S, Jin KN, et al. Development and validation of a deep learning-based automated detection algorithm for major thoracic diseases on chest radiographs. JAMA Netw Open 2019;2(3):e191095.
26. Smith KP, Kang AD, Kirby JE. Automated interpretation of blood culture Gram stains by use of a deep convolutional neural network. J Clin Microbiol 2018; 56(3):e01521-17.
27. Xiong Y, Ba X, Hou A, et al. Automatic detection of *Mycobacterium tuberculosis* using artificial intelligence. J Thorac Dis 2018;10(3):1936–40.
28. Hinson JM Jr, Bradsher RW, Bodner SJ. Gram-stain neutrality of *Mycobacterium tuberculosis*. Am Rev Respir Dis 1981;123(4 Pt 1):365–6.
29. Brown-Elliott BA, Griffith DE, Wallace RJ Jr. Diagnosis of nontuberculous mycobacterial infections. Clin Lab Med 2002;22(4):911–25, vi.
30. Kuroda H, Hosokawa N. Gram-ghost bacilli. J Gen Fam Med 2019;20(1):31–2.
31. World Health Organization. Ethics guidance for the implementation of the end TB strategy. Geneva (Switzerland): World Health Organization; 2017.
32. World Health Organization. High-priority target product profiles for new tuberculosis diagnostics: a report of a consensus meeting. Geneva (Switzerland): World Health Organization; 2014.
33. Fukuda T, Matsumura T, Ato M, et al. Critical roles for lipomannan and lipoarabinomannan in cell wall integrity of mycobacteria and pathogenesis of tuberculosis. mBio 2013;4(1):e00472-12.
34. Bjerrum S, Schiller I, Dendukuri N, et al. Lateral flow urine lipoarabinomannan assay for detecting active tuberculosis in people living with HIV. Cochrane Database Syst Rev 2019;(10):CD011420.
35. World Health Organization. Lateral flow urine lipoarabinomannan assay (LF-LAM) for the diagnosis of active tuberculosis in people living with HIV. Policy update. Geneva (Switzerland): World Health Organization; 2019.
36. Bjerrum S, Broger T, Székely R, et al. Diagnostic accuracy of a novel and rapid lipoarabinomannan test for diagnosing tuberculosis among people with human immunodeficiency virus. Open Forum Infect Dis 2020;7(1):ofz530.
37. Broger T, Sossen B, du Toit E, et al. Novel lipoarabinomannan point-of-care tuberculosis test for people with HIV: a diagnostic accuracy study. Lancet Infect Dis 2019;19(8):852–61.
38. Paris L, Magni R, Zaidi F, et al. Urine lipoarabinomannan glycan in HIV-negative patients with pulmonary tuberculosis correlates with disease severity. Sci Transl Med 2017;9(420).
39. Liu C, Zhao Z, Fan J, et al. Quantification of circulating *Mycobacterium tuberculosis* antigen peptides allows rapid diagnosis of active disease and treatment monitoring. Proc Natl Acad Sci U S A 2017;114(15):3969–74.
40. Liu C, Lyon CJ, Bu Y, et al. Clinical evaluation of a blood assay to diagnose paucibacillary tuberculosis via bacterial antigens. Clin Chem 2018;64(5):791–800.
41. Berry MP, Graham CM, McNab FW, et al. An interferon-inducible neutrophil-driven blood transcriptional signature in human tuberculosis. Nature 2010; 466(7309):973–7.
42. Turner CT, Gupta RK, Tsaliki E, et al. Blood transcriptional biomarkers for active pulmonary tuberculosis in a high-burden setting: a prospective, observational, diagnostic accuracy study. Lancet Respir Med 2020;8(4):407–19.
43. Gupta RK, Turner CT, Venturini C, et al. Concise whole blood transcriptional signatures for incipient tuberculosis: a systematic review and patient-level pooled meta-analysis. Lancet Respir Med 2020;8(4):395–406.

44. Scriba TJ, Penn-Nicholson A, Shankar S, et al. Sequential inflammatory processes define human progression from *M. tuberculosis* infection to tuberculosis disease. PLoS Pathog 2017;13(11):e1006687.

45. Fernández-Carballo BL, Broger T, Wyss R, et al. Toward the development of a circulating free DNA-based in vitro diagnostic test for infectious diseases: a review of evidence for tuberculosis. J Clin Microbiol 2019;57(4):e01234-18.

46. Murugesan K, Hogan CA, Palmer Z, et al. Investigation of preanalytical variables impacting pathogen cell-free DNA in blood and urine. J Clin Microbiol 2019; 57(11):e00782-819.

47. Oreskovic A, Brault ND, Panpradist N, et al. Analytical comparison of methods for extraction of short cell-free DNA from urine. J Mol Diagn 2019;21(6):1067–78.

48. Halse TA, Edwards J, Cunningham PL, et al. Combined real-time PCR and rpoB gene pyrosequencing for rapid identification of *Mycobacterium tuberculosis* and determination of rifampin resistance directly in clinical specimens. J Clin Microbiol 2010;48(4):1182–8.

49. Lin SY, Probert W, Lo M, et al. Rapid detection of isoniazid and rifampin resistance mutations in *Mycobacterium tuberculosis* complex from cultures or smear-positive sputa by use of molecular beacons. J Clin Microbiol 2004;42(9): 4204–8.

50. Ajbani K, Lin SY, Rodrigues C, et al. Evaluation of pyrosequencing for detecting extensively drug-resistant *Mycobacterium tuberculosis* among clinical isolates from four high-burden countries. Antimicrob Agents Chemother 2015;59(1): 414–20.

51. Engström A, Morcillo N, Imperiale B, et al. Detection of first- and second-line drug resistance in *Mycobacterium tuberculosis* clinical isolates by pyrosequencing. J Clin Microbiol 2012;50(6):2026–33.

52. Centers for Disease Control and Prevention. Availability of an assay for detecting *Mycobacterium tuberculosis*, including rifampin-resistant strains, and considerations for its use - United States, 2013. MMWR Morb Mortal Wkly Rep 2013; 62(41):821–7.

53. Van Deun A, Aung KJ, Bola V, et al. Rifampin drug resistance tests for tuberculosis: challenging the gold standard. J Clin Microbiol 2013;51(8):2633–40.

54. Singhal R, Anthwal D, Kumar G, et al. Genotypic characterization of 'inferred' rifampin mutations in GenoType MTBDR*plus* assay and its association with phenotypic susceptibility testing of *Mycobacterium tuberculosis*. Diagn Microbiol Infect Dis 2020;96(4):114995.

55. Makhado NA, Matabane E, Faccin M, et al. Outbreak of multidrug-resistant tuberculosis in South Africa undetected by WHO-endorsed commercial tests: an observational study. Lancet Infect Dis 2018;18(12):1350–9.

56. Nathavitharana RR, Hillemann D, Schumacher SG, et al. Multicenter noninferiority evaluation of Hain GenoType MTBDRplus version 2 and Nipro NTM+MDRTB line probe assays for detection of rifampin and isoniazid resistance. J Clin Microbiol 2016;54(6):1624–30.

57. Mathys V, van de Vyvere M, de Droogh E, et al. False-positive rifampicin resistance on Xpert® MTB/RIF caused by a silent mutation in the rpoB gene. Int J Tuberc Lung Dis 2014;18(10):1255–7.

58. European Centre for Disease Prevention and Control. ERLN-TB expert opinion on the use of the rapid molecular assays for the diagnosis of tuberculosis and detection of drug resistance. Stockholm (Sweden): ECDC; 2013.

59. Shea J, Halse TA, Lapierre P, et al. Comprehensive whole-genome sequencing and reporting of drug resistance profiles on clinical cases of *Mycobacterium tuberculosis* in New York state. J Clin Microbiol 2017;55(6):1871–82.
60. Walker TM, Kohl TA, Omar SV, et al. Whole-genome sequencing for prediction of *Mycobacterium tuberculosis* drug susceptibility and resistance: a retrospective cohort study. Lancet Infect Dis 2015;15(10):1193–202.
61. Doyle RM, Burgess C, Williams R, et al. Direct whole-genome sequencing of sputum accurately Identifies drug-resistant *Mycobacterium tuberculosis* faster than MGIT culture sequencing. J Clin Microbiol 2018;56(8).
62. Colman RE, Schupp JM, Hicks ND, et al. Detection of low-level mixed-population drug resistance in *Mycobacterium tuberculosis* using high fidelity amplicon sequencing. PLoS One 2015;10(5):e0126626.
63. Olaru ID, Patel H, Kranzer K, et al. Turnaround time of whole genome sequencing for mycobacterial identification and drug susceptibility testing in routine practice. Clin Microbiol Infect 2018;24(6):659.e5-7.
64. World Health Organization. The use of next-generation sequencing technologies for the detection of mutations associated with drug resistance in *Mycobacterium tuberculosis* complex: technical guide. Geneva (Switzerland): World Health Organization; 2018.
65. Miotto P, Tessema B, Tagliani E, et al. A standardised method for interpreting the association between mutations and phenotypic drug resistance in *Mycobacterium tuberculosis*. Eur Respir J 2017;50(6):1701354.
66. Somoskovi A, Salfinger M. How can the tuberculosis laboratory aid in the patient-centered diagnosis and management of tuberculosis? Clin Chest Med 2019; 40(4):741–53.
67. Kranzer K, Kalsdorf B, Heyckendorf J, et al. New World Health Organization treatment Recommendations for multidrug-resistant tuberculosis: are we well enough prepared? Am J Respir Crit Care Med 2019;200(4):514–5.
68. Colangeli R, Jedrey H, Kim S, et al. Bacterial factors that predict relapse after tuberculosis therapy. N Engl J Med 2018;379(9):823–33.
69. World Health Organization. WHO consolidated guidelines on drug-resistant tuberculosis treatment. Geneva (Switzerland): World Health Organization; 2019.
70. de Vos M, Ley SD, Wiggins KB, et al. Bedaquiline microheteroresistance after cessation of tuberculosis treatment. N Engl J Med 2019;380(22):2178–80.
71. Somoskövi A, Bruderer V, Hömke R, et al. A mutation associated with clofazimine and bedaquiline cross-resistance in MDR-TB following bedaquiline treatment. Eur Respir J 2015;45(2):554–7.
72. Fowler PW, Gibertoni Cruz AL, Hoosdally SJ, et al. Automated detection of bacterial growth on 96-well plates for high-throughput drug susceptibility testing of *Mycobacterium tuberculosis*. Microbiology 2018;164(12):1522–30.
73. Cambau E, Viveiros M, Machado D, et al. Revisiting susceptibility testing in MDR-TB by a standardized quantitative phenotypic assessment in a European multi-centre study. J Antimicrob Chemother 2015;70(3):686–96.
74. Alcaide F, Amlerova J, Bou G, et al. How to: identify non-tuberculous *Mycobacterium* species using MALDI-TOF mass spectrometry. Clin Microbiol Infect 2018;24(6):599–603.
75. Rodriguez-Temporal D, Perez-Risco D, Struzka EA, et al. Evaluation of two protein extraction protocols based on freezing and mechanical disruption for identifying nontuberculous mycobacteria by matrix-assisted laser desorption ionization-time of flight mass spectrometry from liquid and solid cultures. J Clin Microbiol 2018; 56(4):e01548-17.

76. Rotcheewaphan S, Lemon JK, Desai UU, et al. Rapid one-step protein extraction method for the identification of mycobacteria using MALDI-TOF MS. Diagn Microbiol Infect Dis 2019;94(4):355–60.

77. Brown-Elliott BA, Fritsche TR, Olson BJ, et al. Comparison of two commercial matrix-assisted laser desorption/ionization-time of flight mass spectrometry (MALDI-TOF MS) systems for identification of nontuberculous mycobacteria. Am J Clin Pathol 2019;152(4):527–36.

78. O'Connor JA, O'Reilly B, Corcoran GD, et al. A comparison of the Hain Genotype CM reverse hybridisation assay with the Bruker MicroFlex LT MALDI-TOF mass spectrometer for identification of clinically relevant mycobacterial species. Br J Biomed Sci 2020;77(3):152–5.

79. Rodriguez-Sanchez B, Ruiz-Serrano MJ, Marin M, et al. Evaluation of matrix-assisted laser desorption ionization-time of flight mass spectrometry for identification of nontuberculous mycobacteria from clinical isolates. J Clin Microbiol 2015;53(8):2737–40.

80. Buckwalter SP, Olson SL, Connelly BJ, et al. Evaluation of matrix-assisted laser desorption ionization-time of flight mass spectrometry for identification of *Mycobacterium* species, *Nocardia* species, and other aerobic actinomycetes. J Clin Microbiol 2016;54(2):376–84.

81. Genc GE, Demir M, Yaman G, et al. Evaluation of MALDI-TOF MS for identification of nontuberculous mycobacteria isolated from clinical specimens in mycobacteria growth indicator tube medium. New Microbiol 2018;41(3):214–9.

82. Marekovic I, Bosnjak Z, Jakopovic M, et al. Evaluation of matrix-assisted laser desorption/ionization time-of-flight mass spectrometry in identification of nontuberculous mycobacteria. Chemotherapy 2016;61(4):167–70.

83. van Eck K, Faro D, Wattenberg M, et al. Matrix-assisted laser desorption ionization-time of flight mass spectrometry Fails to identify nontuberculous mycobacteria from primary cultures of respiratory samples. J Clin Microbiol 2016; 54(7):1915–7.

84. Body BA, Beard MA, Slechta ES, et al. Evaluation of the Vitek MS v3.0 matrix-assisted laser desorption ionization-time of flight mass spectrometry system for identification of *Mycobacterium* and *Nocardia* species. J Clin Microbiol 2018; 56(6):e00237-18.

85. Girard V, Mailler S, Welker M, et al. Identification of mycobacterium spp. and nocardia spp. from solid and liquid cultures by matrix-assisted laser desorption ionization-time of flight mass spectrometry (MALDI-TOF MS). Diagn Microbiol Infect Dis 2016;86(3):277–83.

86. Kehrmann J, Schoerding AK, Murali R, et al. Performance of Vitek MS in identifying nontuberculous mycobacteria from MGIT liquid medium and Lowenstein-Jensen solid medium. Diagn Microbiol Infect Dis 2016;84(1):43–7.

87. Leyer C, Gregorowicz G, Mougari F, et al. Comparison of Saramis 4.12 and IVD 3.0 Vitek MS matrix-assisted laser desorption ionization-time of flight mass spectrometry for identification of mycobacteria from solid and liquid culture media. J Clin Microbiol 2017;55(7):2045–54.

88. Miller E, Cantrell C, Beard M, et al. Performance of Vitek MS v3.0 for identification of *Mycobacterium* species from patient samples by use of automated liquid medium systems. J Clin Microbiol 2018;56(8):e00219-18.

89. Epperson LE, Timke M, Hasan NA, et al. Evaluation of a novel MALDI Biotyper algorithm to distinguish *Mycobacterium intracellulare* from *Mycobacterium chimaera*. Front Microbiol 2018;9:3140.

90. Pranada AB, Witt E, Bienia M, et al. Accurate differentiation of *Mycobacterium chimaera* from *Mycobacterium intracellulare* by MALDI-TOF MS analysis. J Med Microbiol 2017;66(5):670–7.
91. Ceyssens PJ, Soetaert K, Timke M, et al. Matrix-assisted laser desorption ionization-time of flight mass spectrometry for combined species identification and drug sensitivity testing in mycobacteria. J Clin Microbiol 2017;55(2):624–34.
92. Mougari F, Loiseau J, Veziris N, et al. Evaluation of the new GenoType NTM-DR kit for the molecular detection of antimicrobial resistance in non-tuberculous mycobacteria. J Antimicrob Chemother 2017;72(6):1669–77.
93. Winslow C-EA. The Life of Hermann M. Biggs, physician and statesman of the public health. Philadelphia: Lea & Febiger; 1929.

Food Safety Genomics and Connections to One Health and the Clinical Microbiology Laboratory

Marc W. Allard, PhD*, Jie Zheng, PhD, Guojie Cao, PhD,
Ruth Timme, PhD, Eric Stevens, PhD, Eric W. Brown, PhD

KEYWORDS

- Whole genome sequencing • Foodborne pathogen isolates • Data sharing
- Ontology • Genetic diversity • Outbreak detection • Contamination

KEY POINTS

- Whole genome sequencing of pathogens fits a one health perspective because their genomes are compared easily regardless of where or what host the pathogen was isolated from.
- Public health agencies rely on interlinking the events to understand the root causes of contamination events to prevent them from reoccurring in the future.
- One health methods embrace interoperability of data sharing with the goal of full integration of the public health evidence that has been gathered by the disparate agencies.
- Generally, the sooner that data are available the more rapidly a pattern of linkage is established and acted on through public health activities.

INTRODUCTION

One health refers to the full integration of the often separately treated subjects of human, animal, and environmental health. Human health is the concern of the health care system, of physicians, clinics, and hospitals. Governments connect to clinical patients through a variety of public health means through state departments of health and the National Institutes of Health, Centers for Disease Control and Prevention, Food and Drug Administration (FDA), and US Department of Agriculture. Animal health and safety is largely the realm of veterinarians that monitor animal health, diagnosis, and treatments. Environmental health of clean air and clean water are

Funding: Work was funded by internal research funding from the US Food and Drug Administration (FDA).
US Food and Drug Administration, Center for Food Safety and Applied Nutrition, 5001 Campus Drive, College Park, MD 20740, USA
* Corresponding author.
E-mail address: Marc.Allard@fda.hhs.gov

regulated by diverse federal and state agencies. Additionally, there are several other groups that more broadly monitor plant and animal diseases. Thus, it is not surprising that the different federal and state agencies often have different priorities and may also differ in their approaches to surveillance, monitoring, testing, and reporting. One health emphasizes that human, animal, and environmental health are interconnected in complex ways and that effects to one sector may cause perturbations to another. Although it is clear that the world is interconnected, it is often not clear how exactly public health is interconnected because of the diversity and complexity of interactions. In addition, the different public health entities are required to find specific solutions to some of these problems and so there should be no surprise that systems are often not only poorly integrated but may lack structural interoperability. Data may be stove-piped into silos and not digitized so they are not easily shared, and thus different groups may not even be aware that the other sectors have data of direct value to their own interests and priorities. When examined from a higher one health perspective it is often clear retrospectively that systems are related, but it is much rarer that de novo predictions from one health interactions are used to prevent public health consequences. Fresh water contaminated with animal waste including foodborne pathogens is incorporated into fresh cut vegetables when exposed to that water, and when that contaminated produce is eaten, sickens a portion of the vulnerable population. Some of those sick individuals end up in the clinics and hospitals with forms of gastroenteritis. Public health agencies rely on interlinking the events to understand the root causes of contamination events to prevent them from reoccurring in the future.

A larger goal is to understand global public health risks and intervene through preventative controls that limit pathogen exposure. One way to understand pathogens is to study them in all of the places where they reside including human, animals, and the environment. One health methods embrace interoperability of data sharing with the goal of full integration of the public health evidence that has been gathered by the disparate agencies. The goal is to integrate and synthesize, to develop new understandings of risk, and then to broadly disseminate that information so that others can benefit from that knowledge to prevent illness in their location.[1,2] To build a one health systems approach one criterion is to convince all stakeholders to collect and share data. A second criteria is to harmonize and validate the data to be collected and shared.[3] Another is to share data transparently, early, and globally to allow linkages to be seen by other stakeholders in a timely fashion. Generally, the sooner that data are available the more rapidly a pattern of linkage is established and acted on through public health activities. The metadata describing the genomic pathogen data are also valuable. For example, clinical laboratories have detailed information about the condition and treatment of the patient, their medical history, the course of treatment, and response to drugs yet these data are rarely anonymized and shared with public health authorities or the public more broadly. Determining what is risky based on severity of the illness might help public health authorities prioritize response, focus research into the riskiest foods, and develop preventative control strategies or treatments to reduce their recurrence and severity.

Whole genome sequencing (WGS) of viral and bacterial pathogens is a natural fit to a one health perspective because their genomes are compared easily regardless of where or what host the pathogen was isolated from. A genome provides a huge amount of data that can be analyzed for numerous applications. Roughly, 5 million base pairs make up a typical *Salmonella* genome. For example, the same genomic data can produce a phylogeny documenting a cluster of emerging pathogens that links food, environmental, and clinical isolates representing an emerging outbreak, contamination, or a spreading hospital-acquired infection.[4,5] The same genomic data can be screened for the presence of genes and allelic variants known to produce antimicrobial resistance (AMR,[6,7]). WGS provides multiple solutions and genetic evidence to answer numerous applications that the one health paradigm wishes to monitor and address. WGS naturally integrates one health disciplines when the diverse public health entities share their genomic data and metadata in a common database. Sharing data and metadata coordinates surveillance efforts across the various disciplines.

One such WGS database is the FDA GenomeTrakr data,[8,9] which consists of a series of bioprojects where data are stored at the National Center for Biotechnology Information (NCBI). In addition to long-term storage, quality assurances, and controls of the genomic data, the NCBI Pathogen Detection portal builds daily phylogenetic trees to document and uncover the most closely related isolates ($\leq$50 single-nucleotide polymorphisms [SNPs]) and also documents the presence/absence of known genes that cause AMR.[10]

AMR monitoring of animal, food, and environmental isolates may be used to predict trends or inform policy relevant to clinical practice,[11-13] discover new genes providing AMR,[14] and document existing genes and their distributions.[15] The NCBI Pathogen Detection and their AMRFinder and AMRFinderPlus databases and tools have been compiled to provide rapid determination of the presence of AMR genes[6] for all publicly released human pathogens currently tracked. NCBI and their collaborators including the FDA National Antimicrobial Resistance Monitoring System continue to expand these data sets and compile novel genes, including phenotype (antibiogram) to genotype predictions of more than 98%.[16]

These databases include more than half a million WGS isolates from food, animal, clinical, and environmental origins. The close association of isolates in a phylogenetic tree that share common ancestry directly documents the one health concept that these pathogens may be directly connected to one another.[17,18] Sharing a recent common ancestor and belonging to a common clade is direct evidence that these isolates are closely connected but further investigation may be needed to fully characterize that relationship.[19-21]

FDA foodborne disease outbreak and compliance investigations are often described as a three-legged stool of investigation. The first leg of the stool often comes from the laboratory, where WGS provides genetic evidence of a phylogenetic cluster that links food, environmental, and clinical isolates. By focusing on the most closely related isolates at the tips of the phylogenetic tree, WGS clusters a subset of the isolates that are monophyletic and share a recent common ancestor. These subclusters often are used to separate outbreak signals from background noise, to unravel the complexities of foodborne contaminations, support epidemiologic and site investigations, support infectious control, and to improve public health. Not only does WGS focus the investigations on the physical evidence of a closely related subcluster, but it also unravels the complexity of a polyclonal outbreak made up of several lineages, by breaking the investigation into smaller solvable parts. Each lineage within a polyclonal outbreak or contamination event is treated as an independent pathogen and piece of evidence tying a specific food commodity, or firm, to a clinical case. For the three legs of the stool of a foodborne investigation, the epidemiologic leg may determine whether the clinical cases have been exposed to a common food contaminant found at a firm. The FDA inspection of the firm is the leg that may provide positive cultures of the foodborne pathogens contaminating the facility. FDA relies on field inspectors to recover the diversity of pathogens present in a contaminated facility. For FDA compliance, it is the inspection results that help determine whether a contamination event is polyclonal or not, although multiple

WGS clusters may each independently point back to the same firm being responsible for the contaminant exposure. It is important to integrate the three legs of the investigation to support an outbreak or contamination event. The power and prediction of the full investigation comes from integrating the various relevant evidence including laboratory, epidemiologic, and field investigations. Losing any one leg reduces the predictive power of the others. These tenants and strategies of infectious control and root cause investigation are critical elements to a successful investigation whether the contaminated area is within a hospital network or part of a food production chain.

Genomic methods are always as good or superior to lower resolution subtyping methods.[22] Thus, more data are always better when the goal is source tracking for infectious control and root cause investigation. The success of WGS use within the United States is evidence of the superior performance of these methods and is one of many reasons why states and federal agencies have adopted WGS. Most of the examples that are critical of WGS- and SNP-based approaches are caused by mixing up the context of information with some perceived inherent limitation of sequencing. This perceived lack of information integration has nothing to do with any limitations of WGS.[23,24] On the contrary, WGS is best suited to integrate all case information, provided it is being used. More data from WGS provide higher resolution, which more clearly defines a contamination case definition and the explicit genetic changes that have occurred among the isolates sequenced. Reduced resolution generally increases false inclusion by collapsing nodes that are particularly problematic for ecological and epidemiologic models when clinical and environmental isolates are included in clusters that were not exposed to the same contaminant. The powerful resolution provided by WGS can separate clinical cases that were not exposed to the same contaminated food or facility.[19,21] The high resolution provided by SNP-based analysis of WGS often resolves all isolates down to the tips of the tree. If exposure data suggest a common contaminant and/or food vehicle, and those data are supported by WGS, then that node on the phylogenetic tree can be set as the case definition. Often there is clear evidence for a cluster break, either based on the number and position of SNPs that define a lineage, the bootstrap score for the node, or genetic evidence that separates one lineage to other sublineages close by.[25] False inclusion has confounded studies of infectious control and hospital-acquired infections when sequence types of lower resolution make cases look like they are related but WGS higher resolution documents differences.[11–13] Often what looks like a large problem is multiple contaminations or infections occurring at the same time.

IMPACT OF ISOLATE DIVERSITY ON WHOLE GENOME SEQUENCING CLUSTER ANALYSIS?

The level of foodborne pathogen diversity observed from an inspection of a food facility does not change the process of WGS analysis or interpretation for compliance investigations.[25] An isolate from each positive swab is grown to pure culture, sequenced, and uploaded to the GenomeTrakr database and analyzed at the NCBI Pathogen Detection Web site. All lineages that are phylogenetically clustered with a close common ancestor are carefully examined and based on those results additional investigations may occur. The current maximum threshold for linkage at the NCBI Pathogen Detection tools is less than or equal to 50 SNPs, a self-imposed limit to reduce the bioinformatic costs of analysis, and greater than these levels isolates generally are more distantly related and not directly connected to the contamination event in question. Finding greater than expected sequence divergence (>50 SNPS) within a "clonal" lineage generally does not support a close common ancestor but rather a more distant relationship. There is no specific time interval limitation imposed on the clustering, allowing all isolates in the publicly released database to be included for possible forensic linkage and cluster detection. Although no time limits are imposed on analysis, often it is difficult to make formal investigational linkages for isolates whose collection dates are separated by more than a year. Any lineage that links food or environmental isolates to clinical isolates is of additional concern because this is hypothetical evidence that the foodborne pathogen has contaminated the food supply causing illness. Whether one lineage or multiple lineages link to clinical cases[23,24] does not confound WGS results, interpretation, or the decisions made at Center of Food Safety and Applied Nutrition Office of Compliance investigations. The strategy of examining each lineage separately unravels the complexity of what is observed during inspection. Each lineage is additional evidence on the scope of the contamination event and may provide additional details concerning the root cause of the contamination. Although there is some observed diversity on what level of genetic variation (eg, SNP differences) suggests whether isolates share a close common ancestor, most contamination event clusters fit into the general recommendations that we have observed for interpreting WGS outbreak investigations,[25] which is less than or equal to 20 SNPs using the CFSAN SNP pipeline[17] and monophyly of the clade with strong bootstrap support.

The genetic evidence from the laboratory is strongest when supported by additional pieces of evidence from the three-legged stool of investigation: epidemiologic evidence of a shared exposure of a contaminated food that caused the illness; and actual site investigations from inspection authorities to determine the root cause of a contamination event. For example, foodborne pathogens isolated from a creek near a tomato farm, are closely related to a turtle collected near that fresh water, and clinical patients that got sick from eating contaminated tomatoes grown on the farm (**Fig. 1, Table 1**). This case and figure are an example of how the three-legged stool of investigation are combined to support linkages by including isolates from clinical, animal, and environmental in one analysis with isolates often collected independently by separate agencies. Not only does the WGS phylogenetic evidence document the one health connections but it also suggests that there is a risk associated with agricultural water sources in this area of the country where produce is grown. Good agricultural practices can outline the risks associated with agricultural water and can provide guidance to farmers on appropriate uses of agricultural water to prevent foodborne contamination of crops.[26–28] Knowledge discovered

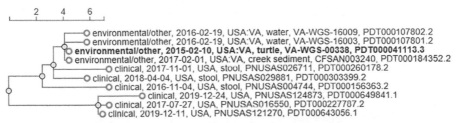

Fig. 1. Phylogenetic results of *Salmonella* clustering environmental isolates, including creek sediment, water, turtle, and human stool, NCBI Pathogen Detection Cluster PDS000051343.129 (as of June 17, 2020). The *number line* corresponds to SNPs, where the branch length is proportional to the number of SNPs present. Detailed SNP differences also are available at the NCBI Pathogen Detection site by searching for either strain IDs or SNP Cluster IDs.

Table 1
Metadata of environmental and clinical isolates of *Salmonella*

Strain	Isolate	Create Date	Location	Isolation Source	Isolation Type	BioSample
VA-WGS-00338	PDT000041113.3	2/10/2015	United States:VA	Turtle	Environmental/other	SAMN03112864
VA-WGS-16003	PDT000107801.2	2/19/2016	United States:VA	Water	Environmental/other	SAMN04431100
VA-WGS-16009	PDT000107802.2	2/19/2016	United States:VA	Water	Environmental/other	SAMN04431106
PNUSAS004744	PDT000156363.2	11/4/2016	United States	Stool	Clinical	SAMN05956750
CFSAN003240	PDT000184352.2	2/1/2017	United States:VA	Creek sediment	Environmental/other	SAMN03463751
PNUSAS016550	PDT000227787.2	7/27/2017	United States		Clinical	SAMN07372786
PNUSAS026711	PDT000260178.2	11/1/2017	United States	Stool	Clinical	SAMN07840830
PNUSAS029881	PDT000303399.2	4/4/2018	United States	Stool	Clinical	SAMN08865572
PNUSAS121270	PDT000643056.1	12/11/2019	United States		Clinical	SAMN13525431
PNUSAS124873	PDT000649841.1	12/24/2019	United States		Clinical	SAMN13675605

Sequences are deposited at NCBI.

using WGS evidence directly links food, human, animal, and environmental isolates and helps the understanding of the sources and mechanisms of pathogen contamination and helps guide preventive controls to minimize or prevent pathogens from contaminating food on the farm.

The farm is just one environment where pathogens reside but there is a world of diversity that also should be monitored, such as the food processing environment[29] or hospitals.[11] NCBI pathogen detection[10] currently monitors one yeast and 31 bacterial human pathogens but does not yet track virus, parasite, and many other plant- or animal-specific pathogens. The original focus of this project was on foodborne bacterial pathogens to support food safety and public health, but this is rapidly expanding to include other human pathogens. For example, a large state department of health might monitor roughly two dozen pathogens for that state, and more work needs to be done so that all other genomes, many isolates or samples collected by hospitals, are uploaded and shared globally and in real time. Sharing the data and acting on the data is a great way to have a big impact in public health outcomes. The sooner that investigators see a pathogen and its link to illness, and environmental reservoirs the sooner that interventions can take place to remove the risk and install preventative controls to limit the pathogen's return.[30] State and federal governments, along with public health agencies, should be encouraged to share all allowable genomic data and metadata descriptions that they collect. International World Wide Web–based tools also must be made available to assist in the rapid phylogenetic analysis of the data. By sharing and communicating across a one health network more pathogens are identified and characterized sooner reducing the burden of public health of sickness and suffering.

The Global Microbial Identifier consortium[31] envisions a global system of DNA genome databases for microbial and infectious disease identification and diagnostics. The Global Microbial Identifier is a not-for-profit international consortium of more than 270 scientists from 55 countries in support of a framework for coordinating the sequencing data collection and analysis of microorganisms, and the open sharing of sequence data. Such a system will benefit those tackling individual problems at the frontline, including clinicians, veterinarian, policymakers, regulators, and industry. By enabling access to this global resource, a professional response on health threats will be within reach of all countries with basic laboratory infrastructure.

In addition to sharing the genomic data, careful consideration should be made for sharing the metadata that describes the genomes.[32,33] Investigators have documented the great value added by including detailed metadata for each isolate.[21,34] Investigators are encouraged to include all legally allowable metadata. They should also consider supplying curated ontologies that provide detailed descriptive hierarchies using standardized language to improve communication and more fully characterize the metadata of the isolate sequenced.[3,32] Ontologies that are machine readable allow for additional artificial intelligence analysis for increased predictions from the genomic data. Risk assessment and risk management investigators have used food ontologies to improve software predictions of foodborne pathogen risk assessment and risk management.[33] AMR monitoring has been able to predict AMR and minimum inhibitory concentration scores using ontologies and machine learning.[35] The zoonotic source attribution of Salmonella has been predicted successfully for some domestic animal investigations using these techniques.[36] FDA investigators are exploring the use of additional food ontologies, such as Interagency Food Safety Analytics Collaboration for food attribution[32] and FoodOn as an alternative ontology for attribution,[37] along with detailed ontologies for epidemiology, pathogens, environmental, hospital, and food process sampling. Adding more machine-readable metadata that is linked to the WGS data is one strategy that will allow for a new era for modern food safety, precision medicine, and public health through timely predictions, improving the understanding of underlying risks, which will allow the food industry to improve their preventive controls making food safer and reducing the incidence of foodborne contamination.

The digitization of metadata combined with WGS will provide powerful rapid tools to improve and integrate one health objectives to improve food safety and reduce its burden on public health. There have already been seen numerous WGS examples of the power to predict country of origin,[34] growing region,[19,21] and even implicated egg farms[19] using phylogenetics. As metadata ontologies are adopted and improved for these foodborne pathogens, it is likely that artificial intelligence and machine learning will bring additional future predictions to support contamination and outbreak investigations.

Estimates on the economic burden of illness within Canada and the United States have been performed for *Salmonella*.[38] These authors estimate that with the adoption of WGS for rapid response and action to impact foodborne illness, the burden of illness in Canada could be reduced by up to one-third of the total burden of illness, which would save millions of dollars in Canada and billions of dollars annually for US foodborne pathogens.[39] The global impact would produce even greater savings because most nations have burdens of foodborne illness at levels somewhere between Canada and the United States with the total global foodborne illness burden estimated at more than 110 billion dollars annually. The economic argument alone should be enough to motivate governments to invest in one health and WGS technologies, surveillance activities, improved capacity for sequencing for public health laboratories, and to share the data globally and in real-time to reduce the burden of illness locally and globally.

By making the foodborne pathogen genomes publicly available in the NCBI Pathogen Detection Web site, state and federal public health agencies allow other countries in the world to share and compare the pathogens that they are collecting. These real-time databases allow for one health global comparisons to track global travel and trade of contaminated products. To date we have observed closely related WGS clusters (10 or fewer SNPs) linked to illnesses, including isolates from contaminated food or the environment, from 72 countries including Australia, Austria, Brazil, Canada, Chile, China, Dominican Republic, Ecuador, Egypt, Ethiopia, Germany, India, Indonesia, Italy, Kenya, Mexico, Peru, the Philippines, Switzerland, Thailand, Turkey, Uganda, Vietnam, and the United Kingdom. State and federal laboratories upload their genomic data to NCBI Pathogen detection to compare their local isolates with publicly released global data. Any closely related genomics cluster may help solve an outbreak or contamination event. If the data are not made publicly available, then investigations will miss these important signals and possible connections. We have seen more and more international clusters where isolates from two or more nations share a close common ancestor either from international travel or international trade of contaminated foods. It is becoming more commonplace for state and federal laboratories to contact their international peers when phylogenetic clusters are observed. The best way to see all available WGS signals is to upload all foodborne pathogen genomes into the NCBI Pathogen Detection Web site and watch for the most closely related emerging clusters. National and international laboratories who do not embrace a one health approach and who do not share their data globally and in real-time risk missing phylogenetic signals that may have led them to solve an outbreak or contamination event sooner.[40] The sooner that the contaminant is removed from the food supply chain the fewer people will be impacted by that event and the greater the reduction in the burden to public health.

AVAILABILITY OF DATA AND MATERIALS' SECTION

All data are available by searching the biosample numbers at the NCBI. The phylogenetic relationships among the strains in comparison with others isolated worldwide and SNP Cluster nomenclature were obtained at the NCBI Pathogen Detection URL.

ACKNOWLEDGMENTS

The authors thank our partners at US Food and Drug Administration (FDA). The authors also thank the many collaborators in the GenomeTrakr network, CDC PulseNet, USDA-FSIS, who provide their data for broad use and applications, and the data support that we all receive at the FDA and the NCBI.

DISCLOSURE

The authors have nothing to disclose.

REFERENCES

1. Ladner JT, Grubaugh ND, Pybus OG, et al. Precision epidemiology for infectious disease control. Nat Med 2019;25:206–11.
2. RE Timme, MS Leon, MW Allard. Utilizing the public GenomeTrakr database for foodborne pathogen traceback. Foodborne Bacterial Pathogens, 201-212.
3. Timme RE, Wolfgang WJ, Balkey M, et al. Optimizing open data to support one health: best practices to ensure interoperability of genomic data from microbial pathogens. Preprints 2020. https://doi.org/10.20944/preprints202004.0253.v1.
4. Ashton PM, Nair S, Peters TM, et al. Identification of Salmonella for public health surveillance using whole genome sequencing. PeerJ 2016;4:e1752.
5. Pecora N, Zhao X, Nudel K, et al. Diverse vectors and mechanisms spread New Delhi metallo-β-lactamases among carbapenem-resistant enterobacteriaceae in the greater Boston area. Antimicrob Agents Chemother 2019;63. e02040–18.
6. Feldgarden M, Brover V, Haft DH, et al. Validating the NCBI AMRFinder tool and resistance gene database using antimicrobial resistance genotype-phenotype correlations in a collection of NARMS isolates. Antimicrob Agents Chemother 2019;63(11):e00483-19.
7. McDermott PF, Tyson GH, Kabera C, et al. Whole-genome sequencing for detecting antimicrobial resistance in nontyphoidal Salmonella. Antimicrob Agents Chemother 2016;60:5515–20.
8. Allard MW, Strain E, Melka D, et al. Practical value of food pathogen traceability through building a whole-genome sequencing network and database. J Clin Microbiol 2016;54:197.
9. Timme RE, Sanchez Leon M, Allard MW. Utilizing the public GenomeTrakr database for foodborne pathogen Traceback. In: Bridier A, editor. Foodborne bacterial pathogens. Methods in molecular biology, vol. 1918. New York: Humana Press; 2019. p. 201–12.
10. NCBI pathogen detection. 2019. Available at: https://www.ncbi.nlm.nih.gov/pathogens/. Accessed September 2, 2020.
11. Pecora ND, Li N, Allard M, et al. Genomically informed surveillance for carbapenem-resistant enterobacteriaceae in a health care system. mBio 2015;6(4). e01030-15.
12. Pecora N, Zhao X, Nudel K, et al. Diverse vectors and mechanisms spread New Delhi metallo-β-lactamases among carbapenem-resistant Enterobacteriaceae in

the Greater Boston area. Antimicrob Agents Chemother 2019;63. https://doi.org/10.1128/AAC.02040-18. e02040-18.

13. Pecora ND, Li N, Allard M, et al. 2015. Genomically informed surveillance for carbapenem-resistant enterobacteriaceae in a health care system. mBio 6(4):e01030-15. doi:10.1128/mBio.01030-15.

14. Zhao S, Mukherjee S, Li C, et al. Cloning and expression of novel aminoglycoside phosphotransferase genes from Campylobacter and their role in the resistance to six aminoglycosides. Antimicrob Agents Chemother 2018;62. https://doi.org/10.1128/AAC.01682-17. e01682-17.

15. Resistome tracker 2020 program FDA CVM NARMS. Available at: https://www.fda.gov/animal-veterinary/national-antimicrobial-resistance-monitoring-system/global-salmonella-resistome-data. Accessed September 2, 2020.

16. Karp BE, Tate H, Plumblee JR, et al. National antimicrobial resistance monitoring system: two decades of advancing public health through integrated surveillance of antimicrobial resistance. Foodborne Pathog Dis 2017;545–57. https://doi.org/10.1089/fpd.2017.2283.

17. Davis S, Pettengill JB, Luo Y, et al. CFSAN SNP pipeline: an automated method for constructing SNP matrices from nextgeneration sequence data. PeerJ Comput Sci 2015;1:e20.

18. Timme RE, Strain E, Baugher J, et al. Phylogenomic pipeline validation for foodborne pathogen disease surveillance. J Clin Microbiol 2019. https://doi.org/10.1128/JCM.01816-18.

19. Allard MW, Luo Y, Strain E, et al. On the evolutionary history, population genetics and diversity among isolates of Salmonella enteritidis PFGE pattern JEGX01.0004. PLoS One 2013;8(1):e55254.

20. Hoffmann M, Zhao S, Pettengill J, et al. Comparative genomic analysis and virulence differences in closely related Salmonella enterica serotype Heidelberg isolates from humans, retail meats, and animals. Genome Biol Evol 2014;6(5):1046–68.

21. Lienau EK, Strain E, Wang C, et al. Identification of a salmonellosis outbreak by means of molecular sequencing. N Engl J Med 2011;364(10):981–2.

22. Kubota KA, Wolfgang WJ, Baker DJ, et al. PulseNet and the changing paradigm of laboratory-based surveillance for foodborne diseases. Public Health Rep 2019. https://doi.org/10.1177/0033354919881650.

23. Besser JM, Carleton HA, Trees E, et al. Interpretation of whole-genome sequencing for enteric disease surveillance and outbreak investigation. Foodborne Pathog Dis 2019;16:7.

24. Gerner-Smidt P, Besser J, Concepción-Acevedo J, et al. Whole genome sequencing: bridging one-health surveillance of foodborne diseases. Front Public Health 2019;27(7):172.

25. Pightling AW, Pettengill JB, Luo Y, et al. Interpreting whole-genome sequence analyses of foodborne bacteria for regulatory applications and outbreak investigations. Front Microbiol 2018;9:1482.

26. Bell R, Zheng J, Burrows E, et al. Ecological prevalence, genetic diversity and epidemiological aspects of Salmonella isolated from tomato agricultural regions of the Virginia Eastern Shore. Front Microbiol 2015;6:415.

27. Walters SP, Thebo AL, Boehm AB. Impact of urbanization and agriculture on the occurrence of bacterial pathogens and stx genes in coastal waterbodies of central California. Water Res 2011;45(4):1752–62.

28. Zheng J, Allard S, Reynolds S, et al. Colonization and internalization of *Salmonella enterica* in tomato plants. Appl Environ Microbiol 2013. https://doi.org/10.1128/AEM.03704-12.

29. Wang Y, Pettengill JB, Pightling A, et al. Genetic diversity of *Salmonella* and *Listeria* isolates from food facilities. J Food Prot 2018;81(12):2082–9.

30. Allard MW, Stevens EL, Brown EW. All for one and one for all: the true potential of whole-genome sequencing. Lancet Infect Dis 2019b;19:683–4.

31. Global Microbial Identifier. 2019. Available at: https://www.globalmicrobial identifier.org/. Accessed September 2, 2020.

32. Richardson LC, Bazaco MC, Parker CC, et al. An updated scheme for categorizing foods implicated in foodborne disease outbreaks: a tri-agency collaboration. Foodborne Pathog Dis 2017;14(12):701–10.

33. Sanaa M, Pouillot R, Garces-Vega FJ, et al. GenomeGraphR: a user-friendly open-source web application for foodborne pathogen whole genome sequencing data integration, analysis, and visualization. BioRxiv 2018. https://doi.org/10.1101/495309.

34. Hoffmann M, Luo Y, Monday SR, et al. Tracing origins of the *Salmonella* Bareilly strain causing a food-borne outbreak in the United States. J Infect Dis 2016; 213(4):502–8.

35. Nguyen M, Long SW, McDermott PF, et al. Using machine learning to predict antimicrobial MICs and associated genomic features for nontyphoidal *Salmonella*. J Clin Microbiol 2019;57. e01260-18.

36. Zhang S, Li S, Gu W, et al. Zoonotic source attribution of *Salmonella enterica* serotype Typhimurium using genomic surveillance data, United States. Emerg Infect Dis 2019;25(1):8.

37. FoodOn. 2019. Available at: https://foodon.org/. Accessed September 2, 2020.

38. Jain S, Mukhopadhyay K, Thomassin PJ. An economic analysis of salmonella detection in fresh produce, poultry, and eggs using whole genome sequencing technology in Canada. Food Res Int 2019;116:802–9.

39. Minor T, Lasher A, Klontz K, et al. The per case and total annual costs of foodborne illness in the United States. Risk Anal 2015;35(6):1125–39.

40. Allard MW, Strain E, Rand H, et al. Whole genome sequencing uses for foodborne contamination and compliance: discovery of an emerging contamination event in an ice cream facility using whole genome sequencing. Infect Genet Evol 2019;73: 214–20.

Update in Infectious Disease Diagnosis in Anatomic Pathology

Alvaro C. Laga, MD, MMSc

KEYWORDS

- Infectious • Pathology • Special stains • Inflammatory pattern • Pitfalls • Detection

KEY POINTS

- Anatomic pathology is an important resource for detection of microorganisms in tissue sections and may be the first indication of an otherwise unsuspected infection.
- Inflammatory patterns (eg, suppurative, granulomatous, necrotizing) are adequate to suggest infection in general, but are nonspecific and suboptimal to accurately point toward a specific pathogen or class of pathogens.
- Common pitfalls in anatomic pathology diagnosis of infectious disease include inadequate interpretation of special stains and immunohistochemistry, diagnosing infections as tumor or malignancy, and mistaking tissue components, products of reactive processes and foreign objects for microorganisms.
- Targeted molecular testing of tissue specimens with microorganisms detected by hematoxylin and eosin and histochemical stains increases the yield of specific identification.

INTRODUCTION

Anatomic pathology is an important resource for detection and exclusion of infectious diseases in tissue specimens.[1] Pathologists investigate the possibility of infection in tissues when clinicians enlist infection as a possible diagnosis and/or when there is an inflammatory reaction or "structures" suggestive of infection or microorganism (**Fig. 1**). Although infectious disease pathology is a subspecialty in anatomic pathology, the low volume of specimens relative to other disciplines (eg, dermatopathology, gastrointestinal pathology) does not allow for having anatomic pathologists dedicated solely to infectious disease pathology in the vast majority of institutions. Consequently, as Guarner[2] has astutely observed, infectious disease pathologists are pathologists with an interest in infectious diseases to whom colleagues show cases deemed potentially infectious, and frequently have another function or area of expertise to justify employment (eg, microbiology laboratory director, neuropathologist,

Department of Pathology, Brigham and Women's Hospital, Harvard Medical School, 75 Francis Street, Amory-3, Boston, MA 02115, USA
E-mail address: alagacanales@bwh.harvard.edu

Clin Lab Med 40 (2020) 565–585
https://doi.org/10.1016/j.cll.2020.08.012
0272-2712/20/© 2020 Elsevier Inc. All rights reserved.

labmed.theclinics.com

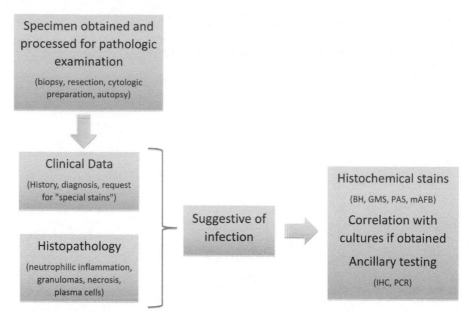

Fig. 1. Investigation of infection by the pathologist.

gastrointestinal pathologist, dermatopathologist). Pathologists consult infectious disease pathologists when they need help evaluating and interpreting special stains or when they find something unusual and consider it could be a microorganism.[2]

Detection of a microorganism (ie, bacteria, fungi, parasite) in tissue sections is frequently the beginning of a workup and only occasionally sufficient for a final diagnosis with definitive microbiologic identification. Close correlation with cultures and ancillary testing in the microbiology laboratory is of paramount importance in arriving at a diagnosis and identify with certitude causative pathogen(s). Whereas microbiology pertains to the study of microscopic organisms, such as viruses, bacteria, fungi, and parasites, infectious disease pathology focuses on pathologic processes caused by such microorganisms, considering the host response to infection at the cellular level. At our institution, the microbiology laboratory performs approximately 500,000 tests per year. In contrast, there are approximately 700 intradepartmental consults to the infectious disease pathology consult service in anatomic pathology, and an estimated additional 200 cases in which anatomic pathologists detect and/or diagnose infection but do not consult infectious disease pathology. This review discusses the adequacy and limitations of histopathology in the diagnosis of infectious diseases, describes potential pitfalls, and discusses the appropriate use of molecular diagnostics in formalin-fixed, paraffin-embedded tissues (FFPE).

INFECTION AND THE ANATOMIC PATHOLOGIST

The presence of inflammation in tissue sections is frequently the first indication of the possibility of infection. Nonetheless, it is by itself a nonspecific finding and noninfectious inflammatory diseases need also be considered in clinical context. The inflammatory patterns seen in tissue specimens associated with infection are dependent on the time of biopsy in the evolution of the process and the immune status of the host. **Table 1** summarizes selected infectious agents and the spectrum of

Table 1
Selected inflammatory patterns with typical and underrecognized microorganism associations

Inflammatory Pattern	Organisms Commonly Associated	Organisms Uncommonly Associated	Recommended Testing (FFPE)
Neutrophilic inflammation	Pyogenic bacteria (eg, *Staphylococcus, Streptococcus*)	Nontuberculous mycobacteria, *Blastomyces* spp., *Sporothrix* spp.	BH, Fite, GMS, PAS
Necrotizing granulomas	*Mycobacterium tuberculosis*	*Coccidioides* spp., *Mycobacterium marinum*, MAC	Fite, PCR if positive
Non-necrotizing granulomas	Mycobacteria, fungi	*Treponema pallidum*	Spirochete IHC
Diffuse necrosis	Bacteria, mycobacteria	HSV, VZV	IHC
Stellate necrosis	*Bartonella henselae* (cat-scratch disease)	*Francisella tularensis, Yersinia pestis*	Warthin-Starry, PCR
Fibrin ring granulomas	*Coxiella burnetii*	CMV, EBV, Hepatitis A and C, *Leishmania*	IHC, PCR
Eosinophilic and granulomatous	Nematodes	*Basidiobolus* and *Conidiobolus*	GMS, PAS

Abbreviations: BH, Brown-Hopps stain; CMV, cytomegalovirus; EBV, Epstein-Barr virus; GMS, Grocott methenamine silver stain; IHC, immunohistochemistry; MAC, *M avium intracellulare* complex; PAS, periodic acid–Schiff stain; PCR, polymerase chain reaction.

inflammatory reactions that may be encountered, including nonclassical morphologic patterns that may be underrecognized. There are limited cellular host responses to a wide variety of infectious agents, including bacteria, viruses, fungi, and parasites. The inflammatory reactions to microorganisms include neutrophilic inflammation with or without abscess formation, mononuclear infiltrates with or without plasma cells, granulomas, with or without necrosis, and diffuse necrosis as the sole finding.

At variance with general perception, it is well established that biopsies of nontuberculous mycobacterial lesions with so-called "rapid growers" and those affecting immunocompromised patients may manifest with suppurative inflammation with micro abscess formation and necrosis, many times without well-formed granulomas.[3,4] It is therefore important to obtain an acid-fast stain on biopsies from immunocompromised patients and suppurative inflammation. Correlation with clinical parameters, cultures, and polymerase chain reaction (PCR) when appropriate, are necessary for accurate diagnosis at the species level. The presence of multinucleate giant cells and foci of prominent neutrophilic infiltrate around clear vacuoles resembling adipose tissue may be clues that should alert the pathologist to perform an acid-fast stain **(Fig. 2)**.

Granulomatous inflammation is the hallmark of mycobacterial infection.[5] The presence of necrosis in granulomatous inflammation is particularly associated with tuberculosis, but may also be seen with nontuberculous mycobacteria, such as *Mycobacterium avium complex* and *Mycobacterium heckershornense*.[6,7] Conversely, tuberculosis may present without granulomas in immunocompromised patients.[8] Accordingly, the presence of acid-fast bacilli (AFB) in necrotizing granulomatous inflammation is not synonymous with tuberculosis. Necrotizing granulomatous

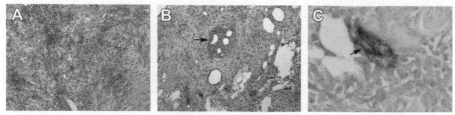

Fig. 2. Patient with myelodysplastic syndrome and new onset erythematous nodules on legs. (*A*) Interstitial neutrophilic infiltrate in the reticular dermis. (*B*) Microscopic abscesses with clear vacuoles (*arrow*) are an important clue to nontuberculous mycobacterial infection in immunocompromised patients. Note the absence of granulomas (*C*). Abundant acid-fast bacilli are evident on AFB stain (*arrow*). A concurrent culture and PCR identified *Mycobacterium avium intracellulare*.

inflammation may also be seen with fungal organisms such as *Coccidioides* spp. (**Fig. 3**) among others, and even viruses can produce necrotizing granulomatous inflammation, such as in herpes simplex virus (HSV).[9] It should be emphasized that suppurative inflammation with or without scattered giant cells or granulomas is neither specific for atypical mycobacteria and may be observed in other infectious processes such as nocardiosis (**Fig. 4**) and deep fungal infection. When evaluating biopsies from immunocompromised hosts, pathologists should remember that suppurative inflammation is not always due to classic pyogenic bacteria (ie, *Streptococcus* or *Staphylococcus*) and to include nontuberculous mycobacterial infection and *nocardia* in the differential diagnosis.

So-called chronic inflammation is characterized by the presence of mononuclear cells (macrophages, lymphocytes, and sometimes plasma cells) and is generally thought to be of slow onset of days to weeks and the consequence of persistence of antigenic stimuli including microorganisms.[10] Spirochetal infections elicit chronic inflammation. *Borrelia burgdorferi,* the causal agent of Lyme disease, commonly presents with *erythema chronicum migrans*, a characteristic cutaneous eruption reminiscent of a large bullseye at the site of a tick bite. The histopathology of erythema migrans is a tightly woven perivascular infiltrate of lymphocytes around the superficial and deep cutaneous vascular plexuses termed gyrate erythema, but it is nonspecific. The diagnosis of Lyme disease, however, requires serologic confirmation of acute infection or demonstration of the bacteria in tissue samples by PCR, as cultures from blood or skin samples are of low yield.[11] *Treponema pallidum,* the causal agent

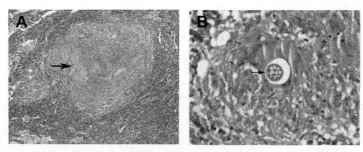

Fig. 3. Young patient with right upper lobe mass and pneumonia. (*A*) Necrotizing granulomas indistinguishable from those of tuberculosis are present (*arrow*). (*B*) Careful examination reveals spherules with endospores (*arrow*), virtually diagnostic of coccidioidomycosis.

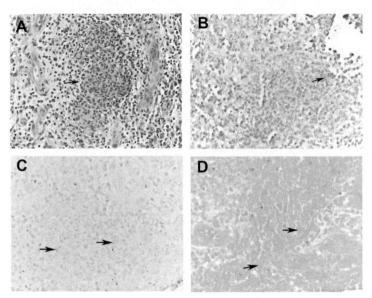

Fig. 4. Patient with multiple myeloma treated by stem-cell transplant with erythematous papules on right hand and arm in sporotrichoid distribution. (*A*) Occasional granulomas with neutrophilic inflammation (*arrow*) are evident on a punch biopsy. (*B*) Scant long, branching acid-fast bacteria are noted on a modified AFB stain (*arrow*, Fite-Faraco stain). These bacteria are gram-positive (*arrows*) (*C*) and also apparent on GMS stain (*arrows*) (*D*).

of syphilis, commonly elicits mononuclear inflammation, characteristically with frequent plasma cells. Syphilis is noteworthy because it may mimic a variety of inflammatory conditions including psoriasis, lichenoid dermatitis, hepatitis, lymphoma, and interstitial nephritis, among others, and therefore has been dubbed "the great mimicker" (**Fig. 5**).[12] The presence of perivascular plasma cells is characteristic of primary syphilis in the skin, but it has been estimated that 25% of cases of secondary syphilis do not have a conspicuous plasma cell infiltrate on biopsy and they are variable in the other 75%.[13–15] Moreover, the presence of perivascular plasma cells is nonspecific, and although commonly associated with syphilis, may be seen in mucosal and scalp biopsies, among others. Infectious processes such as the patch stage of Kaposi sarcoma also have characteristically frequent perivascular plasma cells.[15]

When considering infection based on clinical context and presence of inflammation in a tissue sample, so-called special stains are frequently obtained. The author's recommendation is to keep an open mind and request Gram, acid-fast (AFB), methenamine silver (MSS) and Periodic acid–Schiff (PAS) stains as an initial step. They are widely available, cheap, and can be performed simultaneously increasing the chance of finding microorganisms. It should be emphasized that careful evaluation at high magnification (×40), ideally on at least on 2 separate occasions or also reviewed by an experienced pathologist, and request for additional levels and repeat stains should be considered when there is a high index of suspicion for infection (**Fig. 6**).

MOLECULAR TESTING OF FORMALIN-FIXED PARAFFIN-EMBEDDED TISSUES FOR PATHOGEN DETECTION

Biopsies and surgical resections are frequently performed to establish a diagnosis of malignancy and characterize it to guide treatment. However, not infrequently, the tissue

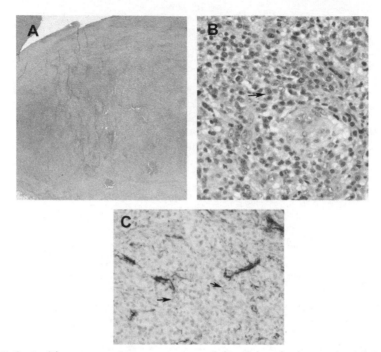

Fig. 5. Patient with upper respiratory symptoms and neck lymphadenopathy. (*A*) Excisional lymph node biopsy shows diffuse effacement of the nodal architecture. (*B*) Higher magnification shows a polymorphous infiltrate with frequent plasma cells, but no evidence of lymphoproliferative disease. (*C*) Immunohistochemistry using an anti-spirochete antibody shows marked immunoreactivity and corkscrew morphology (*arrows*), consistent with syphilis (confirmed by serologic testing).

samples do not reveal malignancy on histopathologic analysis but rather show inflammation in a pattern suggestive of infection. Ideally, when clinicians obtain biopsies or perform surgery, fresh samples should be procured concurrently with those submitted in formalin for histopathologic analysis if infection is a possibility. These samples may be kept frozen for subsequent testing or submitted to the microbiology laboratory if investigation of infection is warranted once the specimen is analyzed. In practice, triaging and allocation of specimens for microbiology testing requires coordination among the treating physician obtaining the tissue, the pathologist, and the microbiology laboratory and thus is rarely done. Consequently, specimens are most frequently placed in formalin for routine histopathology processing eliminating the possibility of culture. In such instances, PCR (targeted quantitative PCR [qPC] or broad-range 16S ribosomal RNA [rRNA]) offers an alternative for pathogen identification. The best choice will depend on clinical context and sample available (eg, from sterile niche vs not). The strengths and weaknesses of both PCR modalities are presented and contrasted with those of cultures and histopathology in **Table 2** and discussed as follows.

TARGETED POLYMERASE CHAIN REACTION

qPCR (also known as real-time PCR) may be used when a result is needed faster than culture would provide (eg, slow-growing organisms such as *Mycobacterium tuberculosis*) or when a fastidious or not easily cultured organism is suspected (eg, *Kingella*

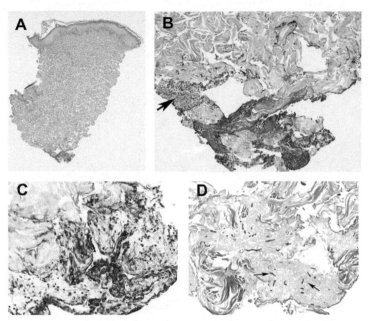

Fig. 6. Patient with neutropenia secondary to chemotherapy for myeloid leukemia. (*A*) At scanning magnification, no inflammation or overt abnormality is evident. (*B*) At the deep aspect of the biopsy, there is minimal neutrophilic inflammation (*black arrow*) and crush artifact (*white arrow*). (*C*) No fungal elements are present on the PAS stain. (*D*) However, the GMS stain shows fragmented septate hyphae (*arrows*), later identified as *Geotrichum candidum* by culture and matrix assisted laser desorption ionization-time of flight mass spectrometry (MALDI-TOF).

kingae or *Bartonella henselae*, respectively). As implied in the name, qPCR allows detection of bacterial load using fluorescent probes for quantification in real time. The measured fluorescence at the time of assay is compared with a prespecified threshold level at which the assay is considered positive. This threshold level is defined as the number of (PCR) cycles needed to reach this threshold and is known as the cycle threshold value (CT value). The CT value is inversely proportional to the initial amount of DNA in the sample. The lower the initial amount of DNA, the higher CT value and vice versa. Samples are considered strongly positive with CT values in the low 20s, and only borderline positive when CT values are in the high 30s. This quantitative aspect can also be exploited to monitor treatment efficacy. One advantage of qPCR in clinical practice is that it can detect bacterial DNA, irrespective of the presence of viable bacteria. This may be beneficial in cases in which antibiotics have been already administered when the specimen is obtained, which may contribute to false-negative culture results.[16] It also should be noted that qPCR is more sensitive than broad-range 16S rRNA PCR (discussed as follows), but it requires a priori knowledge of, or high index of clinical suspicion for, a specific microorganism.[17]

BROAD-RANGE BACTERIAL 16S RIBOSOMAL RNA POLYMERASE CHAIN REACTION AND SEQUENCING

Broad-range bacterial PCR amplification and sequencing of the amplified product offers an alternative for bacterial identification in FFPE tissue samples when bacterial

Table 2
Strengths and weaknesses of histochemical stains, cultures and PCR (qPCR and Broad-Range 16S rRNA)

Method	Strengths	Weaknesses
Histochemical stains	Cheap, widely available, fast turnaround, correlative with host response	Low sensitivity, nonspecific, no susceptibility data
Cultures	Cheap, widely available, susceptibility testing	Slow, not specific at species level, only living bacteria, some pathogens not easily cultured
Targeted PCR (qPCR)	Fastest method of identification at species level, viable and nonviable bacteria, high sensitivity	Not widely available, requires a priori knowledge or suspicion of pathogen to test for (narrow spectrum), limited susceptibility testing
Broad-range 16S rRNA PCR	Wide spectrum without a priori knowledge of pathogen to test for viable and nonviable bacteria, couple with sequencing allows detection at species level. May help when high index of suspicion for infection but negative culture and stains	Lower sensitivity compared with targeted PCR, more prone to contamination, no susceptibility testing

Abbreviations: PCR, polymerase chain reaction; qPCR, quantitative PCR; rRNA, ribosomal RNA.

infection is suspected, but there is no clear candidate pathogen and cultures have not been procured. The preponderance of evidence suggests that specimens in which bacteria can be visualized under the microscope have a higher yield. Good examples of suitable specimens include cardiac valves with bacteria highlighted by the Gram stain and skin or lung biopsies with AFB. Furthermore, recent studies suggest that the number of bacteria, as assessed in semiquantitative fashion by microscopy, is directly correlated with the yield of PCR amplification and subsequent identification by sequencing. A positive result is indicative of the presence of nucleic acid of the specified organism in the specimen tested. In the appropriate clinico-pathologic context, this may enable diagnosis and appropriate treatment. Results must be interpreted in context, however, as environmental or nucleic acid contamination of the specimen may produce a false-positive result. A negative result indicates no detectable bacterial nucleic acids in the specimen. This can be falsely negative due to sampling error, presence of nucleic acids in quantities below the threshold of detection of the assay, and variability of sequencing primers. It should be noted that, as the name implies, this test only detects bacteria (including mycobacteria in some reference laboratories), but not fungi, parasites, or viruses.[18–20]

BROAD-RANGE FUNGAL 28S RIBOSOMAL RNA AND INTERNAL TRANSCRIBED SPACERS POLYMERASE CHAIN REACTION AND SEQUENCING

The incidence of invasive fungal infections (IFI) has increased significantly largely due to an increase in immunosuppressive therapies for cancer and autoinflammatory diseases.[21–23] Nonetheless, the diagnosis of IFI is difficult due to lack of specific clinical manifestations, low sensitivity, and long turnaround time of cultures (30%–60%), and low sensitivity and specificity of histopathology (**Fig. 7**).[24,25] Broad-range (also called panfungal) PCR sequencing allows rapid identification of fungi in clinical specimens including tissue sections. Assays typically target multiple regions of rRNA, including the 18S rRNA, D1 and D2 regions of the 28S rRNA, 5.8S rRNA, and the internal transcribed spacers 1 and 2 (ITS1 and ITS2). Similarly to bacterial PCR amplicon sequencing from FFPE, studies have shown a positive correlation and higher yield of identification when testing samples in which fungal elements are first detected by microscopy or histopathology. A recent study found no significant difference in identification yields between FFPE, fresh tissue, and body fluids. Of interest, the same study found a significantly higher diagnostic yield in open resection tissue specimens compared with core needle biopsies and fine needle aspirates.[24]

As discussed previously, testing of specimens from nonsterile sources should be avoided, and potential commensal or contaminant species should be considered when unusual species are identified. Correlation of sequencing results with histopathologic findings to assess potential false-positive results. Another limitation is that the D2 and ITS2 regions do not allow identification at the species level for all fungi, and therefore, sequence analysis of additional genes is necessary for some species.[26]

PITFALLS
Adequate Use and Interpretation of Histochemical and Immunohistochemical Stains

The presence and morphologic features of bacteria, fungi, and protozoa are difficult to discern in routine hematoxylin and eosin (H&E)-stained sections, if at all detected in many cases. Histochemical stains commonly referred to as "special stains" or "bug stains," have long been used by pathologists to facilitate identification of bacteria, mycobacteria, fungi, and protozoa in tissue sections. Although the main biochemical principles underlying so-called special stains have been known for many years, several procedures and variations of each staining method (eg, Gram, acid-fast, methenamine silver) have been described, and some familiarity with the protocols, especially those used in one's laboratory is needed for adequate interpretation and trouble shooting.

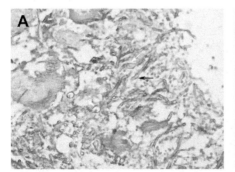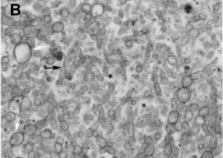

Fig. 7. Patient with solid organ transplant, fever of unknown origin, and new onset erythematous nodules. Hyaline septate hyphae (*black arrow*), some with globose swellings (*white arrows*) are present. Pathologists may be tempted to make a diagnosis of fusariosis in such cases on the basis of the presence of globose swellings, but it is important to remember that other hyaline molds have similar morphology in tissue sections. (*A*) *Aspergillus flavus* by culture and (*B*) *Lomentospora prolificans* by PCR. Broad-range fungal sequencing is useful in such cases to make a diagnosis at the species level.

The Gram method of differentially staining bacteria has had several modifications to optimize the quality of staining in tissue sections. One method commonly used is the one described by Brown and Hopps in 1973.[27] Using this technique, Gram-positive bacteria stain blue-purple and Gram-negatives red. The most common problem with this and other adaptations of the Gram stain to tissue sections is that not infrequently gram-negative bacteria stain faintly or not at all, thus making their detection suboptimal. Another problem relates to the overdiscoloration of Gram-positive bacteria, particularly cocci, which then appear red and are erroneously interpreted as gram-negative (**Fig. 8**). Brown and Hopps emphasized in their original work that "in order to obtain reliable results, the procedure should be followed precisely as described" and noted that faulty staining was the result of not following the protocol instructions precisely.[27] Accordingly, it should be no surprise that the Brown-Hopps stain is frequently unreliable for detection of gram-negative bacteria because it is commonly done by machine in automated fashion, making difficult to follow the procedure "precisely as described." Last, in the current practice environment, with molecular testing ever more accessible, many have learned to practice with suboptimal tissue Gram stains circumventing the problem by using PCR (as discussed previously) without any effort toward staining optimization. This is unfortunate, because adequate staining enables detection and helps better plan the need for ancillary testing and most appropriate

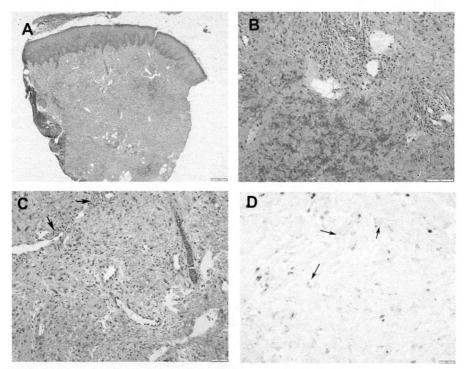

Fig. 8. Patient on treatment for acute myeloid leukemia and pustule on hand. (*A*) On scanning magnification, there is minimal inflammation. (*B*) Hemorrhage and (*C*) scant perivascular lymphocytic inflammation (*arrows*) would be interpreted as not suggestive of bacterial infection by many. (*D*) A Gram stain highlights gram-negative bacilli (*arrows*), subsequently identified as *Kluyvera* spp. by culture. So-called special stains (in this case a Brown-Hopps stain) are a valuable aid when evaluating biopsies from immunocompromised patients.

test. Studies suggest that the number of bacteria in tissue sections, as assessed semi-quantitatively by tissue Gram stain, has direct correlation with PCR amplification and subsequent identification.[28]

The methenamine silver nitrate technique, originally described by George Gomori at the University of Chicago in 1946 for detection of glycogen and mucin, was shown to be optimal for detecting fungal yeast and hyphal forms in tissue sections by Robert Grocott in 1955 when trying to optimize the available methods at the time for the purpose of microscopic photography of fungal structures.[29,30] It is commonly known as an "MSS" (methenamine silver stain) or "GMS" (Grocott methenamine stain) and colloquially referred to as a "fungal stain." Besides fungi, GMS stains the pathogenic algae (*Prototheca* and *Chlorella*), cysts of free-living ameba, the spore coat of microsporidian parasites, and bacteria including *Actinomyces* spp, *Nocardia* spp, most species of Mycobacteria and nonfilamentous bacteria with a polysaccharide capsule, such as *Klebsiella pneumoniae* and *Streptococcus pneumoniae*. In contrast to the tissue Gram stain, the most common issue in infectious disease pathology with this stain is the overzealous interpretation and mistaking of background signal as a fungal element. Elastic fibers, granulocytes, and other exogenous bodies and debris commonly present in tissue sections stain homogenously black and stand out from the background mimicking yeast or hyphae. Besides morphology, size and homogeneous staining (vs only the cell wall in fungi) are important criteria that may help distinguishing artifacts. It is most commonly used to investigate fungal infection and stains yeast and hyphal forms of many different species including *Aspergillus* spp, *Candida* spp, *Coccidioides* spp, *Paracoccidioides* spp, and *Fusarium* spp, among others. It should be noted that MSS staining of Mucorales is variable and sometimes weak or even negative. The reason for this in not known, but in contrast to other human pathogenic fungi (eg, *Candida* and *Aspergillus*), little is known about Mucorales cell wall remodeling in different growth conditions and during tissue invasion.[31,32] One caveat perpetuated by the general idea that GMS is a fungal stain, is mistaking bacterial cocci for small yeast forms, which appear slightly larger on MSS than on H&E or Brown-Hopps stains, but still smaller than small dimorphic fungi, such as *Histoplasma capsulatum*. Likewise, gram-negative bacilli in the Fusobacteriaceae and Leptotrichiaceae families may be mistaken for hyphae, because they are frequently undetected in tissue Gram stains (see previously) and form filamentous chains with joining sections mimicking septae. Knowing that bacteria can be identified by MSS and the smaller size should pose no difficulty in at least avoiding misclassification as hyphae, if difficult ascertaining as bacteria (**Fig. 9**).

The PAS method was originally used (between 1939 and 1944) and described in 1946 by Shabadash as a method to stain glycogen, although most textbooks and references on the subject credit R.D. Hotchkiss.[33,34] The PAS stain, formerly known as the Hotchkiss McManus stain, was first demonstrated to distinctly highlight in bright red the wall of several fungi, including yeast and hyphae, by Kligman and Mescon in 1950.[35] The underlying biochemical principle for this reaction is similar to that of the MSS and relates to the creation of aldehyde binding sites for the silver or Schiff reagent ions from polysaccharides in the fungal cell wall after oxidation with an acid. However, the staining in tissues is not specific to fungal elements, as polysaccharides in tissue components also stain (eg, glycogen, basement membranes, reticular fibers). The addition of diastase is an extra step often used to counteract glycogen staining, facilitating visualization of fungi. Although seldom done nowadays in clinical practice, the use of a stronger oxidizing agent such as chromic acid instead of periodic acid has been shown to enhance fungal staining, likely by destroying aldehydes in tissues that have fewer polysaccharides than the fungal cell wall, rich in 1,2 glycols. This has been

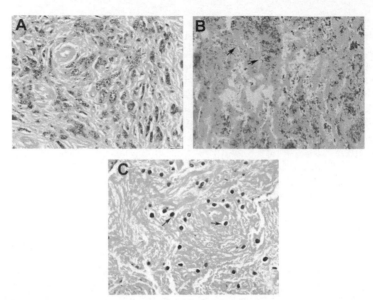

Fig. 9. The GMS stain is not specific for fungi, and also highlights bacteria, including myco-bacteria ([A] *Mycobacterium leprae*; [B] *Streptobacillus moniliformis, arrows*), and cysts of free-living ameba ([C] *Acanthamoeba* spp., *arrows*).

termed a "CAS" stain, and is similar to the Gridley method, which adds aldehyde fuchsin after strong oxidation to enhance staining of fungal elements.[36] It has been debated whether both PAS and GMS stains should be obtained when mycotic disease is investigated in tissue sections; in the opinion of this author and many others, it is optimal to get both. Despite being apparently wasteful and redundant, there are reasons to do so. First, when both stains are obtained, there is additional and thus better sampling, because each stain is done on a separate section, increasing the yield. This may seem trivial and although some studies have suggested GMS is more sensitive and therefore should be the stain of choice for detecting fungus, others suggest this difference may be a matter of sampling. One study comparing the utility of PAS versus GMS stain for detection of onychomycosis found that in cases in which fungal organisms were observed only on a GMS stain obtained after an initial negative PAS, a second PAS stain obtained after the positive GMS also documented fungi.[37] The investigators of this study concluded that PAS and GMS stains are similar and suggested that the sensitivity of both methods can be increased by preparing 2 slides from different levels of the paraffin block. Second, anecdotal evidence suggests that the PAS stain may not stain degenerated fungal elements, in contrast to the GMS. Last, each staining method (GMS and PAS) has different staining artifacts that may mimic fungal elements, and thus having the opposite stain helps making this determination. The PAS stain, for example, highlights calcific bodies sometimes found in granulomas mimicking buddying yeasts when close to each other (**Fig. 10**A, B). In this situation, having a GMS is of value because the chromic acid used as an oxidizer in this protocol (vs periodic acid in PAS) dissolves calcium, eliminating this artifact. Another problem with the PAS stain relates to it highlighting in distinct manner the walls of small capillaries, mimicking branching, septate hyphae to a tee. Again, a negative GMS stain is extremely valuable in this situation, because it will be negative, and the vast majority of hyphae are colored by the GMS method

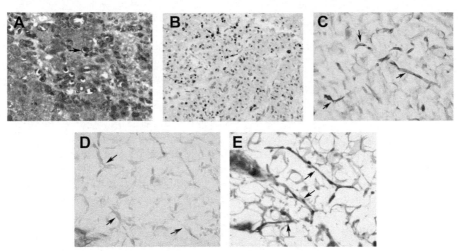

Fig. 10. (A) Calcific bodies, in this photograph corresponding to Michaelis-Guttman bodies (*arrow*) of Malakoplakia may be mistaken for fungal spores on the basis of PAS-positivity. (B) A Von-Kossa stain for calcium (*arrows*), or a negative GMS (not shown) should be helpful in making the distinction. (C) A PAS stain highlights elongated filamentous structures (*arrows*) in the subcutis, some with septa, morphologically compatible with hyphae. (D) However, these structures are not highlighted by a GMS stain (*arrows*), which would be most unusual for fungal filaments. (E) A CD31 immunohistochemical stain, which is a marker of endothelial cells, highlights these hyphae-like structures (*arrows*), and confirms they are capillaries and not hyphae.

(**Fig. 10**C–E). For these reasons, obtaining both stains is ideal; it can be accomplished in the same time frame, without significant additional cost, and with the benefits detailed previously.

A method to stain *M tuberculosis* was originally developed by Koch in March of 1882.[38] Koch's[38] staining method underwent several modifications aiming to improve the technique by using more stable compounds, and 16 months later there was a standardized method of staining the tubercle bacillus. A decade later, this method became widely recognized as the Ziehl-Neelsen (ZN) method, despite being the product of complementary work by Koch, Ehrlich, Ziehl, Rindfleisch, and Neelsen (in chronologic order).[39] Despite being a successful method, the ZN stain was modified by numerous researchers. Notably, Kinyoun described a method optimized for detecting tubercle bacilli in sputum, known as the "cold staining" technique, because it is performed at room temperature. These 2 protocols, ZN and Kinyoun, known as AFBs, remain a pillar in the diagnosis of tuberculosis and are still used by pathologists and microbiologists worldwide today.[40] AFB stains are relatively simple, cost-effective and much faster than cultures. However, AFB staining has numerous issues leading to false-negative, and rarely, false-positive results. The sensitivity of AFB stains is estimated to be between 20% and 60%.[41,42] The processing and thickness of the samples, conservation, duration, and concentration of the primary stain (carbol-fuchsin) and counterstain (methylene blue), and expertise of technical and medical staff have been shown to impact the sensitivity and specificity of AFB stains.[43–45] A common problem in our clinical practice relates to the sensitivity of the AFB stain in tissues. In our group's experience, the ZN and Kinyoun stain sensitivities are suboptimal and lower than that of the modified AFB stains (Fite and Nocardia) for the detection of tuberculous and nontuberculous mycobacteria (Crothers JW et al. AJCP 2020; in press). This seems to be the case in other laboratories in the United States where staining is done by a machine in automated fashion, and not manually by an experienced technician (**Fig. 11**).

Infectious Pseudomalignancies

Pathologists spend most of their time ruling in or ruling out neoplasia.[2] This is both understandable and commendable, because histopathology is the gold standard for diagnosis and classification of benign and malignant tumors, and accurate diagnoses are necessary for adequate treatment. Moreover, the ever-present shadow of litigation, further incentivizes pathologists "not to miss" a diagnosis of malignancy, which would have negative consequences to both the patient and the pathologist. An unintended sequel of all this is the overdiagnosis of malignancy, which is not unique to infectious processes that can mimic malignant tumors and can also occur when benign neoplasms and reactive processes are misclassified as cancer.

A list of pathogens, histologic patterns and the neoplasms they may mimic is presented in **Table 3**. A common scenario germane to infectious disease pathology is misclassification of pseudoepitheliomatous hyperplasia secondary to infection as invasive squamous cell carcinoma. This can occur as a response to bacterial, fungal,

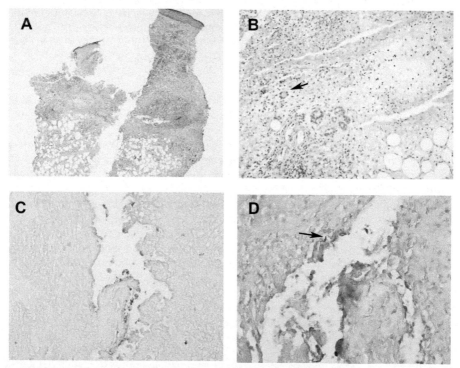

Fig. 11. Skin biopsy from a patient receiving a "biologic" for rheumatoid arthritis. (*A*) There is necrotizing inflammation in the dermis and subcutis. (*B*) Granulomatous inflammation with sparse giant cells (*arrow*) is noted. (*C*) A ZN AFB stain is negative. (*D*) After the culture turned positive for *Mycobacterium chelonae*, a Fite-Faraco stain was obtained, highlighting acid-fast bacteria (*arrow*), confirming infection and not contamination. Of note, both the ZN and Fite-Faraco stains were repeated with similar results, pointing to a systematic error.

Table 3
Selected infectious pseudoneoplasms and associated microorganisms

Pseudoneoplasm	Associated Microorganism(s)
Pseudoepitheliomatous hyperplasia mimicking squamous cell carcinoma	Bacteria (eg, *Staphylococcus*, *Treponema pallidum*), Leishmania, Fungi (eg, spp. in chromoblastomycosis, *Scopulariopsis brevicaulis*)
Hemangioma, hemangioendothelioma, angiosarcoma	*Bartonella bacilliformis*, *Bartonella quintana*
Spindle cell sarcoma, melanoma	Nontuberculous mycobacteria in immunocompromised patients (eg, *M avium intracellulare* complex)
Colonic adenocarcinoma, sarcoma	*Basidiobolus ranarum*
Lymphoma	*Borrelia burgdorferi*, *Treponema pallidum*

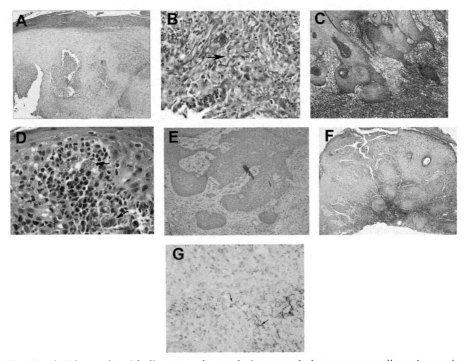

Fig. 12. Florid pseudoepitheliomatous hyperplasia may mimic squamous cell carcinoma in cases of fungal infection. (*A*) Endophytic squamous proliferation suggestive of squamous cell carcinoma. (*B*) Septate hyphae (*arrow*) are highlighted by PAS stain obtained in the same case, identified as *Scopulariopsis brevicaulis* by PCR. (*C*) Leishmaniasis. Atypical endophytic squamous proliferation, at first glance compatible with squamous cell carcinoma. (*D*) Parasitized macrophages with amastigotes are seen (*arrows*) (*Leishmania tropica* by culture and PCR). (*E*) Furunculosis caused by methicillin-resistant *Staphylococcus aureus* (by culture) in a patient with multiple lesions that resolved after treatment. (*F*) Syphilis. Endophytic squamous tumor highly suggestive of well-differentiated squamous cell carcinoma. (*G*) Spirochete immunohistochemistry demonstrates abundant spirochetes (*arrows*) in the same case (*F*), characteristic of syphilis.

and protozoan infections (**Fig. 12**). Although not always discernible, exuberant prolif-eration of squamous epithelium around preexisting hair follicles, as well as the pres-ence of suppurative inflammation, multinucleate giant cells and granulomas, should be a clue to the pathologist to consider infection in the differential diagnosis and inves-tigate with histochemical stains. A less common problem arises when vaso-formative lesions caused by infections with *Bartonella* spp are diagnosed as vascular tumors, benign and malignant.[46]

Many times, infectious processes present with mass lesions, and are treated definitively with presumptive diagnoses such as colon cancer, sarcoma or lym-phoma, which turn out to be an infection. One example of this is basidiobolomycosis mimicking colon cancer, which is a histologically distinct fungal infection caused by *Basidiobolus ranarum*, but difficult for the unaware to accept as an infectious pro-cess because it mimics colon cancer to a tee clinically and radiologically.[47–50] Sup-purative granulomatous inflammation with large numbers of eosinophils is characteristic, and large coenocytic hyphae with she Splendore-Höeppli similar to those of zygomycetes can be detected on H&E, PAS, and GMS stains (**Fig. 13**). Another example, which is infrequent, but most common in patients with human im-munodeficiency virus (HIV) infection when encountered is the so-called mycobacte-rial spindle cell pseudotumor (**Fig. 14**). This presents as a mass anywhere in the body (eg, nasal cavity, lymph node, skin and soft tissues, retroperitoneum) and can be easily misdiagnosed as a mesenchymal neoplasm or a melanoma because of diffuse S100 immunoreactivity given the lesion is composed of histiocytes.[51,52] Once considered, the diagnosis is straightforward, as there are numerous acid-fast bacilli that are readily identified on AFB stains. Mycobacterial spindle cell pseudotumor is caused by nontuberculous mycobacteria, most frequently *Mycobacterium avium complex* (MAC), but other species have been implicated. As discussed previously, diagnosis at the species level requires isolation by culture or identification by PCR from FFPE sections.

Another caveat worth considering is the possibility of concomitant infection in bi-opsies showing a neoplasm. This may be a problem for pathologists evaluating sam-ples from patients with history of a particular neoplasm or cancer, in which the evaluation may be "framed" to rule in or rule out recurrence of the known malignancy.

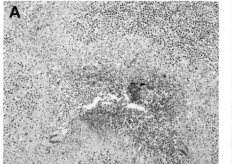
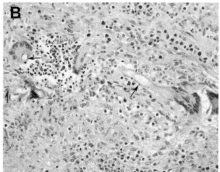

Fig. 13. A 58-year-old man presented with acute colonic obstruction and underwent colec-tomy for presumptive adenocarcinoma based on imaging. (*A*) Histologic sections revealed a transmural inflammatory mass with granulomas, numerous eosinophils and Splendore-Höeppli phenomenon (*arrow*). (*B*) Large, nonseptate hyphal structures were also noted (*ar-rows*). These findings are characteristic of basidiobolomycosis (*Basidiobolus ranarum*).

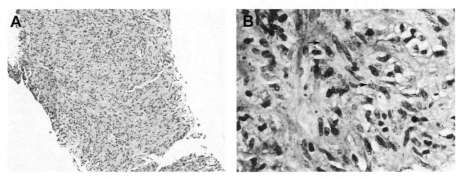

Fig. 14. A patient with HIV underwent resection of a retroperitoneal mass. (*A*) A diffuse infiltrate of spindle cells were suspected to represent sarcoma on frozen section. (*B*) An AFB stain shows numerous acid-fast bacilli (*arrows*), characteristic of the spindle cell mycobacterial pseudotumor.

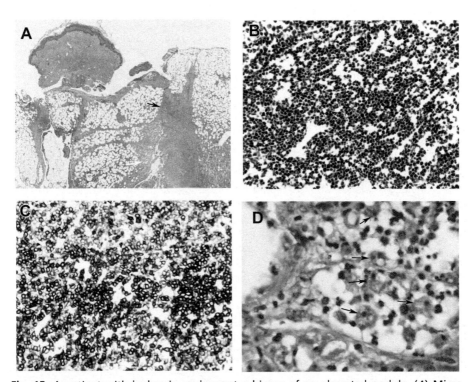

Fig. 15. A patient with leukemia underwent a biopsy of an ulcerated nodule. (*A*) Microscopic examination revealed a monomorphic infiltrate (*black arrow*) and necrosis (*white arrow*). Immunohistochemistry confirmed the mononuclear infiltrate to be recurrent leukemia ([*B* and *C*] BSAP and CD5, respectively). After the patient progressed despite treatment, a repeat review revealed numerous trophozoites of acanthamoeba (*arrows*) within the necrotic debris (*D*).

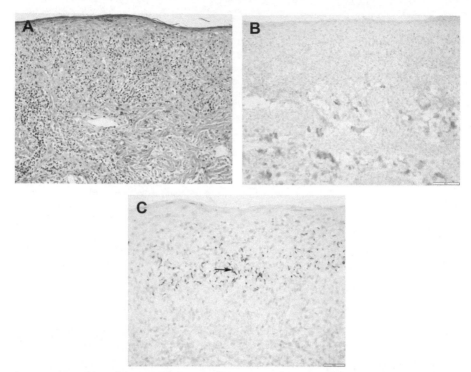

Fig. 16. A patient with a long history of waxing and waning skin rashes underwent a biopsy. (*A*) Examination revealed a lichenoid pattern with frequent plasma cells suggestive of syphilis. (*B*) Immunohistochemistry was pursued and confirmed the diagnosis, but appeared negative the next day when the case was discussed at conference. (*C*) A repeat immunohistochemical stain was obtained and showed spirochetes in the epidermis (*arrow*), confirming a diagnosis of secondary syphilis. The fast-red chromogen used with alkaline phosphatase is known to be prone to fading.

When this circumstance conspires with the presence of an infrequent organism, the possibility of detection and/or identification is greatly diminished (**Fig. 15**).

Last, immunohistochemistry has been increasingly used in the diagnosis of infection. A good example is the spirochete antibody for the diagnosis of syphilis. Studies have shown increased sensitivity of spirochete immunohistochemistry compared with the traditional silver impregnation technique of Warthin and Starry.[53,54] The immunohistochemical reaction is clean, with no background and allows identification of the characteristic corkscrew morphology of treponemes, making it extremely user friendly. In the skin, the use of a red chromogen is preferred to avoid confusion of brown peroxidase with melanin in the basal cell layer. It is important to know, however, that the red chromogen used with alkaline phosphatase is prone to fading if the tissues are exposed to xylene for too long, creating a chance of a false-negative diagnosis (**Fig. 16**).

SUMMARY

Histopathology is an important resource for detection of microorganisms in tissue sections. Identification of microorganisms at the species level generally requires correlation with cultures and/or PCR, with a few notable exceptions (*Coccidioides,*

Rhinosporidium, *Prototheca*, amebas). Histochemical stains (Brown-Hopps, GMS, PAS, and AFB) are useful in highlighting bacteria, fungi, and mycobacteria but are nonspecific. PCR testing for bacterial or fungal identification is of higher yield when performed on specimens with organisms detected by histopathology, and correlation of sequencing results with morphologic findings is valuable to assess contamination versus disease. Pathologists should be aware of the possibility of infection mimicking malignancy.

DISCLOSURE

The author has nothing to disclose.

REFERENCES

1. Procop G, Wilson M. Infectious disease pathology. Clin Infect Dis 2001;32: 1589–601.
2. Guarner J. Incorporating pathology in the practice of infectious disease: myths and reality. Clin Infect Dis 2014;59:1133–41.
3. Gable AD, Marsee DK, Milner DA, et al. Suppurative inflammation with microabscess and pseudocyst formation is a characteristic histologic manifestation of cutaneous infections with rapid-growing *Mycobacterium* species. Am J Clin Pathol 2008;130:514–7.
4. Li JJ, Beresford R, Fyfe J, et al. Clinical and histopathological features of cutaneous nontuberculous mycobacterial infection: a review of 113 cases. J Cutan Pathol 2017;44:433–43.
5. Co DO, Hogan LH, Kim SI, et al. Mycobacterial granulomas: keys for a long-lasting host-pathogen relationship. Clin Immunol 2004;113:130–6.
6. Florido M, Appelberg R. Granuloma necrosis during mycobacterium avium infection does not require tumor necrosis factor. Infect Immun 2004;72:6139–41.
7. Carpenter RJ, Graf PCF. Pott's disease? AIDS-associated mycobacterium heckenshornense spinal osteomyelitis and diskitis. J Clin Microbiol 2015;53:716–8.
8. Coelho ID, Romaozinho C, Texeira AC, et al. A rare manifestation of tuberculosis in a renal transplant patient: a case report. Transplant Proc 2019;51:1618–20.
9. Martinez-Mera C, Hospital MG, Lopez-Negrete E, et al. Atypical herpes simplex presenting necrotizing granulomas in an immunocompromised patient. Am J Dermatopathol 2020;42:305–6.
10. Kumar V, Abbas A, Aster J. Acute and chronic inflammation. In: Kumar V, Abbas A, Aster J, editors. Robbins and Cotran pathologic basis of disease. 9th edition. Philadelphia: Elsevier Saunders; 2015. p. 69–111.
11. Aguero-Rosenfeld ME, Wang G, Schwartz I, et al. Diagnosis of lyme borreliosis. Clin Microbiol Rev 2005;18:484–509.
12. Peeling RW, Hook EW 3rd. The pathogenesis of syphilis: the Great Mimicker, revisited. J Pathol 2006;208:224–32.
13. McCalmont T, Macerenco R. Syphilis: it's around and ready for (Mis)Diagnosis. J Cutan Pathol 2008;35:95 [abstract].
14. Abell E, Marks R, Jones EW. Secondary syphilis: a clinico-pathological review. Br J Dermatol 1975;93:53–61.
15. LeBoit PE. Dermatopathologic findings in patients infected with HIV. Dermatol Clin 1992;10:59–71.
16. Valones MA, Guimaraes RI, Brandao LA, et al. Principles and applications of polymerase chain reaction in medical diagnostic fields: a review. Braz J Microbiol 2009;40:1–11.

17. Patel A, Harris KA, Fitzgerald F. What is broad-range 16S rDNA PCR? Arch Dis Child Educ Pract Ed 2017;102:261–4.
18. Harris KA, Hartley JC. Development of broad-range 16S rDNA PCR for use in the routine diagnostic clinical microbiology service. J Med Microbiol 2003;52:685–91.
19. Woo PC, Lau SK, Teng JL, et al. Then and now: use of 16S rDNA gene sequencing for bacterial identification and discovery of novel bacteria in clinical microbiology laboratories. Clin Microbiol Infect 2008;14:908–34.
20. Neofytos D, Horn D, Anaissie E, et al. Epidemiology and outcome of invasive fungal infection in adult hematopoietic stem cell transplant recipients: analysis of Multicenter Prospective Antifungal Therapy (PATH) Alliance Registry. Clin Infect Dis 2009;48:265–73.
21. Pappas PG, Alexander BD, Andes DR, et al. Invasive fungal infections among transplant recipients : results of the Transplant-Associated Infection Surveillance Network (TRANSNET). Clin Infect Dis 2010;50:1101–11.
22. Corzo-Leon DE, Satlin MJ, Soave R, et al. Epidemiology and outcome of invasive fungal infections in allogeneic hematopoietic stem cell transplant recipients in the era of antifungal prophylaxis: a single-centre study with focus on emerging pathogens. Mycoses 2015;58:325–6.
23. Rickerts V, Mousset S, Lambrecht E, et al. Comparison of histopathological analysis, culture, and polymerase chain reaction assays to detect invasive mold infections from biopsy specimens. Clin Infect Dis 2007;44:1078–83.
24. Terrand J, Lichterfeld M, Warraich I, et al. Diagnosis of invasive septate mold infections. A correlation of microbiological culture and histologic or cytologic examination. Am J Clin Pathol 2003;119:854–8.
25. Gomez CA, Budvytiene I, Zemek AJ, et al. Performance of targeted fungal sequencing for culture-independent diagnosis of invasive fungal disease. Clin Infect Dis 2017;65:2035–41.
26. Clinical and Laboratory Standards Institute. Interpretive criteria for identification of bacteria and fungi by DNA target sequencing. Approved guideline. MM18-A, vol. 28. Wayne (PA): CLSI; 2008.
27. Brown RC, Hopps HC. Staining of bacteria in tissue sections: a reliable gram stain method. Am J Clin Pathol 1973;60:234–40.
28. Solomon IH, Lin C, Horback KL, et al. Utility of histologic and histochemical screening for 16S ribosomal RNA gene sequencing of formalin-fixed, paraffin-embedded tissue for bacterial endocarditis. Am J Clin Pathol 2019;152:431–7.
29. Gomori G. A new histochemical test for glycogen and mucin. Am J Clin Pathol 1946;10:177–9.
30. Grocott R. A stain for fungi in tissue sections and smears using Gomori's methenamine-silver nitrate technic. Am J Clin Pathol 1955;25:975–9.
31. Ribes JA, Vanover-Sams CL, Baker DJ. Zygomycetes in human disease. Clin Microbiol Rev 2000;13:236–301.
32. Lecointe K, Cornu M, Leroy J, et al. Polysaccharides cell wall architecture of Mucorales. Front Microbiol 2019;10:469.
33. Hotchkiss RD. A microchemical reaction resulting in the staining of polysaccharide structures in fixed tissue preparations. Arch Biochem 1948;148(16):131–41.
34. Aterman K, Norkin S. The periodic acid – Schiff reaction. Nature 1963;197:1306.
35. Kligman AM, Mescon H. The periodic acid-Schiff stain for the demonstration of fungi in animal tissue. J Bacteriol 1950;60:415–21.
36. Gridley MF. A stain for fungi in tissue sections. Am J Clin Pathol 1953;23:303–7.
37. Reza Kermanshahi T, Rhatigan R. Comparison between PAS and GMS stains for the diagnosis of onychomycosis. J Cutan Pathol 2010;37:1041–4.

38. Koch R. Die aetiology der tuberkulose. Berl Klinischen Wochenschr 1882;15: 221–30.
39. Bishop PJ, Neuman G. The history of the Ziehl-Neelsen stain. Tubercle 1970;51: 196–206.
40. Kinyoun JJ. A note on Uhlenhuths method for sputum examination, for tubercle bacilli. Am J Public Health (N Y) 1915;5:867–70.
41. Siddiqi K, Lambert ML, Walley J. Clinical diagnosis of smear-negative pulmonary tuberculosis in low-volume income countries: the current evidence. Lancet Infect Dis 2003;3:288–96.
42. Aber VR, Allen BW, Mitchison DA, et al. Laboratory studies in isolated positive cultures and the efficiency of direct smear examination. Tubercle 1980;61: 123–33.
43. Alausa KO, Osoba AO, Montefiore D, et al. Laboratory diagnosis of tuberculosis in a developing country 1968-1975. Afr J Med Med Sci 1977;6:103–8.
44. Angra P, Becx-Bleumink M, Gilpin C, et al. Ziehl-Neelsen staining: strong red on weak blue, or weak red under string blue? Int J Tuberc Lung Dis 2007;11:1160–1.
45. Petersen KF, Urbanczik R. Microscopic and cultural methods for the laboratory diagnosis of tuberculosis. A short historical review (In German). Zentralbl Bakteriol Mikrobiol Hyg A 1982;251:308–25.
46. Arias-Stella J, Lieberman PH, Garcia Caceres U, et al. Verruga peruana mimicking malignant neoplasms. Am J Dermatopathol 1987;9:279–91.
47. Omar Takrouni A, Heitham Schammut M, Al-Otaibi M, et al. Disseminated intestinal basidiobolomycosis with mycotic aneurysm mimicking obstructing colon cancer. BMJ Case Rep 2019;29:e225054.
48. Mohammadi R, Ansari Chaharshoghi M, Khorvash F, et al. An unusual case of gastrointestinal basidiobolomycosis mimicking colon cancer; literature and review. J Mycol Med 2019;29:75–9.
49. Ilyas MI, Jordan SA, Nfonsam V. Fungal inflammatory masses masquerading as colorectal cancer: a case report. BMS Res Notes 2015;8:32.
50. Nemenqani D, Yaqoob N, Khoja H, et al. Gastrointestinal basidiobolomycosis: an unusual infection mimicking colon cancer. Arch Pathol Lab Med 2009;133: 1938–42.
51. Rahmani M, Alroy J, Zoukhri D, et al. Mycobacterial pseudotumor of the skin. Virchows Arch 2013;463:843–6.
52. Yeh I, Evan G, Jokinen CH. Cutaneous mycobacterial spindle cell pseudotumor: a potential mimic of soft tissue neoplasms. Am J Dermatopathol 2011;33:e66–9.
53. Hoang MP, High WA, Molberg KH. Secondary syphilis: a histologic and immunohistochemical evaluation. J Cutan Pathol 2004;31:595–9.
54. Martin-Ezquerra G, Fernandez-Casado A, Barco D, et al. Treponema pallidum distribution patterns in mucocutaneous lesions of primary and secondary syphilis: an immunohistochemical and ultrastructural study. Hum Pathol 2009;40: 624–30.

Blood Banking and Transfusion Medicine Challenges During the COVID-19 Pandemic

Andy Ngo, MD, Debra Masel, MT, (ASCP) SBB, Christine Cahill, RN, MS,
Neil Blumberg, MD, Majed A. Refaai, MD*

KEYWORDS

- COVID-19 • Blood banking • Transfusion medicine • Blood shortage
- Blood wastage • FDA donation policies • Convalescent plasma

KEY POINTS

- COVID-19 has had a negative impact on blood collection.
- The Centers for Disease Control, blood centers, and American Red Cross have developed new policies to protect donors and the blood supply.
- Blood management has become more important with decreasing supply as well as management of blood bank personnel.
- Convalescent plasma, although touted as a possible treatment, has limited literature on its efficacy.

INTRODUCTION

Within 3 months of the first diagnosed case, the outbreak of acute respiratory disease caused by the novel coronavirus (SARS-CoV-2), also known as COVID-19, rapidly grew into a global pandemic. The eruption of this virus, reportedly, may have been linked to a seafood and wildlife market in Wuhan, Hubei Province, China.[1,2] Person-to-person spread is thought to occur via respiratory droplet contact (≤6 feet), skin contacts, and even the transmission through air while speaking. Despite the extraordinary universal attempts to limit the spread of this virus, new cases are diagnosed on a daily basis throughout the world and have dramatically affected, among other health care disciplines, the blood bank and transfusion medicine. Because of the growing prevalence and highly infectious nature of COVID-19, new policies and guidelines

Department of Pathology and Laboratory Medicine, Transfusion Medicine Unit, University of Rochester, Strong Memorial Hospital - Blood Bank, 601 Elmwood Avenue, Box 608, Rochester, NY 14642, USA
* Corresponding author.
E-mail address: Majed_Refaai@URMC.Rochester.edu

Clin Lab Med 40 (2020) 587–601
https://doi.org/10.1016/j.cll.2020.08.013
labmed.theclinics.com

have started to develop in transfusion medicine practices. In this article the authors address the myriad of ways that COVID-19 has affected blood banking and transfusion medicine, including the safety of both blood donors and blood product recipients, the management and distribution of blood products during a pandemic, and the use of blood product–derived therapeutics.

CLINICAL MANIFESTATIONS OF COVID-19

Common symptoms of COVID-19 infection, which typically appear within 2 to 14 days after exposure, include fever, sore throat, cough, shortness of breath, chills, muscle pain, headache, and sensory changes such as loss of smell or taste. Nausea, vomiting, diarrhea, skin rash, delirium, and dizziness have also been reported.[3,4] In advanced cases, mild-to-severe lower respiratory tract infection can be seen and may progress to critical status, as a result of the cytokine storm, requiring intubation and mechanical ventilation. Acute respiratory failure and a widespread thromboembolic disease are also common in these critical cases.[5,6] However, conservative estimates of 30% to as high as 96% of infected individuals may manifest mild to no symptoms, posing huge challenges in containing this pandemic crisis and protecting blood donors.[7]

In one of the earlier studies of COVID-19 patients, Guan and colleagues[8] reported that in addition to the usual viral route of respiratory droplets, the virus could be transmitted by saliva, urine, and stool.[9] Extracted data of 1099 patients with laboratory-confirmed COVID-19–related acute respiratory distress syndrome (ARDS) showed a predominant male gender (58%), median age of 47 years with most common symptoms of fever (88%) and cough (68%). The median incubation period was found to be 3 days with a range of 0 to 24 days. Only 1.2% of patients reported to have a direct contact with wildlife and 31% had been to Wuhan city, whereas the majority (72%) had contact with people from Wuhan city. At time of admission, ground-glass opacity was the typical (56.4%) radiological finding on chest computed tomography (CT). Interestingly, a significant number of severe cases were diagnosed by clinical symptoms and real-time reverse transcriptase polymerase chain reaction (RT-PCR) with normal radiological findings. Multivariate analysis revealed that severe pneumonia was an independent factor associated with either intensive care unit (ICU) admission, mechanical ventilation, or death (hazard ratio, 9.80; 95% confidence interval, 4.06–23.67).[8]

COVID-19 DIAGNOSIS

Ideally, testing every blood donor for COVID-19 would be the best practice; however, at least for the time being, this task cannot realistically be accomplished. To date, 7 recognized types of coronavirus strains that can infect humans have been identified, including *Alpha coronavirus* (229E and NL63) and *Beta coronavirus* (OC43 and HKU1). The rare but more severe types are called MERS-CoV, which lead to Middle East respiratory syndrome (MERS), and SARS-CoV, responsible for severe acute respiratory syndrome (SARS) endemic.[10]

Laboratory confirmation of COVID-19 infection is based on detection of unique sequences of viral RNA by RT-PCR. Sputum samples provide better detection than throat samples, whereas lower respiratory tract samples are superior to those from the upper respiratory tract.[11] The presence of SARS-CoV-2 RNA in the blood is a marker of severe illness based on 113 studies.[12] Additional laboratory findings in COVID-19 infection include lymphopenia (83%); neutrophilia; and elevated levels of serum alanine aminotransferase, aspartate aminotransferase, lactate dehydrogenase, C-reactive protein (CRP), ferritin, and D-dimer.[13] Substantial increase in CRP, ferritin, and D-dimer levels were found to be associated with severe infection.[14] In addition, significant association has been recognized between lymphopenia and high levels of D-dimer with mortality.[15,16]

Bilateral air-space consolidation is typically seen on chest radiograph; however, findings may be unremarkable early in the disease. Chest CT images usually demonstrate bilateral, peripheral ground glass opacities, which is nonspecific to COVID-19 infection.

MANAGEMENT OF COVID-19

An effective COVID-19 vaccine would be the ultimate solution for all of the concerns surrounding blood bank industry. However, currently there is no vaccine available to protect against SARS-CoV-2. Likewise, no prophylactic therapy has yet been proved to be effective in patients who have been exposed to SARS-CoV-2 nor a clearly successful treatment of those who develop the infection.[17] Patients who are confirmed positive for COVID-19 and present with mild symptoms are usually managed by self-isolation at home for up to 14 days, which is also the minimal deferral period recommended by many blood centers.[7–10] In advanced cases, hospitalization may be required for clinical observation and supportive management with fluid and oxygen resuscitations, anticoagulation, empirical antibiotics in case of a secondary infection, and nonsteroidal antiinflammatory agents in some cases. Critical cases may require ICU admission for possible intubation and mechanical ventilation. Corticosteroids and immunosuppressive agents are usually not recommended except when required for other indications or in a cytokine storm. Extracorporeal membrane oxygenation can be considered but is associated with a high mortality rate.

Complications of COVID-19 infection include pneumonia, respiratory failure, ARDS, sepsis and septic shock, cardiomyopathy and arrhythmia, acute kidney injury, bacterial infections, thromboembolism, gastrointestinal bleeding, polyneuropathy, and death.

The only means we have for reducing infection in the general population and protecting blood donors relies on recommended infection control. Measures, such as proper hand and environmental hygiene, and appropriate use of personal protective equipment along with maintaining the social distancing (at least 6 feet) are necessary to prevent COVID-19 spreading. Early detection, triage, and isolation of potentially infectious patients are also important considerations. A combination of these measures is the basis of current blood donation protocols, which will hopefully protect and maintain our blood supply.

BLOOD DONATION AND BLOOD PRODUCTS

There are multiple Federal Drug Administration (FDA) criteria a blood donor must meet before donating blood products. These parameters range from physical requirements, such as age, weight, temperature, blood pressure, and pulse, to a background check of the donor's sexual, medical, and travel history. Any discrepancies or issues that arise during the interview process and the physical examination could temporarily or permanently defer the donor from the blood donation system.[18]

Following the start of the COVID-19 outbreak in the United States, additional screening questions and requirements were implemented. Although not standardized across all blood collection organizations, the American Red Cross implemented new deferral policies in February 2020 before regional and national shutdown. All donors with a recent travel history to China, Hong Kong, Macau, Iran, Italy, and South Korea were deferred for 28 days. Donors diagnosed or suspected to have COVID-19 or had contact with a COVID-19–positive patient were also deferred for 28 days despite the absence of any data or evidence as of yet that SARS-CoV-2 can be transmitted through blood products.[19]

Several measures were adopted by all blood donation centers and blood drives to prevent transmission of SARS-CoV-2. Measures included temperature screening for all donors and staff before entry into the donation centers, social distancing (>6 feet) when possible, disinfecting machines and surfaces between donations, having donors and staff wear face masks, use of hand sanitizer before and during the donation process, and increased spacing between beds. These preventative practices echoed the Centers of Disease Control (CDC) guidelines and were similarly implemented in other blood donation centers.[20–23]

As these policies were put into place, blood donations began to decrease as the COVID-19 pandemic grew and blood drive cancellation increased. Regionally, one of the hospitals affected was University of Washington Medical Center, which reported a blood supply shortfall as early as February 29, 2020.[24] Nationally blood collections dropped and in a press release by the American Red Cross on March 17, 2020, approximately 2700 Red Cross blood drives were canceled across the country, resulting in 86,000 fewer donations. Evidently, more than 80% of their usual blood supply comes from these blood drives.[25] Of note, as per the American Association of Blood Banks (AABB), 33,000 units of blood are needed daily to meet patient need before the pandemic.[26]

As a result, hospitals needed to develop strategies to adapt to these blood supply shortages. Mitigation strategies that were proposed included additional criteria for transfusion orders review with more stringent guidelines. Splitting platelet units into 2 doses each were also considered to minimize platelet shortage. Hospitals increasingly adopted these measures over the course of a few weeks starting in March 2020.[27]

On April 2, 2020, the FDA issued new blood donation guidance to address the need for blood and blood components. They no longer required collections to be discarded due to errors in vital signs or donation intervals and added a 72-hour window to allow a donor to respond to questions about eligibility and component suitability.[28] The FDA changed deferral guidelines and a previous guidance that deferred many donors for up to 12 months due to various reasons was revised to a deferral of 3 months (**Table 1**).[29] In addition, donors who were previously permanently deferred between 1980 to 1986 due to spending more than 3 months in specified European countries were allowed to be reconsidered for donation. Exceptions and alternatives were also issued under 21 CFR 640.120(b) to address blood and blood component shortages.[30]

Concurrently, the CDC and Centers for Medicare and Medicaid Services recommended rescheduling elective surgeries as needed and shifting elective urgent inpatient surgical procedures to outpatient settings when feasible. The American College of Surgeons similarly recommended the same guidelines.[31] They stated surgeries should be reviewed with "a plan to minimize, postpone, or cancel electively scheduled operations, endoscopies, or other invasive procedures."[32] These policies were initiated by hospitals such as University of Washington Medical Center where elective surgeries and procedures were postponed starting March 7, 2020. During that time, blood usage and blood demand reached parity at Washington Medical Center.[24] This decrease in elective surgery was echoed in many hospitals, with one report citing a 71.7% decrease in surgical volume.[33]

Nationally, elective surgery cancellation and blood mitigation strategies became ubiquitous as seen by the AABB survey. The week of March 23, 2020, most of the hospitals reported they were no longer performing elective surgeries, with only 10.6% of

Table 1 Updated blood collection policies and Federal Drug Administration regulatory changes	
New Screening Measures and Changes	**Deferral**
Persons who traveled in COVID-19 endemic areas [a] Persons diagnosed with COVID-19, contact with people with the virus, and those suspected of having it [a]	14–28 d[a]
For male donors who would have been deferred for having sex with another man For female donors who would have been deferred for having sex with a man who had sex with another man For those with recent tattoos and piercings For those who have traveled to malaria-endemic areas (and are residents of malaria nonendemic countries): the agency is changing the recommended deferral period from 12 to 3 mo. In addition, the guidance provides notice of an alternate procedure that permits the collection of blood and blood components from such donors without a deferral period, provided the blood components are pathogen-reduced using an FDA-approved pathogen reduction device.	From 12 mo to 3 mo
For those who spent time in certain European countries or on military bases in Europe who were previously considered to have been exposed to a potential risk of transmission of Creutzfeldt-Jakob disease or variant Creutzfeldt-Jakob disease, the agency is eliminating the recommended deferrals and is recommending allowing reentry of these donors.	From indefinite deferral to no deferral

[a] Policy of various blood centers.[20–23]
Data from Refs.[19–23,29]

hospitals still conducting elective surgeries.[34] Blood usage mitigation techniques as mentioned earlier became more prevalent.[27] In fact, blood wastage increased the following week, March 30th, with 25% of hospitals reporting increased blood wastage due to cancellation of elective surgeries and nonurgent medical procedures.[35] Wastage peaked the week of May 4 at 54% and the subsequent week, May 11, decreased to 52% as many hospitals started to resume elective procedures (**Fig. 1**).[36,37]

PATIENT BLOOD MANAGEMENT DURING COVID-19 PANDEMIC
General Principles

Blood transfusion is considered one of the most common hospital procedures performed in the United States. The safety of blood products and the appropriateness of transfusion are significant and timely issues. Over the last 3 decades, studies have shown that transfusion of one red blood cell (RBC) unit increases wound complications by 4%, hospital length of stay (LOS) by 1.5 days, and mortality by 0.9%.[38–40] In nonbleeding patients, restricting blood transfusions by using a hemoglobin trigger of less than 7 g/dL significantly reduces cardiac events, rebleeding, bacterial infections, and total mortality.[41] Other blood components carry similar risks. Plasma is frequently misused, and its benefits are overestimated particularly in nonbleeding patients. In a retrospective cohort study, Warner and colleagues[42] found that prophylactic administration of plasma in the critically ill was not associated with improved clinical outcomes. Similar studies on prophylactic preprocedure platelet transfusion showed an increase in risk of thrombosis and mortality.[43]

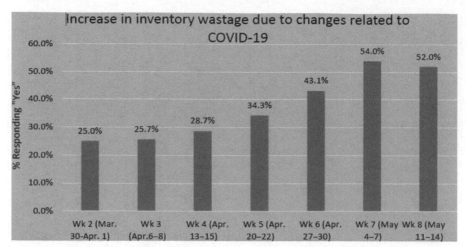

Fig. 1. As elective surgical cases were canceled and blood utilization decreased in much of the United States, a trend of increased wastages was seen. (*From* AABB. COVID-19 weekly hospital transfusion services survey: week 8 snapshot. Available at: http://www.aabb.org/research/hemovigilance/bloodsurvey/Docs/AABB-COVID-19-Impact-Survey-Snapshot-Week-8.pdf.)

Patient blood management (PBM) is a multidisciplinary, evidence-based strategy in which the need for blood products is managed in order to provide better patient outcomes and appropriate stewardship of a limited resource while reducing health care costs (**Table 2**). The primary goal of PBM program is to ensure optimal decision support using evidence-based guidelines and transfusing the most appropriate blood products with a minimum dose required for the clinical situation.[44] In addition, pharmaceutical products such as desmopressin and antifibrinolytics (such as Amicar or Tranexamic acid) have been shown to reduce bleeding.[45–48] Prothrombin complex concentrates and vitamin K may also be effective in warfarin reversal and correcting international normalized ratio.[49–51] Iron supplements, oral or intravenous preparations, and erythropoiesis-stimulating agents are proved to be useful in repleting iron stores and thus increasing hemoglobin levels.[52] PBM and bloodless medicine programs is now a priority throughout national and international health systems (**Fig. 2**).[53] Hospitals and academic medical centers across the nation are beginning to develop bloodless medicine and PBM programs in response to the favorable evidence.

PATIENT BLOOD MANAGEMENT STRATEGIES USED IN COVID-19 PANDEMIC

During the 2020 COVID-19 pandemic, blood supply shortages were observed worldwide, including the United States. The major blood suppliers and hospitals across the country issued emergency pleas for donations and reports significant numbers of blood drives were canceled due to school and workplace closures, which resulted in thousands of fewer blood donations typically collected.[19] In Beijing, China during the 2003 SARS epidemic, blood products shortages necessitated importation of blood products from other Chinese provinces to supply needs for clinical use in patients.[54,55] Similarly, the COVID-19 pandemic has had a major ripple effect on the number of eligible blood donors, blood supply, and on blood safety.

Therefore, PBM strategies are imperative in order to manage shortages during natural disaster or disease pandemics as well as long-term socioeconomic effects

Table 2
University of Rochester Medical Center evidence-based transfusion guideline

Product	Clinical Indication	Transfusion Trigger
Red blood cells	Anemia	Hct <21%; Hgb <7 g/dL
	Anemia with acute coronary syndromes	Hct <24%; Hgb <8 g/dL
Platelets	High risk of bleeding	Platelet count <10,000
	Fever or sepsis	Platelet count<20,000
	Acute bleeding	Platelet count<50,000
	Intracranial hemorrhage	Platelet count<100,000
	Documented platelet dysfunction	Per platelet function test
Plasma	Urgent need for warfarin reversal	INR >1.7
	Clinical coagulopathy	Based on relevant laboratory and TEG values
	Acute bleeding	To maintain the RBC to plasma ratio of our MTP
	Plasma exchange for TTP	
	Factor V or XI deficiency	
Cryoprecipitate	Low fibrinogen level	<150 and bleeding
	Documented dysfibrinogenemia	Clinically significant bleeding without obvious causation
	Uremic coagulopathy unresponsive to DDAVP	
	Factor VIII deficiency	

Abbreviations: DDAVP, desmopressin; Hct, hematocrit; Hgb, hemoglobin; INR, international normalized ratio; MTP, massive transfusion policy; TEG, thromboelastography; TTP, thrombotic thrombocytopenic purpura.

following these crises. Implementation of the most recent evidence-supported transfusion guidelines and eliminating unnecessary transfusions are considered the main goals of PBM programs during major disasters. Some effective strategies are as follows:

- Evaluation of appropriateness of transfusion orders and further discussion with clinical team if needed.
- Use of other pharmaceutical products such as desmopressin, antifibrinolytics, vitamin K, prothrombin complex concentrates, or intravenous iron if appropriate.

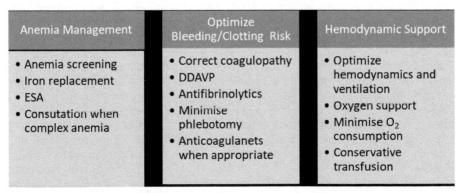

Anemia Management	Optimize Bleeding/Clotting Risk	Hemodynamic Support
• Anemia screening • Iron replacement • ESA • Consutation when complex anemia	• Correct coagulopathy • DDAVP • Antifibrinolytics • Minimise phlebotomy • Anticoagulanets when appropriate	• Optimize hemodynamics and ventilation • Oxygen support • Minimise O_2 consumption • Conservative transfusion

Fig. 2. Patient blood management strategies.

- Blood-sparing strategies during surgery such as implementation of normovolemic or hemodilution measures or usage of cell salvage.
- Staff education and open communication is imperative.

CHALLENGES OF MANAGING RESUMPTION OF NORMAL HOSPITAL SURGICAL OCCUPANCY

Although the demand for blood products during the COVID-19 pandemic has decreased due to postponement of elective surgeries, hospitals must have an emergency blood management plan. This plan should be in place and ready to be implemented during and following any natural crisis in order to maintain sustainability of a safe blood supply. As hospitals resume elective surgery and see increases in non-COVID-19 admissions, long-term shortages beyond the pandemic peak persist. At this time, blood collection centers and donors are still required to avoid large gatherings and follow all safety measures. Thus, a significant blood supply shortage may be present beyond the pandemic peak. In addition, due to the prolonged incubation period (up to 14 days) of SARS-CoV-2 and the potential of asymptomatic carriers, recruitment of blood donors as well as maintaining safety in the blood collection process remains a major concern.

EFFECT OF COVID-19 PANDEMIC ON TRANSFUSION SERVICE AND BLOOD BANK OPERATIONS

Being prepared to face a pandemic ensures that blood products are available to those patients requiring transfusion support, and a robust plan helps to protect the safety and health of the transfusion service professionals needed to perform testing and prepare blood products.[56] The effects of any pandemic on transfusion service and blood bank operations are 2-fold the work force and the blood supply.

Although many employees were encouraged or required to work remotely during the COVID-19 pandemic, this is not an option for laboratory professionals working in an academic medical center transfusion service and blood bank. To provide necessary transfusion support and to prepare and modify blood products, blood bank employees must be physically present in the laboratory at all times. Thus, for employees' safety and to prevent the spread of infection, repeated cleaning and disinfection of the work environment should be undertaken in conjunction with universal masking of employees and meticulous handwashing. To promote social distancing, separating staff by off-setting shift hours across the operation will more evenly distribute the staff across a 24-hour period. Depending on the physical layout of the work area it may be possible to set up workstations in different areas of the laboratory so that the staff is physically separated from each other as much as possible. That being said, plans must be in place to continue operations if multiple staff members become infected and cannot work. Because of the extensive regulations surrounding blood bank testing and competency requirements, cross-training technologists from other areas in the clinical laboratory on short notice tends not to be a viable option. A plan must be in place at the institutional level to postpone elective surgeries and other elective procedures that rely on transfusion support if staffing levels become critically low due to employee absenteeism and quarantine.

The second concern that transfusion services and blood banks may experience during a pandemic is the blood products supply. Blood collection mainly depends on volunteer blood donors at collection centers. During such a crisis blood donation can be greatly reduced as a result of donors becoming infected, unable to donate, or avoiding public gatherings.[57] Several conservation options should be considered by the transfusion service in order to conserve a rapidly dwindling blood supply along with additional measures promoted by a PBM program, when available.

- The blood type of trauma patients should be determined as rapidly as possible so that transfusion can be performed using type-specific RBC, thereby conserving the supply of group "O" RBC, a universal donor type. Group "O−" RBC should be reserved for women of childbearing age (<50 years) and female children. All other group "O" individuals should receive group "O+" RBC.
- If platelet availability is constrained, units can be split into 2 doses. At the authors' facility they found that one-half unit of platelets is sufficient to provide clinical benefit to most patients. However, based on the patient's clinical condition, a full dose can be transfused if required.
- Because of decreased blood utilization as a result of elective procedures withholding, reducing standing orders and managing blood product standing orders with the blood supplier is essential to minimize waste, particularly in multisite hospital systems with transfusion services located at each hospital. Transferring RBC to the highest transfusion volume facility in the health care system could be an option as well to reduce wastage.
- Inventory levels of reagents and supplies must be closely monitored. The transfusion service must work closely with the supply chain to ensure that critical reagents and supplies are available throughout the pandemic to perform critical testing. This may involve placing orders to bring levels to a level sufficient to perform testing for 3 months or more if availability or delivery could potentially be a problem.
- To assist the blood supplier, facilities could host additional blood drives either at the facility itself (if there is sufficient room to ensure adequate social distancing) or supporting drives in a larger venue (such as a mall closed due to the pandemic or a government building not currently or minimally occupied).
- If the hospital blood bank is FDA registered or licensed, the collection of convalescent plasma could be undertaken to provide a possible course of treatment either alone or in combination with other treatments to infected patients.[58]

Although blood conservation measures may be necessary, there likely will be a decrease in demand for RBC resulting from canceling elective surgical procedures. In the COVID-19 pandemic a reduction in blood orders from our blood supplier reduced spending at our facility by approximately 50%. Blood bank serologic testing was reduced by approximately 30% during the same time period but without the associated decrease in budget due to the advanced purchase of reagents and supplies. Close monitoring of testing volumes, blood product purchases, and waste is important to determine how the pandemic will affect cost projections.

CONVALESCENT PLASMA
Blood-Based Therapeutics for COVID-19

Unlike other subspecialties in pathology and laboratory medicine, transfusion medicine/blood banking is almost exclusively focused on therapeutics, including hands on treatment of patients. Thus it is understandable that physicians, nurses, and medical technologists in this area of medicine have been focused on possible treatment approaches for COVID-19. In the absence of effective and safe antiviral treatments, the strategy of transfusing convalescent plasma has long attracted interest and has been used in treatment of infectious disease, most recently in viral diseases.[59] The interest is due to the abundant evidence that humoral immunity plays a role in resolution of viral infection and prevention of reinfection after primary infection or vaccination. Convalescent plasma has a long history but almost no quality evidence for its efficacy and safety, as its use has often been reserved for last ditch efforts in desperately ill patients. In addition, much of the history of its use antedates the recognition that randomized trials are needed for ultimate proof of efficacy and safety due to the highly variable course of many illnesses, including COVID-19.[60]

In the current pandemic, early case reports of convalescent plasma usage reported that some patients who were seriously ill, requiring ICU care and mechanical ventilation,[61] cleared virus more rapidly than expected and made sufficient recovery and shorter LOS. Thousands of units of plasma, almost all untested for antiviral neutralizing titers, have been transfused in the United States using FDA-approved emergency investigational new drug and expanded access protocols.[62] Many small randomized trials and a few larger multicenter trials are underway a few months into the epidemic in the United States. These include some trials in patients with critical illness, using primary endpoints for efficacy such as ability to be weaned from mechanical ventilation, discharge from hospital, and survival. Other trials target prevention of infection in exposed individuals or prevention of hospitalization in newly SARS-CoV-2 RNA–positive individuals with mild or moderate symptoms. In most cases, given the uncertainty of whether antibody is protective, no specific titer or neutralizing titer of antibody in the plasma is specified. In other trials, high titers of antibody are required (eg, reactive at >1:320). Donors must meet standard FDA and state safety requirements for blood donation and be either RNA negative or greater than 28 days past clinical recovery in order to donate.[63] Donation can be by manual plasmapheresis or machine apheresis, with the former considerably less efficient but less costly.

There are many unresolved issues concerning convalescent plasma efficacy and safety, for example,[59] does antibody clearance of virus lead to clinical improvement in moderately to severely ill patients?,[60] does antibody prevent clinical deterioration in recently infected, asymptomatic or mildly symptomatic patients?, and[61] are there mid- to longer-term consequences of transfusing allogeneic plasma? Many statements have been made that allogeneic plasma transfusion is a common therapy with only rare acute complications (acute lung injury, volume overload, hemolysis, anaphylaxis, etc.). However, recent observational literature in critically ill patients demonstrate that allogeneic plasma transfusion is associated with nosocomial bacterial infection,[64] organ failure, and thrombosis.[65] The role of transfusing ABO "compatible plasma," an accepted practice, in worsening the risk of bleeding,[66] infection/sepsis,[67] organ failure,[67] and mortality[66] is not proved, but transfusion of ABO compatible, but not identical, plasma is likely not immunologically neutral. Immune complexes between antibody and soluble antigen form after transfusion and, at least in model systems, can activate monocytes, interfere with platelet and coagulation factor function, and may injure endothelial cells.[68]

A likely more efficacious and safer product than convalescent plasma being considered for use in COVID-19 disease and its prevention is hyperimmune immunoglobulin G (IgG). Intravenous IgG (IVIgG) made from multiple donors with detectable titers of anti-SARS-CoV-2 antibody would be expected to be more potent and carry fewer risks than convalescent allogeneic plasma that has not been processed.[69] However, it will be many months before such products are routinely available and much less proven effective and safe in patients. One clear cut benefit of IVIgG is a reduced risk of some adverse immune effects (acute lung injury, hemolysis, organ failure) because no single donor is heavily represented. Infectious disease transmission, although uncommon, after plasma that has been tested for HIV, hepatitis C, etc. is in general not a risk with use of IVIgG preparations. Both convalescent plasma and hyperimmune IgG may carry risks of antibody enhancement of viral infection.[70]

Finally, although not a blood product, humanized monoclonals to proteins and glycoproteins that are necessary for viral entry and replication hold some promise as preventive and therapeutic strategies in COVID-19.

BLOOD SAFETY DURING COVID-19
Steps Taken to Protect Blood Supply

In general, blood donors must be healthy on the day of donation and meet existing FDA donor screening measures. Typically, these measures should prevent individuals with any respiratory symptoms or infection from donation. Donors are also instructed to contact the blood collection center if any signs or symptoms developed within the next few days of donation. The collected blood or blood components will then be discarded and any distributed products will be recalled. Nevertheless, to date no transfusion-transmitted COVID-19 cases have been reported.

RISK OF BLOOD PRODUCTS CONTAMINATION WITH COVID-19

Overall, respiratory viruses are not known to be transmitted via blood transfusions. Thus far, there are no reported cases of transfusion-transmitted COVID-19 nor any type of the other coronaviruses. As a precaution measure to the blood safety, particularly after the rapid increase in COVID-19 infection rates in China, Chang and colleagues[71] screened all donations collected at the Wuhan Blood Center over 2 months (January through March 2020). RT-PCR testing for SARS-CoV-2 RNA was performed on pools of 6 to 8 plasma samples. Out of the screened 2430 donations, one donor tested positive for SARS-CoV-2. This donor was positive for COVID-19 previously and was quarantined appropriately in a cabin hospital in Wuhan until 2 consecutive negative throat swab results 3 days apart were obtained. At the time of donation, the donor displayed no symptoms. However, his plasma SARS-CoV-2 was still detectable. Later on, in a retrospective testing of 4995 donations collected between December 2019 and January 2020, plasma samples of 3 more healthy donors from Wuhan were also found to be positive for SARS-CoV-2. However, specific IgG and IgM against SARS-CoV-2 by enzyme-linked immunosorbent assay were negative, indicating the possibility of infection in the early stage. The investigator concluded that because of the asymptomatic COVID-19 cases, screening donors for SARS-CoV-2 will be critical to ensure blood safety.

Hence, to date there are no FDA requirements in place to screen blood donors or test blood components for COVID-19. Individuals with COVID-19 infection do not meet the blood donation guidelines.

DISCLOSURE

Dr. Majed A. Refaai has received consulting fees and/or research funding from CSL Behring, Octapharma, Bayer, Instrumentation Laboratory, and iLine microsystems and has received speaking fees from CSL Behring.The other Authors have nothing to disclose.

REFERENCES

1. Wu F, Zhao S, Yu B, et al. A new coronavirus associated with human respiratory disease in China. Nature 2020;579(7798):265–9.

2. Paules CI, Marston HD, Fauci AS. Coronavirus infections—more than just the common cold. JAMA 2020;323(8):707–8.
3. Sultan S, Altayar O, Siddique SM, et al. AGA Institute rapid review of the gastrointestinal and liver manifestations of COVID-19, meta-analysis of international data, and recommendations for the consultative management of patients with COVID-19. Gastroenterology 2020;159(1):320–34.e27.
4. Huang C, Wang Y, Li X, et al. Clinical features of patients infected with 2019 novel coronavirus in Wuhan, China. Lancet 2020;395(10223):497–506.
5. Chan JF, Yuan S, Kok KH, et al. A familial cluster of pneumonia associated with the 2019 novel coronavirus indicating person-to-person transmission: a study of a family cluster. Lancet 2020;395(10223):514–23.
6. Coronavirus (COVID-19). 2020. Available at: https://www.cdc.gov/coronavirus/2019-ncov/index.html. Accessed May 28, 2020.
7. Oran DP, Topol EJ. Prevalence of Asymptomatic SARS-CoV-2 Infection: A Narrative Review [published online ahead of print, 2020 Jun 3]. Ann Intern Med 2020. M20-3012. https://doi.org/10.7326/M20-3012.
8. Guan WJ, Ni ZY, Hu Y, et al. Clinical characteristics of coronavirus disease 2019 in China. N Engl J Med 2020;382(18):1708–20.
9. Nomoto H, Ishikane M, Katagiri D, et al. Cautious handling of urine from moderate to severe COVID-19 patients. Am J Infect Control 2020;48(8):969–71.
10. Killerby ME, Biggs HM, Haynes A, et al. Human coronavirus circulation in the United States 2014-2017. J Clin Virol 2018;101:52–6.
11. Wang W, Xu Y, Gao R, et al. Detection of SARS-CoV-2 in different types of clinical specimens. JAMA 2020;323(18):1843–4.
12. Chen W, Lan Y, Yuan X, et al. Detectable 2019-nCoV viral RNA in blood is a strong indicator for the further clinical severity. Emerg Microbes Infect 2020;9(1):469–73.
13. Pascarella G, Strumia A, Piliego C, et al. COVID-19 diagnosis and management: a comprehensive review. J Intern Med 2020;288(2):192–206.
14. Liu T, Zhang J, Yang Y, et al. The role of interleukin-6 in monitoring severe case of coronavirus disease 2019. EMBO Mol Med 2020;12(7):e12421.
15. Tan L, Wang Q, Zhang D, et al. Lymphopenia predicts disease severity of COVID-19: a descriptive and predictive study. Signal Transduct Target Ther 2020;5(1):33.
16. Zhang L, Yan X, Fan Q, et al. D-dimer levels on admission to predict in-hospital mortality in patients with Covid-19. J Thromb Haemost 2020;18(6):1324–9.
17. Jean SS, Lee PI, Hsueh PR. Treatment options for COVID-19: the reality and challenges. J Microbiol Immunol Infect 2020;53(3):436–43.
18. CFR - code of federal regulations title 21. 2019. Available at: https://www.accessdata.fda.gov/scripts/cdrh/cfdocs/cfcfr/cfrsearch.cfm?fr=630.10. Accessed May 15, 2020.
19. What to know about the coronavirus and blood donation. 2020. Available at: https://www.redcrossblood.org/donate-blood/dlp/coronavirus–covid-19–and-blood-donation.html. Accessed May 15, 2020.
20. Coronavirus and blood donation. 2020. Available at: https://www.mbc.org/coronavirus-blood-donation/. Accessed May 15, 2020.
21. COVID-19 and the blood supply. 2020. Available at: https://www.carterbloodcare.org/covid-19-and-the-blood-supply/. Accessed May 15, 2020.
22. COVID Info. 2020. Available at: https://www.vitalant.org/COVID-Info. Accessed May 15, 2020.
23. COVID-19 response. 2020. Available at: https://www.bloodcenter.org/donate/donor/covid19-response/. Accessed May 15, 2020.

24. Pagano MB, Hess JR, Tsang HC, et al. Prepare to adapt: blood supply and transfusion support during the first 2 weeks of the 2019 novel coronavirus (COVID-19) pandemic affecting Washington State. Transfusion 2020;60(5):908–11.

25. American red cross faces severe blood shortage as coronavirus outbreak threatens availability of nation's supply. 2020. Available at: https://www.redcross.org/about-us/news-and-events/press-release/2020/american-red-cross-faces-severe-blood-shortage-as-coronavirus-outbreak-threatens-availability-of-nations-supply.html. Accessed May 15, 2020.

26. Message to blood donors during the COVID-19 pandemic. AABB: Bethesda, MD; 2020. p. 2.

27. COVID-19 impact on hospital practices: week 1-4 survey snapshot. AABB: Bethesda, MD; 2020. Available at: http://www.aabb.org/research/hemovigilance/bloodsurvey/Docs/AABB-COVID-19-Impact-Survey-Snapshot-Week-1-4.pdf. Accessed May 15, 2020.

28. Alternative Procedures for Blood and Blood Components during the COVID-19 Public Health Emergency. U.S. Department of Health and Human Services Food and Drug Administration Center for Biologics Evaluation and Research. p. 8. Available at: https://www.fda.gov/regulatory-information/search-fda-guidance-documents/alternative-procedures-blood-and-blood-components-during-covid-19-public-health-emergency. Accessed May 15, 2020.

29. Coronavirus (COVID-19) update: FDA provides updated guidance to address the urgent need for blood during the pandemic. 2020. Available at: https://www.fda.gov/news-events/press-announcements/coronavirus-covid-19-update-fda-provides-updated-guidance-address-urgent-need-blood-during-pandemic. Accessed May 15, 2020.

30. Alternative procedures for blood and blood components during the COVID-19 public health emergency. 2020. Available at: https://www.fda.gov/regulatory-information/search-fda-guidance-documents/alternative-procedures-blood-and-blood-components-during-covid-19-public-health-emergency. Accessed May 15, 2020.

31. Healthcare facilities: preparing for community transmission. 2020. Available at: https://www.cdc.gov/coronavirus/2019-ncov/hcp/guidance-hcf.html. Accessed May 15, 2020.

32. COVID-19: recommendations for management of elective surgical procedures. 2020. Available at: https://www.facs.org/covid-19/clinical-guidance/elective-surgery. Accessed May 15, 2020.

33. Hemingway JF, Singh N, Starnes BW. Emerging practice patterns in vascular surgery during the COVID-19 pandemic. J Vasc Surg 2020;72(2):396–402.

34. AABB survey COVID-19 impact on care of patients requiring transfusion: week 1 snapshot. 2020. 1. Available at: http://www.aabb.org/research/hemovigilance/bloodsurvey/Docs/AABB-COVID-19-Impact-Survey-Snapshot-Week-1.pdf. Accessed May 16, 2020.

35. AABB survey COVID-19 impact on care of patients requiring transfusion: week 2 snapshot. 2020. 1. Available at: http://www.aabb.org/research/hemovigllance/bloodsurvey/Docs/AABB-COVID-19-Impact-Survey-Snapshot-Week-2.pdf. Accessed May 16, 2020.

36. AABB COVID-19 weekly hospital transfusion services survey: week 7 snapshot. 2020. 1. Available at: http://www.aabb.org/research/hemovigilance/bloodsurvey/Docs/AABB-COVID-19-Impact-Survey-Snapshot-Week-7.pdf. Accessed May 16, 2020.

37. AABB COVID-19 weekly hospital transfusion services survey: week 8 snapshot. 2020. 1. Available at: http://www.aabb.org/research/hemovigilance/bloodsurvey/Docs/AABB-COVID-19-Impact-Survey-Snapshot-Week-8.pdf. Accessed May 16, 2020.

38. Ferraris VA, Davenport DL, Saha SP, et al. Surgical outcomes and transfusion of minimal amounts of blood in the operating room. Arch Surg 2012;147(1):49–55.

39. Bernard AC, Davenport DL, Chang PK, et al. Intraoperative transfusion of 1 U to 2 U packed red blood cells is associated with increased 30-day mortality, surgical-site infection, pneumonia, and sepsis in general surgery patients. J Am Coll Surg 2009;208(5):931–7, 937.e1-2; [discussion: 938–9].

40. Ferraris VA, Ferraris VA, Brown JR, et al. 2011 update to the Society of Thoracic Surgeons and the Society of Cardiovascular Anesthesiologists blood conservation clinical practice guidelines. Ann Thorac Surg 2011;91(3):944–82.

41. Hajjar LA, Vincent JL, Galas FR, et al. Transfusion requirements after cardiac surgery: the TRACS randomized controlled trial. JAMA 2010;304(14):1559–67.

42. Warner MA, Chandran A, Jenkins G, et al. Prophylactic plasma transfusion is not associated with decreased red blood cell requirements in critically ill patients. Anesth Analg 2017;124(5):1636–43.

43. Schmidt AE, Henrichs KF, Kirkley SA, et al. Prophylactic preprocedure platelet transfusion is associated with increased risk of thrombosis and mortality. Am J Clin Pathol 2017;149(1):87–94.

44. Mehra T, Seifert B, Bravo-Reiter S, et al. Implementation of a patient blood management monitoring and feedback program significantly reduces transfusions and costs. Transfusion 2015;55(12):2807–15.

45. Twum-Barimah E, Abdelgadir I, Gordon M, et al. Systematic review with meta-analysis: the efficacy of tranexamic acid in upper gastrointestinal bleeding. Aliment Pharmacol Ther 2020;51(11):1004–13.

46. Myles PS, Smith JA, Forbes A, et al. Tranexamic acid in patients undergoing coronary-artery surgery. N Engl J Med 2017;376(2):136–48.

47. Dunn CJ, Goa KL. Tranexamic acid: a review of its use in surgery and other indications. Drugs 1999;57(6):1005–32.

48. Lim CC, Tan HZ, Tan CS, et al. Desmopressin acetate (DDAVP) to prevent bleeding in percutaneous kidney biopsy: a systematic review. Intern Med J 2020. https://doi.org/10.1111/imj.14774.

49. Refaai MA, Kothari TH, Straub S, et al. Four-factor Prothrombin complex concentrate reduces time to procedure in vitamin K antagonist-treated patients experiencing gastrointestinal bleeding: a post hoc analysis of two randomized controlled trials. Emerg Med Int 2017;2017:8024356.

50. Polito NB, Kanouse E, Jones CMC, et al. Effect of vitamin K administration on rate of warfarin reversal. Transfusion 2019;59(4):1202–8.

51. Mazur H, Young S, McGraw M, et al. 471: efficacy and safety of 4F-PCC VS. FFP for warfarin reversal in emergent surgery/invasive procedure. Crit Care Med 2019;47(1):216.

52. Cho BC, Serini J, Zorrilla-Vaca A, et al. Impact of preoperative erythropoietin on allogeneic blood transfusions in surgical patients: results from a systematic review and meta-analysis. Anesth Analg 2019;128(5):981–92.

53. Tokin C, Almeda J, Jain S, et al. Blood-management programs: a clinical and administrative model with program implementation strategies. Perm J 2009;13(1):18–28.

54. Cai X, Ren M, Chen F, et al. Blood transfusion during the COVID-19 outbreak. Blood Transfus 2020;18(2):79–82.

55. Raturi M, Kusum A. The active role of a blood center in outpacing the transfusion transmission of COVID-19. Transfus Clin Biol 2020;27(2):96–7.
56. AABB Interorganizational Task Force on Pandemic Influenza and the Blood Supply, in Pandemic influenza issues outline. AABB. p. 16. Bethesda, MD;2020.
57. Maintaining a Safe and Adequate Blood Supply during Pandemic Influenza, in Guidelines for Blood Transfusion Services. World Health Organization (WHO). Geneva, Switzerland;2011.
58. Roback JD, Guarner J. Convalescent Plasma to Treat COVID-19: Possibilities and Challenges [published online ahead of print, 2020 Mar 27]. JAMA 2020. https://doi.org/10.1001/jama.2020.4940.
59. Bloch EM, Shoham S, Casadevall A, et al. Deployment of convalescent plasma for the prevention and treatment of COVID-19. J Clin Invest 2020;130(6):2757–65.
60. Dzik S. COVID-19 Convalescent Plasma: Now Is the Time for Better Science [published online ahead of print, 2020 Apr 23]. Transfus Med Rev. 2020;S0887-7963(20)30026-2. http://doi.org/10.1016/j.tmrv.2020.04.002.
61. Zeng F, Chen X, Deng G. Convalescent plasma for patients with COVID-19. Proc Natl Acad Sci U S A 2020;117(23):12528.
62. Joyner M. 2020. Available at: https://www.uscovidplasma.org/#workflow. Accessed May 22, 2020.
63. Available at: https://www.fda.gov/emergency-preparedness-and-response/coronavirus-disease-2019-covid-19/donate-covid-19-plasma.
64. Subramanian A, Berbari EF, Brown MJ, et al. Plasma transfusion is associated with postoperative infectious complications following esophageal resection surgery: a retrospective cohort study. J Cardiothorac Vasc Anesth 2012;26(4):569–74.
65. Bence CM, Traynor MD Jr, Polites SF, et al. The incidence of venous thromboembolism in children following colorectal resection for inflammatory bowel disease: A multi-center study [published online ahead of print, 2020 Feb 20]. J Pediatr Surg. 2020;S0022-3468(20)30121-4. http://doi.org/10.1016/j.jpedsurg.2020.02.020.
66. Refaai MA, Fialkow LB, Heal JM, et al. An association of ABO non-identical platelet and cryoprecipitate transfusions with altered red cell transfusion needs in surgical patients. Vox Sang 2011;101(1):55–60.
67. Inaba K, Branco BC, Rhee P, et al. Impact of ABO-identical vs ABO-compatible nonidentical plasma transfusion in trauma patients. Arch Surg 2010;145(9):899–906.
68. Refaai MA, Cahill C, Masel D, et al. Is it time to reconsider the concepts of "universal donor" and "ABO compatible" transfusions? Anesth Analg 2018;126(6):2135–8.
69. Nguyen AA, Habiballah SB, Platt CD, et al. Immunoglobulins in the treatment of COVID-19 infection: proceed with caution! Clin Immunol 2020;216:108459.
70. Liu L, Wei Q, Lin Q, et al. Anti-spike IgG causes severe acute lung injury by skewing macrophage responses during acute SARS-CoV infection. JCI Insight 2019;4(4):e123158.
71. Chang L, Zhao L, Gong H, et al. Severe acute respiratory syndrome coronavirus 2 RNA detected in blood donations. Emerg Infect Dis 2020;26(7):1631–3.

Measuring the Serologic Response to Severe Acute Respiratory Syndrome Coronavirus 2: Methods and Meaning

Check for updates

Nicole D. Pecora, MD, PhD[a],*, Martin S. Zand, MD, PhD[b]

KEYWORDS

- SARS-CoV-2 • COVID-19 • COVID-19 serology

KEY POINTS

- Early in the coronavirus disease 2019 (COVID-19) pandemic, the release of poorly characterized antibody tests caused concern about the quality of serologic results and a national discussion about test performance.
- The positive predictive value of COVID-19 serologic tests varies with seroprevalence and is a major concern.
- The kinetics of the antibody response to severe acute respiratory syndrome coronavirus 2 (SARS-CoV-2) are characterized by the appearance of immunoglobulin (Ig) G in most individuals by at least 2 weeks after symptom onset, slightly after IgM and IgA.
- There is continued uncertainty about the significance of antibody tests in terms of the degree and durability of immunity.
- The differential and quantitative detection of viral antigens may prove to be important and will require the development of test platforms to answer these nuanced questions.

Funding: This work was supported by the National Institutes of Health Institute of Allergy, Immunology and Infectious Diseases grants R01 AI129518 and R21 AI138500 (M.S. Zand), and the University of Rochester Clinical and Translational Science Award UL1 TR002001 from the National Center for Advancing Translational Sciences of the National Institutes of Health (M. S. Zand). The content is solely the responsibility of the authors and does not necessarily represent the official views of the National Institutes of Health. None of the mentioned funders had any role in study design, data collection and analysis, decision to publish, or preparation of the article.
[a] University of Rochester Medical Center, Rochester, NY, USA; [b] Department of Medicine, Nephrology (SMD), Clinical & Translational Science Institute, Clinical Research University of Rochester Medical Center, School of Medicine and Dentistry, 601 Elmwood Avenue, Box 675, Rochester, NY 14642, USA
* Corresponding author. UR Medicine Central Laboratory, 211 Bailey Road, West Henrietta, NY 14586, USA.
E-mail address: Nicole_pecora@urmc.rochester.edu

INTRODUCTION

The coronavirus disease 2019 (COVID-19) pandemic began in December 2019 with several cases of a pneumonia of unknown cause in Wuhan, China.[1] The causative agent was quickly identified using molecular techniques as the Betacoronavirus severe acute respiratory syndrome coronavirus 2 (SARS-CoV-2).[2] This discovery was followed by a global effort to develop accurate molecular diagnostics at tremendous scale and pace in order to diagnose acute infection and contain spread of the virus. Questions about serologic testing followed soon after.

Early in the pandemic, lack of regulatory restrictions on serologic testing led to a wave of more than 40 antibody tests to detect immunoglobulin (Ig) G and/or IgM binding to SARS-CoV-2 spike (S) and nucleocapsid (NP) proteins.[3–9] Many of these tests were poorly characterized, which caused concern about the quality of serologic data. Several discussions about so-called immunity passports caused further concern about the use of serologic data.[10] In response, the US Food and Drug Administration (FDA) moved to tighten regulation of new commercial serologic tests; more than 30 were subsequently withdrawn from distribution.[11] These events have highlighted the importance of rigorous testing evaluation and scope of use. At the same time, tremendous effort has been focused on understanding the immune response to SARS-CoV-2, both from data coming out of the hardest-hit regions and from previous knowledge gleaned from the study of SARS-CoV-1, Middle East respiratory syndrome (MERS), and circulating human coronaviruses (HCoVs). This knowledge has helped to refine the questions of who to test for antibodies to SARS-CoV-2 and for what purpose they should be tested.[12]

This article reviews the basis of antibody-mediated immunity to SARS-CoV-2 and other coronaviruses (CoVs), with a focus on kinetics and correlates of protection. It then discusses currently available testing options for SARS-CoV-2 antibodies in the context of the rapidly evolving knowledge of disease immunopathogenesis, and how testing may be used to inform a diverse and complicated set of questions.

VIRAL ANTIGENS

SARS-CoV-2 is a member of the family Coronaviridae, which consists of 2 genera that infect mammals: Alphacoronavirus and Betacoronavirus.[13] Strains that are relevant to human infections include the 4 circulating seasonal coronaviruses: 229E and NL63 (both Alphacoronavirus), and OC43, HKU1, MERS-CoV, and SARS-CoV-1 (all Betacoronavirus).[13] All of the CoVs are enveloped RNA viruses with genomes in the range of 30 kilobases (**Fig. 1**). The first portion of the genome consists of open reading frames (ORFs) 1a and 1b, encoding the replicase-transcriptase polyprotein (pp1ab), followed by 4 structural proteins: S, NP, envelope (E), and membrane (M). Studies on SARS-CoV-1 indicated that the structural NP and S proteins are the dominant antigens for host immune responses to SARS-CoV-2.[14,15]

The mature S protein is a ~180 kDa glycosylated homotrimer that protrudes from the viral surface, giving the characteristic halo appearance for which CoVs are named.[16] The extracellular region is organized into the S1 and S2 domains. S1

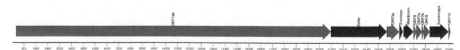

Fig. 1. The SARS-CoV-2 genome: SARS-CoV-2 isolate Wuhan-Hu-1, complete genome (NC_045512). Genes encoding nonstructural proteins are shown in gray. Genes encoding structural proteins S, E, M, and NP are shown in blue. ORF, open reading frame.

comprises the outermost region, contains the receptor-binding domain (RBD) for the target human ACE2 receptor, and initiates host cell entry.[17–20] Studies of SARS-CoV-1 show that receptor binding and proteolytic cleavage at the S1/S2 junction triggers a conformational change in S2 that mediates entry via the membrane fusion peptide sequence.[21] The S protein is moderately conserved among members of the Betacoronaviridae, particularly the S2 region proximal to the viral surface (**Fig. 2**).[22] The S1 region, including the RBD, is less conserved and of great interest as a target for immunoassays because of its prime role in interaction with the human host.[22] Several studies have shown that anti-S antibodies can neutralize virus in cell culture, and efforts toward vaccine development are heavily focused on this protein.[16,17,23–25]

Functional and biochemical studies on the ~50-kDa SARS-CoV-1 and SARS-CoV-2 NP proteins show roles in replication, transcription, and packaging of the genome[26,27] (**Fig. 3**). The high abundance and antigenicity of NP have made it a focus of both diagnostic and vaccine work for SARS-CoV-1 as well as SARS-CoV-2.[28–30] NP sequences show 99% identity with related bat CoVs (RaTG13) and ~90% identity with SARS-CoV-1.[31]

These sequence homologies have implications for antibody testing. By sequence analysis, the normal circulating CoV strain OC43 has moderate homology with SARS-CoV-2 in both the NP and S proteins (**Fig. 4**). Sequence similarities can translate into cross-strain antibody binding, decreasing test specificity when used to determine infection prevalence. In contrast, increased specificity may occur from strain differences on surface sequences that are likely targets of antibody-mediated responses.

ANTIBODY KINETICS

Using a variety of technologies and antigens, the kinetics of the antibody response to SARS-CoV-2 are being explored. The earliest information came from several groups in

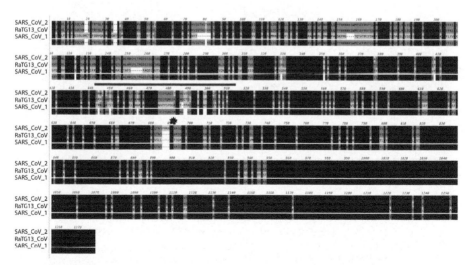

Fig. 2. Alignment of the S protein among closely related betacoronaviruses: peptide sequences from SARS-CoV-2 (NCBI [National Center for Biotechnology Information] YP_009724390), RaTG13-CoV (NCBI QHR63300), and SARS-CoV-1 (NCBI BAE93401) were aligned using ClustalW. Conserved residues (3/3) are shown in dark blue, (2/3) in teal, (1/3) in gray. The S1/S2 cleavage site is indicated by a red star. The receptor-binding motif is designated by the red line.

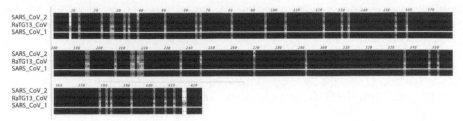

Fig. 3. Alignment of the NP protein among closely related betacoronaviruses: peptide sequences from SARS-CoV-2 (NCBI YP_009724390), RaTG13-CoV (NCBI QHR63300), and SARS-CoV-1 (NCBI BAE93401) were aligned using ClustalW. Conserved residues (3/3) are shown in dark blue, (2/3) in teal, (1/3) in gray.

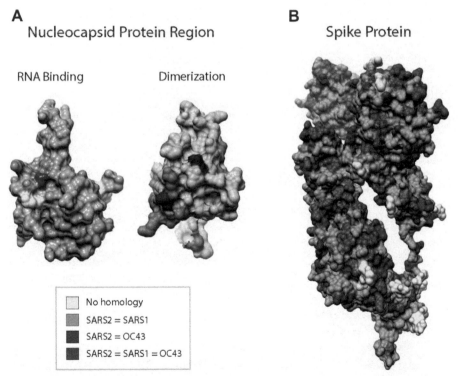

Fig. 4. Conservation of surface amino acids between SARS-CoV-2, SARS-CoV-1, and CoV-OC43: (*A*) space-filling model of the NP protein RNA-binding region (PDB [Protein Data Bank] 6M3M) and dimerization region (PDB 2GIB) from SARS-CoV-1 with sequence conservation mapped on the surface projection from ClustalW alignments between SARS-CoV-1 (NCBI BAE93401), SARS-CoV-2 (NCBI YP_009724390), and CoV-OC43 (NCBI YP_009555245). (*B*) Space-filling model of the full-length SARS-CoV-2 S protein monomer (PDB CVYB) with sequence conservation mapped on the surface projection from ClustalW alignments from SARS-CoV-2 (NCBI YP_009724390), SARS-CoV-1 (NCBI BAE93401), and CoV-OC43 (NCBI YP_009555241).

China who characterized the serologic responses of patients at the beginning of the pandemic using enzyme-linked immunosorbent assays (ELISAs) based either exclusively on the detection of NP alone or on NP in conjunction with the RBD domain of the S protein. These 2 antigens performed equivalently as assay targets, with antibodies becoming detectable in some individuals within the first week of symptom onset.[32–36]

There are conflicting reports regarding the disease course kinetics of anti-NP and anti-S antibody detection, and thus the relative sensitivity of serologic tests. Some reports have shown detection of anti-NP slightly earlier than anti-S antibodies, whereas others have shown the contrary, possibly because of differences in assay format.[36,37] Similarly, human SARS-CoV-1 anti-NP antibodies were detectable by serologic assays slightly earlier than anti-S Ig.[38,39] Additional studies have suggested that assays using more restricted epitopes, namely S1 or RBD, may be more specific than those using the full S protein.[32–34,36,40] Importantly, although antibody responses may be detectable in the first week after symptom onset, a full 2 to 3 weeks is required for a robust response.[9,36,41] Over the course of infection, IgM and IgA appeared earliest, often within 5 days of symptom onset, although IgG appeared in close succession.[32–34,36,40]

With respect to the kinetics of viral RNA (the viral shedding window), antibodies seem to become detectable as the viral load diminishes.[33–35] However, patients with both mild and severe clinical presentations may generate a detectable antibody response before viral clearance.[34,35,42] In contrast, there have been reports that asymptomatic (reverse transcriptase polymerase chain reaction confirmed) individuals may show late onset or even no seroconversion.[35]

TEST VALIDATION

Much of the controversy surrounding SARS-CoV-2 serologic testing has centered on fundamental aspects of test validation, and this was also true for SARS-CoV-1.[43,44] SARS-CoV-2 antibody detection tests have used several platforms, including ELISAs, chemiluminescent, lateral flow, and multiplex methods. All have previously been used to detect antibodies to other viral pathogens.[45] In general, these methods involve solid phase coupling of recombinant S or NP as fully trimerized (S protein), monomeric (NP), or peptide fragments (S1-RBD, linear peptide fragments). The solid phase coupled proteins are incubated with serum to allow immunoglobulin binding, which is detected by a secondary anti-IgG/IgA/IgM reagent. Assay readouts include serum dilution titers, colorimetric absorbance, changes in surface reflectivity, or fluorescence intensity.

Assay validation requires a set of known positive and negative serum samples. Archived samples from the pre-COVID-19 era (eg, pre-2020) can be used for a negative gold standard. There is particular interest in determining the false-positive rate because the presence of antibodies will be interpreted as proof of prior infection. Across multiple studies, specificity of ELISA-format assays has been reported to be between 95% and 100%.[9,32–34,36,41] For studies that include samples from individuals with known HCoV infections (HKU1, NL63, OC43, or 229E), SARS-CoV-1, or MERS-CoV, cross-reactivity was generally found to be low, with the exception of sera taken from individuals infected with SARS-CoV-1. Similarly, several clinical conditions are associated with broadly cross-reactive antibodies, including acute respiratory infections, autoimmune diseases (eg, lupus, rheumatoid arthritis), and other infections (eg, syphilis, Lyme disease). Including such serologic samples from the pre-COVID-19 era is critical for test specificity validation. Defining a known positive gold standard poses some challenges. Given the postinfection kinetics of anti-S and anti-NP antibody, it seems prudent to choose positive validation sera from patients taken at least 2 weeks after SARS-CoV-2 infection confirmed by a nucleic acid test.

For any clinical assay, the trade-off between specificity and sensitivity is a key factor in how it will be ultimately used. For example, if a positive value is to be used as a surrogate marker for infection, with potential translation for immunity, minimizing the false-positive rate is critical. In contrast, other considerations are a focus for a test that is used to monitor antibody kinetics after infection, in vaccine clinical trials, or to monitor convalescent plasma or monoclonal antibody therapy. Here, binary (positive or negative) or titer (ranked categorical) test results are less useful than a continuous readout (ie, absolute antibody concentration; eg, nanograms per milliliter), especially when performing statistical comparisons of vaccine efficacy in clinical trials[46] or determining who should donate convalescent plasma. Identifying antibody subsets poses another challenge for test validation. The acceptable threshold for anti-S1/RBD antibodies may need to be different for convalescent plasma donor screening than for identifying postinfectious immunity.

CURRENT CLINICAL TESTING OPTIONS

Serologic testing for SARS-CoV-2 infection has become available in the United States over the first few months of the pandemic in 2 main formats: point of care and clinical laboratory. Several companies produced rapid, lateral flow–type devices with readouts of total antibody or separate IgM and IgG. Whitman and colleagues[47] performed an assessment of many of these and found widely varying performance: between 81.8% and 100% sensitivity at more than 20 days after symptom onset and 84.3% to 100% specificity. Gradually, established manufacturers have begun releasing product for testing in high-complexity clinical laboratories. At the time of writing, 13 assays by 11 different manufacturers have been granted Emergency Use Authorization (EUA) by the FDA, and these represent a variety of targets and technologies (**Table 1**).[48]

NP-based assays include chemiluminescent immunoassay (CLIA) and electrochemiluminescence immunoassay technologies offered by Abbott and Roche, respectively. Both of these assays measure IgG and seem to be highly specific and sensitive. The Abbott platform has been evaluated independently in a large cohort in Idaho with confirmation of its performance: 99.90% specificity and 100% sensitivity 17 days after symptom onset.[3] Additional technologies with EUA based on detection of NP include a microsphere immunoassay developed by the New York State Department of Health at the Wadsworth. S and S derivative (S1 and RBD)–based assays include a CLIA assay developed by Ortho-Clinical Diagnostics and ELISAs from Euroimmun and Mount Sinai Hospital.[9] False-positive results have been noted for sera from patients infected with HCoV-OC43 in the Euroimmun assay.[41]

IMPLICATIONS FOR IMMUNITY

Some questions where antibody testing can provide clarity include seroprevalence and, on an individual level, whether a person has previously been infected with SARS-CoV-2.[49] This assessment can be straightforward, such as when an individual had clinically suggestive symptoms weeks prior but could not, or did not, get a molecular test. Beyond simply assessing previous infection, there is considerable interest in interpreting serologic test results as correlates of protection against future infection (**Box 1**). When using serologic testing to answer such questions, it is important to consider (1) the durability of the immune response, (2) the neutralization potential of antibodies, and (3) the translation of these findings into an assessment of functional

Table 1
Performance of severe acute respiratory syndrome coronavirus 2 immunoassays with Food and Drug Administration Emergency Use Authorization[a]

Manufacturer	Antigen	Ab Class	Format	Sensitivity (%)	Specificity (%)	Platform
Abbott	NP	IgG	CLIA	100.0	99–99.6	Architect/Alinity
Roche	NP	IgG	ECLIA	100.0	99.8	Elecsys
Ortho	S	IgG, Tot Ab	CLIA	90–100	100.0	Vitros
Diasorin	S1/S2	IgG	CMIA	97.6	99.3	Liaison XL
Euroimmun	S1	IgG	ELISA	90.0	97.8–100	None
Wadsworth	NP	Tot Ab	MIA	88.0	98.8	FlexMap
Mt Sinai	RBD and S	IgG	2-step ELISA	92.5	100.0	None
Cellex	NP and S	IgG and IgM	LFA	93.8[b]	96.0[b]	None
Bio-Rad	NP	Tot Ab	ELISA	92.2	99.6	None
Autobio	S	IgG and IgM	LFA	99[b]	99.0[b]	None

Abbreviations: Ab, antibody; CLIA, chemiluminescent immunoassay; CMIA, chemiluminescent microparticle immunoassay; ECLIA, electrochemiluminescence immunoassay; LFA, lateral flow assay; MIA, microsphere immunofluorescence assay; Tot, total.

[a] Performance was assessed using EUA data and FDA assessment as described (https://www.fda.gov/medical-devices/emergency-situations-medical-devices/eua-authorized-serology-test-performance).

[b] Combined IgM/IgG performance.

in vivo immunity. Critically, there currently are no data regarding the association between the presence and titers of anti–SARS-CoV-2-S or anti—SARS-CoV-2-NP antibodies and protection from reinfection.

The COVID-19 pandemic is still in its early stages, so there has not been the opportunity to assess the longevity of the antibody response, although small cohort studies show that IgG antibodies are detectable for at least 6 weeks after symptom onset,[35,40] whereas IgM is diminished within the first month postinfection.[36,40] A recent study of IgG levels in asymptomatic versus symptomatic individuals found that neutralizing titers were more likely to diminish in the early convalescent phase in those without a history of symptoms.[50] Furthermore, the same study showed that 40.0% of asymptomatic

Box 1
Questions for severe acute respiratory syndrome coronavirus 2 antibody testing

Has the individual been infected (if the molecular result is negative and the patient is likely outside of the window of viral shedding)?

Does the pediatric patient have multisystem inflammatory syndrome?

Are the infection prevention policies and personal protective equipment guidelines adequate for protecting health care workers in the institution?

Can a recovered COVID-19 patient donate plasma for therapeutic use? What is the half-life of anti–SARS-CoV-2 antibodies in a recipient of convalescent plasma?

Does a given serologic response indicate a successful trial vaccine?

Has the individual mounted an adequate response to a vaccine (once one becomes available)?

individuals became seronegative in the convalescent phase versus only 12.9% of those who were symptomatic.[50] Previous reports indicate that individuals infected with SARS-CoV-1 have detectable IgG antibodies for at least 8 to 24 months after symptom onset, whereas IgM and IgA were markedly decreased.[51–53] In contrast, patients infected with HCoV 229E have markedly diminished antibody levels 1 year postinfection.[54] Such results may complicate future interpretation of serologic test results, especially if SARS-CoV-2 infection becomes endemic and seasonal.

Plaque reduction neutralization tests can assess whether infected patients mount a neutralizing antibody response to the virus. Serum or plasma from individuals infected with SARS-CoV-1 or SARS-CoV-2 has been shown in several studies to neutralize viral infectivity in vitro.[24,41,55–57] Several purified neutralizing antibodies have been characterized against epitopes of both SARS-CoV-1 and SARS-CoV-2, most of which are directed against the RBD of the S protein.[14,16,23–25,58] It remains to be seen how these findings can be translated in vivo to natural immunity or therapeutics.

Neutralizing antibodies are the basis for convalescent plasma therapy, which showed promise in treating patients with SARS-CoV-1 and is currently being tested for those with SARS-CoV-2. Monoclonal antibodies directed at the S1-RBD and other antigenic sites are also in development. Both classes of therapies pose opportunities and challenges for clinical serologic testing. Convalescent plasma donors will need to be screened for high anti–SARS-CoV-2 protective titers, although it is not known which antibodies confer protection. Similarly, such tests may be used to monitor post-infusion antibody levels during convalescent plasma treatment, monoclonal antibody therapies, or after vaccination. Further complicating this issue is evidence from SARS-CoV-1 that antibody-dependent enhancement (ADE) of infection may occur, where antibodies facilitate, rather than block, viral infection.[59] Current serologic tests do not distinguish between protective and ADE-inducing antibodies. Such uses of a clinical test will need to be carefully monitored to assure that anti–SARS-CoV-2 antibody tests are suited to these goals.

SUMMARY

Serologic testing is an evolving and complex area of testing for COVID-19. Challenges include test validation and performance, usage, and interpretation across multiple contexts. As knowledge accumulates about the significance of differential and quantitative detection of viral antigens, it will be beneficial to have test platforms that can address questions going beyond a qualitative assessment of previous infection. Careful test validation and appropriate matching to the questions to be answered will help ensure clinical and scientific research rigor and reproducibility. It is likely that the testing landscape for measuring the serologic response to SARS-CoV-2 will evolve rapidly over the next several years. Furthermore, if it is determined that neutralizing antibodies do not confer protection (which may be known within 6–12 months), serologic testing for SARS-CoV-2 may be of purely epidemiologic value and thus less likely to occur in clinical laboratories.

DISCLOSURE

Nicole Pecora has received research support from Luminex.

REFERENCES

1. Zhu N, Zhang D, Wang W, et al. A novel coronavirus from patients with pneumonia in China, 2019. N Engl J Med 2020;382(8):727–33.

2. Coronaviridae Study Group of the International Committee on Taxonomy of Viruses. The species Severe acute respiratory syndrome-related coronavirus: classifying 2019-nCoV and naming it SARS-CoV-2. Nat Microbiol 2020;5(4):536–44.
3. Bryan A, Pepper G, Wener MH, et al. Performance characteristics of the Abbott Architect SARS-CoV-2 IgG assay and seroprevalence in Boise, Idaho. J Clin Microbiol 2020;58(8):e00941-20.
4. Hoffman T, Nissen K, Krambrich J, et al. Evaluation of a COVID-19 IgM and IgG rapid test; an efficient tool for assessment of past exposure to SARS-CoV-2. Infect Ecol Epidemiol 2020;10(1):1754538.
5. Zainol Rashid Z, Othman SN, Abdul Samat MN, et al. Diagnostic performance of COVID-19 serology assays. Malays J Pathol 2020;42(1):13–21.
6. Infantino M, Grossi V, Lari B, et al. Diagnostic accuracy of an automated chemiluminescent immunoassay for anti-SARS-CoV-2 IgM and IgG antibodies: an Italian experience. J Med Virol 2020. https://doi.org/10.1002/jmv.25932.
7. Takita M, Matsumura T, Yamamoto K, et al. Challenges of community point-of-care antibody testing for COVID-19 herd-immunity in Japan. QJM 2020. hcaa182. PMCID: 7313848.
8. Yan Y, Chang L, Wang L. Laboratory testing of SARS-CoV, MERS-CoV, and SARS-CoV-2 (2019-nCoV): Current status, challenges, and countermeasures. Rev Med Virol 2020;30(3):e2106.
9. Amanat F, Stadlbauer D, Strohmeier S, et al. A serological assay to detect SARS-CoV-2 seroconversion in humans. Nat Med 2020;26(7):1033–6.
10. Phelan AL. COVID-19 immunity passports and vaccination certificates: scientific, equitable, and legal challenges. Lancet 2020;395(10237):1595–8.
11. Administration USFaD. What tests should no longer be distributed for COVID-19?. 2020. Available at: https://www.fda.gov/medical-devices/emergency-situations-medical-devices/faqs-testing-sars-cov-2 - nolonger. Accessed May 28, 2020.
12. Abbasi J. The promise and Peril of antibody testing for COVID-19. JAMA 2020; 323(19):1881–3.
13. Cui J, Li F, Shi ZL. Origin and evolution of pathogenic coronaviruses. Nat Rev Microbiol 2019;17(3):181–92.
14. Qiu M, Shi Y, Guo Z, et al. Antibody responses to individual proteins of SARS coronavirus and their neutralization activities. Microbes Infect 2005;7(5–6):882–9.
15. Tay MZ, Poh CM, Renia L, et al. The trinity of COVID-19: immunity, inflammation and intervention. Nat Rev Immunol 2020;20(6):363–74.
16. Du L, He Y, Zhou Y, et al. The spike protein of SARS-CoV–a target for vaccine and therapeutic development. Nat Rev Microbiol 2009;7(3):226–36.
17. Walls AC, Park YJ, Tortorici MA, et al. Structure, function, and antigenicity of the SARS-CoV-2 spike glycoprotein. Cell 2020;181(2):281–92.e6.
18. Shang J, Ye G, Shi K, et al. Structural basis of receptor recognition by SARS-CoV-2. Nature 2020;581(7807):221–4.
19. Wrapp D, Wang N, Corbett KS, et al. Cryo-EM structure of the 2019-nCoV spike in the prefusion conformation. Science 2020;367(6483):1260–3.
20. Wang Q, Zhang Y, Wu L, et al. Structural and functional basis of SARS-CoV-2 entry by using human ACE2. Cell 2020;181(4):894–904.e9.
21. Millet JK, Whittaker GR. Physiological and molecular triggers for SARS-CoV membrane fusion and entry into host cells. Virology 2018;517:3–8.
22. Jaimes JA, Andre NM, Chappie JS, et al. Phylogenetic analysis and structural modeling of SARS-CoV-2 spike protein reveals an evolutionary distinct and proteolytically sensitive activation loop. J Mol Biol 2020;432(10):3309–25.

23. Wu Y, Wang F, Shen C, et al. A noncompeting pair of human neutralizing antibodies block COVID-19 virus binding to its receptor ACE2. Science 2020; 368(6496):1274–8.
24. Tai W, Zhang X, He Y, et al. Identification of SARS-CoV RBD-targeting monoclonal antibodies with cross-reactive or neutralizing activity against SARS-CoV-2. Antiviral Res 2020;179:104820.
25. Wrapp D, De Vlieger D, Corbett KS, et al. Structural basis for potent neutralization of Betacoronaviruses by single-domain Camelid antibodies. Cell 2020;181(5): 1004–15.e15.
26. Surjit M, Lal SK. The SARS-CoV nucleocapsid protein: a protein with multifarious activities. Infect Genet Evol 2008;8(4):397–405.
27. Zeng W, Liu G, Ma H, et al. Biochemical characterization of SARS-CoV-2 nucleocapsid protein. Biochem Biophys Res Commun 2020;527(3):618–23.
28. Che XY, Hao W, Wang Y, et al. Nucleocapsid protein as early diagnostic marker for SARS. Emerg Infect Dis 2004;10(11):1947–9.
29. Ahmed SF, Quadeer AA, McKay MR. Preliminary identification of potential vaccine targets for the COVID-19 coronavirus (SARS-CoV-2) based on SARS-CoV immunological studies. Viruses 2020;12(3).
30. Liu SJ, Leng CH, Lien SP, et al. Immunological characterizations of the nucleocapsid protein based SARS vaccine candidates. Vaccine 2006;24(16):3100–8.
31. Tilocca B, Soggiu A, Sanguinetti M, et al. Comparative computational analysis of SARS-CoV-2 nucleocapsid protein epitopes in taxonomically related coronaviruses. Microbes Infect 2020;22(4–5):188–94.
32. Xiang F, Wang X, He X, et al. Antibody Detection and Dynamic Characteristics in Patients with COVID-19 [published online ahead of print, 2020 Apr 19]. Clin Infect Dis 2020;ciaa461. https://doi.org/10.1093/cid/ciaa461.
33. Guo L, Ren L, Yang S, et al. Profiling early humoral response to diagnose novel coronavirus disease (COVID-19). Clin Infect Dis 2020;71(15):778–85.
34. Zhao J, Yuan Q, Wang H, et al. Antibody responses to SARS-CoV-2 in patients of novel coronavirus disease 2019 [published online ahead of print, 2020 Mar 28]. Clin Infect Dis 2020;ciaa344. https://doi.org/10.1093/cid/ciaa344.
35. Yongchen Z, Shen H, Wang X, et al. Different longitudinal patterns of nucleic acid and serology testing results based on disease severity of COVID-19 patients. Emerg Microbes Infect 2020;9(1):833–6.
36. Liu W, Liu L, Kou G, et al. Evaluation of nucleocapsid and spike protein-based ELISAs for detecting antibodies against SARS-CoV-2. J Clin Microbiol 2020; 58(6):e00461-20.
37. Burbelo PD, Riedo FX, Morishima C, et al. Sensitivity in Detection of Antibodies to Nucleocapsid and Spike Proteins of Severe Acute Respiratory Syndrome Coronavirus 2 in Patients With Coronavirus Disease 2019. The Journal of infectious diseases 2019;222(2):206–13. https://doi.org/10.1093/infdis/jiaa273.
38. Tan YJ, Goh PY, Fielding BC, et al. Profiles of antibody responses against severe acute respiratory syndrome coronavirus recombinant proteins and their potential use as diagnostic markers. Clin Diagn Lab Immunol 2004;11(2):362–71.
39. Woo PC, Lau SK, Wong BH, et al. Differential sensitivities of severe acute respiratory syndrome (SARS) coronavirus spike polypeptide enzyme-linked immunosorbent assay (ELISA) and SARS coronavirus nucleocapsid protein ELISA for serodiagnosis of SARS coronavirus pneumonia. J Clin Microbiol 2005;43(7): 3054–8.
40. Zhang G, Nie S, Zhang Z, et al. Longitudinal Change of Severe Acute Respiratory Syndrome Coronavirus 2 Antibodies in Patients with Coronavirus Disease 2019.

The Journal of infectious diseases 2020;222(2):183–8. https://doi.org/10.1093/infdis/jiaa229.

41. Okba NMA, Muller MA, Li W, et al. Severe acute respiratory syndrome coronavirus 2-specific antibody responses in coronavirus disease 2019 patients. Emerg Infect Dis 2020;26(7):1478–88.

42. Wajnberg A, Mansour M, Leven E, et al. Humoral immune response and prolonged PCR positivity in a cohort of 1343 SARS-CoV 2 patients in the New York City region. medRxiv 2020. 2020.04.30.20085613.

43. Niedrig M, Leitmeyer K, Lim W, et al. First external quality assurance of antibody diagnostic for SARS-new coronavirus. J Clin Virol 2005;34(1):22–5.

44. Meyer B, Drosten C, Muller MA. Serological assays for emerging coronaviruses: challenges and pitfalls. Virus Res 2014;194:175–83.

45. Wang J, Wiltse A, Zand MS. A complex dance: measuring the multidimensional worlds of influenza virus evolution and anti-influenza immune responses. Pathogens 2019;8(4):238.

46. Li D, Wang J, Garigen J, et al. Continuous readout versus titer-based assays of influenza vaccine trials: sensitivity, specificity, and false discovery rates. Comput Math Methods Med 2019;2019:9287120.

47. Whitman JD, Hiatt J, Mowery CT, et al. Test performance evaluation of SARS-CoV-2 serological assays. medRxiv 2020. 2020.2004.2025.20074856.

48. FDA. Available at: https://www.fda.gov/medical-devices/emergency-situations-medical-devices/eua-authorized-serology-test-performance. Accessed May 30, 2020.

49. Huang AT, Garcia-Carreras B, Hitchings MDT, et al. A systematic review of antibody mediated immunity to coronaviruses: antibody kinetics, correlates of protection, and association of antibody responses with severity of disease. medRxiv 2020. 2020.2004.2014.20065771.

50. Long QX, Tang XJ, Shi QL, et al. Clinical and immunological assessment of asymptomatic SARS-CoV-2 infections. Nat Med 2020;26(8):1200–4.

51. Woo PC, Lau SK, Wong BH, et al. Longitudinal profile of immunoglobulin G (IgG), IgM, and IgA antibodies against the severe acute respiratory syndrome (SARS) coronavirus nucleocapsid protein in patients with pneumonia due to the SARS coronavirus. Clin Diagn Lab Immunol 2004;11(4):665–8.

52. Liu W, Fontanet A, Zhang PH, et al. Two-year prospective study of the humoral immune response of patients with severe acute respiratory syndrome. J Infect Dis 2006;193(6):792–5.

53. Wu LP, Wang NC, Chang YH, et al. Duration of antibody responses after severe acute respiratory syndrome. Emerg Infect Dis 2007;13(10):1562–4.

54. Callow KA, Parry HF, Sergeant M, et al. The time course of the immune response to experimental coronavirus infection of man. Epidemiol Infect 1990;105(2):435–46.

55. Wu F, Wang A, Liu M, et al. Neutralizing antibody responses to SARS-CoV-2 in a COVID-19 recovered patient cohort and their implications. medRxiv 2020. 2020.2003.2030.20047365.

56. Perera RA, Mok CK, Tsang OT, et al. Serological assays for severe acute respiratory syndrome coronavirus 2 (SARS-CoV-2), March 2020. Euro Surveill 2020;25(16):2000421.

57. Yuchun N, Guangwen W, Xuanling S, et al. Neutralizing antibodies in patients with severe acute respiratory syndrome-associated coronavirus infection. J Infect Dis 2004;190(6):1119–26.

58. Wang C, Li W, Drabek D, et al. A human monoclonal antibody blocking SARS-CoV-2 infection. Nat Commun 2020;11(1):2251.
59. Wang J, Zand MS. The potential for antibody-dependent enhancement of SARS-CoV-2 infection: Translational implications for vaccine development. *Journal of Clinical and Translational Science*, 1–4. https://doi.org/10.1017/cts.2020.39.

UNITED STATES POSTAL SERVICE®

Statement of Ownership, Management, and Circulation (All Periodicals Publications Except Requester Publications)

1. Publication Title	2. Publication Number	3. Filing Date
CLINICS IN LABORATORY MEDICINE	000 – 713	9/18/2020

4. Issue Frequency	5. Number of Issues Published Annually	6. Annual Subscription Price
MAR, JUN, SEP, DEC	4	$277.00

7. Complete Mailing Address of Known Office of Publication (Not printer) (Street, city, county, state, and ZIP+4®)

ELSEVIER INC.
230 Park Avenue, Suite 800
New York, NY 10169

Contact Person
Malathi Samayan

Telephone (Include area code)
91-44-4299-4507

8. Complete Mailing Address of Headquarters or General Business Office of Publisher (Not printer)

ELSEVIER INC.
230 Park Avenue, Suite 800
New York, NY 10159

9. Full Names and Complete Mailing Addresses of Publisher, Editor, and Managing Editor (Do not leave blank)

Publisher (Name and complete mailing address)

DOLORES MELONI, ELSEVIER INC.
1600 JOHN F KENNEDY BLVD. SUITE 1800
PHILADELPHIA, PA 19103-2899

Editor (Name and complete mailing address)

KATERINA HEIDHAUSEN, ELSEVIER INC.
1600 JOHN F KENNEDY BLVD. SUITE 1800
PHILADELPHIA, PA 19103-2899

Managing Editor (Name and complete mailing address)

PATRICK MANLEY, ELSEVIER INC.
1600 JOHN F KENNEDY BLVD. SUITE 1800
PHILADELPHIA, PA 19103-2899

10. Owner (Do not leave blank. If the publication is owned by a corporation, give the name and address of the corporation immediately followed by the names and addresses of all stockholders owning or holding 1 percent or more of the total amount of stock. If not owned by a corporation, give the names and addresses of the individual owners. If owned by a partnership or other unincorporated firm, give its name and address as well as those of each individual owner. If the publication is published by a nonprofit organization, give its name and address.)

Full Name	Complete Mailing Address
WHOLLY OWNED SUBSIDIARY OF REED/ELSEVIER, US HOLDINGS	1600 JOHN F KENNEDY BLVD, SUITE 1800 PHILADELPHIA, PA 19103-2899

11. Known Bondholders, Mortgagees, and Other Security Holders Owning or Holding 1 Percent or More of Total Amount of Bonds, Mortgages, or Other Securities. If none, check box ▶ ☐ None

Full Name	Complete Mailing Address
N/A	

12. Tax Status (For completion by nonprofit organizations authorized to mail at nonprofit rates) (Check one)
The purpose, function, and nonprofit status of this organization and the exempt status for federal income tax purposes:
☒ Has Not Changed During Preceding 12 Months
☐ Has Changed During Preceding 12 Months (Publisher must submit explanation of change with this statement)

PS Form 3526, July 2014 [Page 1 of 4 (see instructions page 4)] PSN: 7530-01-000-9931   PRIVACY NOTICE: See our privacy policy on www.usps.com.

13. Publication Title			14. Issue Date for Circulation Data Below	
CLINICS IN LABORATORY MEDICINE			JUNE 2020	

15. Extent and Nature of Circulation			Average No. Copies Each Issue During Preceding 12 Months	No. Copies of Single Issue Published Nearest to Filing Date
a. Total Number of Copies (Net press run)			85	68
b. Paid Circulation (By Mail and Outside the Mail)	(1)	Mailed Outside-County Paid Subscriptions Stated on PS Form 3541 (Include paid distribution above nominal rate, advertiser's proof copies, and exchange copies)	33	26
	(2)	Mailed In-County Paid Subscriptions Stated on PS Form 3541 (Include paid distribution above nominal rate, advertiser's proof copies, and exchange copies)	0	0
	(3)	Paid Distribution Outside the Mails Including Sales Through Dealers and Carriers, Street Vendors, Counter Sales, and Other Paid Distribution Outside USPS®	17	15
	(4)	Paid Distribution by Other Classes of Mail Through the USPS (e.g. First-Class Mail®)	0	0
c. Total Paid Distribution (Sum of 15b (1), (2), (3), and (4))		▶	50	41
d. Free or Nominal Rate Distribution (By Mail and Outside the Mail)	(1)	Free or Nominal Rate Outside-County Copies included on PS Form 3541	21	12
	(2)	Free or Nominal Rate In-County Copies Included on PS Form 3541	0	0
	(3)	Free or Nominal Rate Copies Mailed at Other Classes Through the USPS (e.g. First-Class Mail)	0	0
	(4)	Free or Nominal Rate Distribution Outside the Mail (Carriers or other means)	0	0
e. Total Free or Nominal Rate Distribution (Sum of 15d (1), (2), (3) and (4))		▶	21	12
f. Total Distribution (Sum of 15c and 15e)		▶	71	53
g. Copies not Distributed (See Instructions to Publishers #4 (page #3))		▶	14	15
h. Total (Sum of 15f and g)		▶	85	68
i. Percent Paid (15c divided by 15f times 100)		▶	70.42%	77.35%

* If you are claiming electronic copies, go to line 16 on page 3. If you are not claiming electronic copies, skip to line 17 on page 3.

16. Electronic Copy Circulation		Average No. Copies Each Issue During Preceding 12 Months	No. Copies of Single Issue Published Nearest to Filing Date
a. Paid Electronic Copies	▶		
b. Total Paid Print Copies (Line 15c) + Paid Electronic Copies (Line 16a)	▶		
c. Total Print Distribution (Line 15f) + Paid Electronic Copies (Line 16a)	▶		
d. Percent Paid (Both Print & Electronic Copies) (16b divided by 16c × 100)	▶		

☒ I certify that 50% of all my distributed copies (electronic and print) are paid above a nominal price

17. Publication of Statement of Ownership

☒ If the publication is a general publication, publication of this statement is required. Will be printed in the DECEMBER 2020 issue of this publication.   ☐ Publication not required.

18. Signature and Title of Editor, Publisher, Business Manager, or Owner

Malathi Samayan

Malathi Samayan - Distribution Controller

Date 9/18/2020

I certify that all information furnished on this form is true and complete. I understand that anyone who furnishes false or misleading information on this form or who omits material or information requested on the form may be subject to criminal sanctions (including fines and imprisonment) and/or civil sanctions (including civil penalties).

PS Form 3526, July 2014 (Page 3 of 4)   PRIVACY NOTICE: See our privacy policy on www.usps.com.